Practical Wildlife Care
for
Veterinary Nurses, Animal Care Students and Rehabilitators

Les Stocker MBE

Drawings by Tessa Eccles
Photographs by Les Stocker

D1434900

Blackwell
Science

Millpledge

© Les Stocker 2000

Blackwell Science Ltd, a Blackwell Publishing
Company
Editorial Offices:
Osney Mead, Oxford OX2 0EL, UK
  Tel: +44 (0)1865 206206
Blackwell Science, Inc., 350 Main Street,
Malden, MA 02148-5018, USA
  Tel: +1 781 388 8250
Iowa State Press, a Blackwell Publishing
Company, 2121 State Avenue, Ames, Iowa
50014-8300, USA
  Tel: +1 515 292 0140
Blackwell Science Asia Pty, 54 University
Street, Carlton, Victoria 3053, Australia
  Tel: +61 (0)3 9347 0300
Blackwell Wissenschafts Verlag,
Kurfürstendamm 57, 10707 Berlin, Germany
  Tel: +49 (0)30 32 79 060

First published 2000 by Blackwell Science Ltd
Reprinted 2001 (twice), 2002

Library of Congress
Cataloging-in-Publication Data
Stocker, Les
    Practical wildlife care : for veterinary nurses,
animal care students and rehabilitators / Les
Stocker; drawings by Tessa Eccles.
      p. cm.
    Includes bibliographical references (p.).
    ISBN 0-632-05245-7 (pb)
      1. Wildlife rehabilitation. 2. Wildlife
rescue. 3. Wildlife diseases–Treatment. 4. First
aid for animals. I. Title.

SF996.45 .S755 2000
639.9′6–dc21   99-461977

ISBN 0-632-05245-7

A catalogue record for this title is available
from the British Library

Set in 9.5 on 11.5pt Times
by SNP Best-set Typesetter Ltd., Hong Kong
Printed and bound in Great Britain by
the Alden Group, Oxford

For further information on
Blackwell Science, visit our website:
www.blackwell-science.co.uk

Contents

Foreword

A fundamental paradox besets wildlife rehabilitation today – most wildlife rehabilitators have insufficient understanding of veterinary medicine and most veterinarians have little experience with wildlife. Although there are scattered references in the literature describing care and rehabilitation of British wildlife casualties, a comprehensive account of the subject, in a format accessible to the dedicated rehabilitator and professional veterinarian alike, has hitherto not been published. In *Practical Wildlife Care*, Les Stocker has gone a long way towards addressing this problem.

Les Stocker is perhaps the best known and probably the most experienced British wildlife rehabilitator, and under his inspired leadership the Wildlife Hospital Trust (more familiarly known as St Tiggywinkles) has grown from a garden shed to Europe's largest, purpose-built, wildlife hospital. This would be a wonderful achievement in itself, but Les has always believed that to develop rehabilitation techniques without passing the knowledge to others would only achieve half of his self-imposed mission. In writing *Practical Wildlife Care* he has been able to offer the benefit of his long experience to rehabilitators all over the world. Although Les's experience has very largely been with British wildlife, much of the information provided and many of the techniques described are applicable to species from a much wider geographical range.

Throughout the book, a close partnership between rehabilitators and their veterinarians is encouraged - an attitude that has no doubt significantly aided the development of the Wildlife Hospital Trust and one which vets and rehabilitators alike must develop to a greater degree if further advances are to be made in the field. *Practical Wildlife Care* is written in a sufficiently informal style to hold the attention of the interested amateur yet contains enough medical detail to inform the veterinarian. This book should certainly facilitate growth of the essential partnership and stimulate ceaseless debate between the partners!

Practical Wildlife Care takes the reader through the many different phases of the rehabilitation process and provides essential veterinary information about every group of animals likely to be presented to the British rehabilitator. In attempting to be so comprehensive it is clear that the book will not satisfy everybody's thirst for detailed information about his or her chosen speciality. As more is learnt about the rehabilitation of different species, more specialist volumes will no doubt be required.

Rehabilitators and vets in the UK have long been starved of a common sense manual of good practice and I suspect that many will use this book as their first port of call when confronted with a wildlife casualty.

Dr John Lewis
International Zoo Veterinary Group

Preface

Although the overall care and treatment of any animal, including a wild animal, usually falls to the veterinary surgeon, the support of the veterinary nurse or the trained rehabilitator is crucial to manage the number of wild casualties now being found.

Nearly all of the casualties are as a direct result of collision with man or the environment he has created. The truly natural casualty is a rarity but incidences do occur with our innate compassion demanding that these animals are also taken into care.

However, practically all wildlife casualties are the victims of trauma and are suffering from some degree of shock. A knowledge of the physiology of wild animals and an understanding of the metabolic changes that may occur will allow anyone to provide the first-aid and life-saving techniques that will keep the animal alive to benefit from the ever-advancing techniques of veterinary surgery. The purpose of this book is to lay out simply the support services that the veterinary nurse or rehabilitator may provide to assist the veterinary surgeon.

The book is a result of my 20 years of experience in dealing with the idiosyncracies of British wild animals. In that time I have always worked in close cooperation with veterinary surgeons especially for diagnosis, prescription and surgical intervention.

My directive is to rescue the animal, keep it alive and provide first aid and stabilisation. Under the direction of the veterinary surgeon many of the casualties need no more than care and support before rehabilitation and release, whereas others need the surgeon's diagnosis, medication and even surgery. However, after these disciplines the animal is once more returned to my care for its rehabilitation and release.

This book deals with the anomalies of wildlife care and covers the vital disciplines of wildlife care, namely rescue, first aid, rehabilitation and release. The diagnosis of disease is always the province of the veterinary surgeon but I have touched on those diseases that are so regularly seen that routine treatments can easily be directed by a veterinary surgeon. Also included are simple stabilisation techniques that can often be adopted to prevent pain and suffering and provide a long-term treatment of choice.

Although there may be other products available for the treatment of wildlife casualties, those I have mentioned have proven suitable for the many thousands of patients The Wildlife Hospital Trust (St Tiggywinkles) has cared for. However, although at the time of writing the medical information given is correct, the reader should always first verify that the data have not changed. Neither I nor the Publisher can take responsibility for any matters arising from the guidance given in this book.

Over the last 20 years the care and treatment of sick or injured wildlife has become accepted all over the world. Yet all over the world the vast majority of the care has been provided by veterinary nurses and rehabilitators under the direction, where possible, of veterinary surgeons.

Early in the development of St Tiggywinkles I was indebted to Gary and Derek Carthew of Millpledge Pharmaceuticals for their care and advice on many aspects of animal support. Now, nearly 20 years later, I still look to Gary, Graham Cheslyn-Curtis and Millpledge for their support and I am especially grateful for their sponsorship of the colour photographs in this book which makes my experiences even more accessible to veterinary nurses and students.

I believe that if we all work together and take our own responsibilities then wildlife care will not impede the already busy veterinary practices and will lead to more wildlife casualties receiving that vital first aid, expertise and rehabilitation allowing more than ever to survive and be released back into the wild.

Les Stocker MBE
Aylesbury, 2000

Acknowledgements

Working with British wildlife casualties is not just about heroic rescue and tender loving care. Its base is solidly in the first principles and adaptability of veterinary care. Dr John Lewis of the International Zoo Veterinary Group has, over the last 10 years, coped with all the enigmas I have set before him. His reading of this manuscript set a marathon before him and I will be forever grateful for the comments and advice he passed on to me.

The drawings by Tessa Eccles add so much explanation to the book that I am indebted to her for the expertise she has so strikingly applied.

Lisa Frost has been tireless in databasing the manuscript from my hand-written draft and, at times, when even she was swamped, I had to call on Andrea Sims and her team, who run the office at St Tiggywinkles, to help out.

In addition to those mentioned in the Preface, I would also like to also thank: Mel Beeson, of the Swan Sanctuary for information on the latest treatments of lead poisoning; Tony Hutson, of the Bat Conservation Trust, for advice on rabies vaccination; Alan Knight, of the British Divers Marine Life Rescue, for the procedures of sea mammals strandings; Dr Andrew Kitchener for his work on Scottish wildcats and Dr Katherine Whitwell for her research on diseases of the hare.

Finally, I would like to acknowledge the ever-growing numbers of the British public who go out of their way to pick up the casualties and bring them to care.

1
Prime Directives

Wild animals are either mammals, birds, reptiles, amphibians, fish, or invertebrates. All sound familiar; they are exactly the same classes of animals seen in veterinary practices. However, there the similarity ends. Wild casualties may be of a similar structure to companion or domestic animals but they demand a completely different strategy in their care and treatment (Stocker, 1995). It is a demanding strategy especially on veterinary practices that are already overloaded, but to succeed with wildlife casualties it is crucial to set aside time and facilities to cater for their specialised needs.

Of course, wild animals benefit from the first principles of veterinary surgery and they will prosper given the basic disciplines of standard veterinary nursing or animal care procedures such as:

- A sound regime of hygiene practices both for the animals and the handlers
- The measured clinical use of prescribed drugs and the sterile use of multi-dose bottles, needles, syringes and other medical disposables
- The use of sterile utensils, equipment and clean cages and bedding
- The proper disposal of clinical waste especially sharps and bodies
- Adherence to health and safety recommendations
- Proper acquaintance and maintenance of the Control of Substances Hazardous to Health (COSHH) register
- A prohibition of eating, drinking or smoking wherever animals are present

These recognised standard practices should already be in place. They provide a firm base on which to build the different practices demanded by wildlife casualties. The additional practices may appear, at first, onerous and time-consuming but the wild animals will benefit as, indirectly, will their handlers as more animals recover and grow suitable for release into the wild.

All the practices are part of The Wildlife Hospital Trust's (St Tiggywinkles) own code of conduct and although not so stringently adhered to in some other centres, we have found them essential for a well-managed hospital and a consistent success rate. Trying not to make them sound like a list of 'dos and don'ts', you will find that they marry well with standard procedures and when in place will themselves become standard in the wild animal facility.

Starting with the basic principles of wildlife care some of these practices may seem out of place in a veterinary practice or other animal centre but they are essential for good, humane wildlife care which should not even be attempted if you cannot provide the specialities wild animals demand.

The following wildlife recommended practices complement the whole spectrum of a wild animal's stay in captivity right through to its release, if that is possible.

(1) NEVER MIX WILD ANIMALS AND DOMESTIC ANIMALS

The author appreciates that this would put an enormous burden on the facilities of many veterinary practices and animal care establishments, but this is the directive most often flouted with disastrous consequences. A wild animal facility joined on to an existing practice does not need to be a state-of-the-art hospital. It could be just a small room or a basement where only wild animals are kept. Many wildlife rescue centres around the world operate from sheds or caravans in a garden. Without them wildlife rehabilitation would not have made the great strides forward that it has.

There are sound reasons for this aversion to mixing wild and domestic animals and the author knows of some wildlife rescue centres that have suffered terribly by innocently allowing companion animals into their facility.

Disease

The major disaster that really brought the matter to the fore was when over 30 badgers died after contracting canine parvovirus at a rescue centre which allowed people, with dogs, to visit. It was not recorded if the parvovirus was contracted directly from the dogs or from contamination on the visitors' footwear, but it made everybody aware of the potential hazards.

Some wild animals are susceptible to many of the common diseases seen in some of our domestic animals but they do not have the benefit of vaccinations. Most companion animals taken anywhere by anybody should be vaccinated against the familiar diseases. But what if they are not or what if they had been vaccinated with a live virus vaccine and are shedding the virus? Any contact with infected animal material can lead to fatal disease for wild animals. No one knows if viruses shed by vaccinated companion animals into the environment are affecting wild animals but in the close confinement of a practice or rescue facility the likelihood of infection is infinitely greater.

Many diseases emanating from domestic animals have been recorded in wildlife. These include:

- Parvovirus in badgers, can also affect foxes
- Canine distemper in foxes
- Infectious canine hepatitis in foxes
- Feline leukaemia in Scottish wildcats
- Paramyxo virus in pigeons
- Viral haemorrhagic disease in rabbits
- The possibility of Aleutian disease in mustelids

Generally it is not advisable to routinely vaccinate wild animals unless there are extenuating circumstances.

Wild animals, therefore, have to rely on their own immune systems which will not have been exposed to many of these domestic diseases and consequently any disease will quickly run its course unchallenged, culminating in the death of any wild animal unlucky enough to contract it. By keeping wild and domestic animals separate we are at least taking all the precautions possible to prevent that happening.

Stress

Wild animals are programmed to classify some other animals as extremely dangerous. Top of the list are human beings, so when a wild animal is picked up it will become severely stressed. Then if it is taken to within scenting, hearing or seeing distance of another arch enemy its stress levels can run out of control. Add to this the confinement in a cage and the animal is rapidly losing control of its internal homeostatic mechanisms. It panics more and possibly injures itself in its efforts to escape. The animal might well die just from being put into a cage near to a potential enemy. Some of the incidents the author has witnessed, when picking up a casualty, surely highlight the stress these animals must have been going through:

- A wild deer put into a kennel in a room full of dogs. The deer's terror must have been absolute as it could scent, hear and see, as it was in this case, similar animals to those that had injured it in the first place.
- A common or garden blackbird injured by a cat and now put into a cattery full of cats. Small birds are renowned for dying instantly from stress.
- A fox, surely the most nervous of all wildlife casualties, also put into a kennel in a room full of dogs.
- To top all these there is the constant to and fro in a busy centre exposing any wild animal kept there to an ever-changing cavalcade of humans – the worst enemy of all.

Stress is said, in humans, to be the twentieth century disease. This is also the case in the wild animal population even before they are brought into captivity and subjected to even more.

Noise

Working at any treatment facility you cannot fail to hear all the noisy bangs and clangs going on the whole time. Most of them are unavoidable like:

- The stainless steel lids of pots and pans that are impossible to remove quietly
- The buzz and hum of clippers and vacuum cleaners
- The hiss of autoclaves
- The bang of those stainless steel cage doors you try to close quietly
- The incessant ringing of the telephone

Every noise must be like a gunshot to a wild animal who is not used to the closely confined atmosphere of a practice facility.

It is difficult, if not impossible, to counter disease, stress or noise in a close environment but just a bit of peace and quiet in an annex will give a wild casualty that little bit extra it needs to recover.

Familiarity

Another hazard of keeping wild animals near to domestic animals is that they may have become familiar with those animals and lose any fear they might have had. When they are released these wild animals might seek out the company of 'familiar' domestic animals and fall foul of an arch enemy (Plate 1).

Similarly, orphaned wild animals should never be reared by, or be in the company of, companion animals. The same perils will beset these orphans when they are released.

(2) PHOTOPERIOD

Wild animals are very much creatures of habit; if they are diurnal, they are active during the day and if they are nocturnal, they are active at night. However, when we take them into care they move into this glassy world of electric lighting putting yet another stress on an already confused animal.

Yes, operatives need bright lights in order to examine, operate on or even clean animals but once these necessary procedures are completed the lights should be turned off so that the animal is in daylight or night, Do not close the blinds during the day or even at night. Wild animals need the gradual lighting of dawn or the darkening of dusk. It is something familiar in the strange captive world in which they find themselves.

Bird fanciers even fit dimmer switches to their lighting so that their birds are not subjected to the sudden switch on or switch off. Even this may help a wild casualty relax that little bit more and help it recover more quickly.

(3) WHITE COATS

There is no reason why white coats have to be white. Surely any coat, if it is laundered properly, will be just as hygienic. Wild animals taken into care only know that this gleaming white apparition is going to approach and catch hold of it. If the animal was not already stressed this white coat is just another catalyst it could well do without.

With green or dark blue coats there is not that stark contrast that is so alarming and more colour conscious coats would still look respectable to onlookers (Fig. 1.1). Birds get easily stressed by coloured images. Green and blue are far more natural than white and are more readily accepted than the danger colours birds respond to: black, red or yellow.

(4) RECORDS

Written records are even more crucial for the wildlife casualty than they are for domestic animals.

The information which is so important in the animal's treatment can be vital to a medical database and may also produce material useful to biologists and zoologists majoring on British wildlife.

Vital information recorded even as the animal is admitted can have a direct bearing on its treatment and future. Included on a record card (Fig. 1.2), as well as its medical programme, should be:

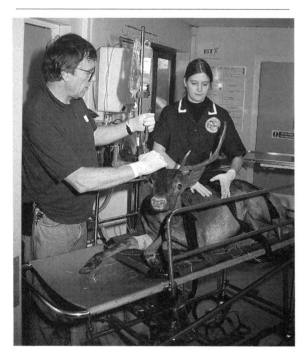

Fig. 1.1 Green or blue coats are much less stark than white coats.

- The name, address and telephone number of whoever found the animal. This is important in case any further information is required and if assistance is needed in getting the animal to an appropriate release site.
- The circumstances of rescue can often assist the veterinary surgeon in coming to a diagnosis, e.g. a bird that has flown into a window that shows no apparent injuries could be suffering from head trauma.
- Any treatments given. Sometimes caring people will have already provided their own version of first-aid care and medication. This may include inappropriate substances, detrimental food and most common of all, a drink of water, brandy, warm milk or herbal remedies that can predispose to inhalation pneumonia.
- It is important to know exactly where the animal was found.
- If it is a territorial or bonding species, like a swan, did it have a mate and were any dependent siblings left behind?

- Lastly, once the animal is admitted, comprehensive records must be maintained of its progress, any medication given or biopsies carried out, and procedures involved and the final outcome of its stay in care.

Finally, all this information should be entered on a database and any findings published as there is still a dearth of worthwhile literature relevant to British wildlife casualties.

(5) PERSONNEL HAZARDS

Any wild animal taken into care will be terrified and feel under threat. It will make every effort to escape and if it has the capability it will fight, bite, scratch, kick and even scream. Some animals do not pose much of a threat to a handler but even a sparrow or a mouse can inflict a painful little bite, while other casualties can cause serious injury. By handling wildlife properly there should be no need to get bitten or injured. Taking the right precautions, concentrating on the animal and being prepared for even a comatose animal to suddenly spring to snapping life will prevent any mishaps. Potentially dangerous animals likely to be presented for care include:

- Badgers, otters, foxes and seals have very powerful jaws and will bite if given the opportunity. Their reactions are much faster than a human being so give them plenty of respect (Fig. 1.3).
- Deer are more predictable. They are extremely strong and will kick, head butt or use their antlers. It takes two people to even think of restraining a fallow buck. Small deer like muntjac or Chinese water deer will attempt to slash with their tusks.
- Birds of prey and some crows will attack with their feet which in the case of birds of prey are armed with razor sharp talons.
- Some birds of prey will bite, as will crows and gulls.
- Sharp-billed birds like herons and some seabirds will stab like lightning at the face. Always restrain the bird's head first of all.
- Squirrels are potentially the most dangerous. They are exceptionally fast and will bite severely.

DATE / / NO	ST TIGGYWINKLES.................................RECORD	I.D.

NAME ADDRESS	CIRCUMSTANCE OF RESCUE
POSTCODE	SOURCE

DAILY TREATMENT	TEETH	SEX	AGE	WEIGHT
	CONDITION			
	LAB. REF. NO.		OUTCOME	

DATE/TIME	WEIGHT	A	D	U	F	TREATMENT	NOTES

□ Please tick this box if you do NOT wish to receive any future mailings about St Tiggywinkles.
I agree that St Tiggywinkles will not be handing this animal back to me:..

Fig. 1.2 A record card carries vital information for treatments and database entry.

They will also scratch with the long claws on their back feet.

- Scottish wild cats are like aggravated feral cats only much stronger and more aggressive.
- The only native poison snake is the adder or viper. These very rarely need rescuing but should still be treated with the utmost caution. Because of all the exotic snakes that have escaped from the pet trade there will be calls to snakes that are not easy to recognise. Treat all strange snakes as potentially venomous as some non-venomous exotic snakes still have a nasty bite.
- Wild boar are now being seen in some of the southern counties. These can be extremely

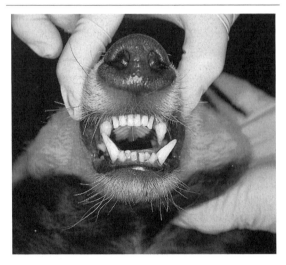

Fig. 1.3 Badgers have powerful jaws and will bite if given the opportunity.

dangerous and are best handled by zoo personnel with experience of the species.

(6) VACCINATIONS

These are important not just for companion animals but also for anybody working with animals. Unfortunately vaccinations are not available for all the zoonotic infections an animal worker might encounter but two vaccinations will stand anyone in good stead if they are exposed to the diseases.

Tetanus

Caused by the toxins of the bacterium *Clostridium tetani*, tetanus is potentially fatal and can be contracted through any open wound. All animal workers should make sure their tetanus immunisation is up to date. Boosters are needed 10 years after the primary course but can be given at 5-year intervals in high-risk vocations like animal care.

Rabies

Although not a problem in this country, rabies has recently been recorded in a Daubenton's bat in the south of England. People handling domestic animals are more likely to encounter rabid animals but everybody working with wild animals should be aware of the possibility of a wild animal contracting the disease from a companion animal. In fact people who are regularly handling bats should refer to the guidelines in Appendix 1.

(7) GLOVES

Although sometimes not used in veterinary practices, disposable latex gloves offer good protection against zoonotic infection when handling wildlife casualties. They are cheap and essential.

Other protection is likely to be needed against hazardous substances that all too regularly affect wildlife. In particular oils, solvents, acids and paints are seen on birds, hedgehogs and other small mammals.

Also the handling of medicines during treatment can lead to absorption through the skin. Latex gloves will prevent this. Particular precautions must be taken if an operative is sensitive to some drug, e.g. has an allergy to penicillin.

(8) ZOONOSES

Anybody who wants to offer care to wildlife casualties is a welcome ally. The negative information, like zoonoses, that is provided is not to be taken as a deterrent but more as words of advice to help wildlife care prosper.

Zoonotic hazards are where animals can infect handlers with a range of conditions ranging from irritating to fatal. However, with the right precautions and standards of practice and hygiene they should not be problem.

Leptospirosis (Weil's disease in humans)

This disease is potentially fatal to humans if prompt medical attention is not sought. In wild animals *Leptospira* bacteria are well entrenched in the brown rat *Rattus norvegicus* which is now at plague proportions in Britain. Transmission is through the urine of infected animals and is reported to be contaminating many of Britain's watercourses.

Wild animals, especially those like the fox, who prey on brown rats are susceptible to the disease. Normal conditions of hygiene should rule out the transmission of infection but typically an animal with leptospirosis infection will show yellowish mucous membranes. Clinical tests will confirm if the animal is positive for leptospirosis. Any suspect animal should be isolated and barrier nursed. Bear in mind that although many foxes present with the typical yellow mucous membranes and a small proportion may be showing leptospirosis, most seem to be suffering from infectious canine hepatitis which is not contagious to humans, and from internal haemorrhage especially after road traffic accidents (Plate 2).

Lyme disease

This is a disease of humans caused by the spirochaete bacterium *Borrelia burghdorferi* and does seem to be on the increase. It is transmitted by ticks from animals, particularly deer. If anybody finds a tick on their body which causes a reaction then the bite should be referred to a general practitioner who will prescribe a course of antibiotics which should overcome any infection. Untreated Lyme disease can be fatal or can lead to arthritis in later life.

Make sure any ticks taken off animals are killed. If not they can travel and climb on to people who will not necessarily feel their bite.

Ringworm

Ringworm can be contracted off many companion animals and usually fluoresces under a Wood's lamp. However, the form of ringworm found on hedgehogs does not fluoresce and is often misdiagnosed. The organism involved is *Trichophyton erinacei* and it can transfer to humans (Stocker, 1987). Infection usually starts with an itching bump on the hand or fingers. It will spread rapidly and should be referred to a general practitioner.

Tuberculosis

In its many forms tuberculosis is a chronic progressive disease and is caused by bacteria of the genus *Mycobacterium* that has three common forms: *M. bovis* which affects ruminants and badgers; *M. avium* which affects birds, mainly pigeons; and *M. tuberculosis* which affects humans. Humans are susceptible to all three forms so the veterinary surgeon will advise if an animal may be harbouring *Mycobacterium*, particularly diseased pigeons. Most people have received their BCG vaccination which might provide some protection but in spite of this all the necessary precautions should be in place, particularly during post-mortems of suspect animals.

Ornithosis

Ornithosis is the non-psitticine term for psittacosis. It is caused by various strains of *Chlamydia* which are rickettsia-like organisms. In wildlife rescue, care should be taken of any of the pigeon family showing ocular or nasal discharge. In particular look out for the 'one-eyed cold', a term applied by pigeon fanciers to birds showing symptoms of the disease. Any bird that arrives with these symptoms should be isolated, barrier-nursed and referred to the veterinary surgeon for diagnosis and instruction.

Mange

In particular sarcoptic mange is the infestation most likely to affect people handling contagious animals. Caused by a mite, *Sarcoptes scabiei*, it can be controlled in foxes, its most likely victims, with ivermectin or doramectin. It can, however, be transmitted to humans where the infestation is known as 'scabies'. Given time it can spread all over the body and from the outset needs intervention by a general practitioner.

Causing similar severe skin irritation is an allergy to sarcoptic mange which seems to flare up within 48 hours of handling an infected animal. This is a very common side effect of meeting sarcoptic mange but can be prevented, as can scabies, by wearing protective clothing, surgical gloves, apron, mask and cap, when handling suspect animals. This allergy usually resolves after about 3 weeks of constant irritation and application of soothing ointments (Stocker, 1994b).

The author has only seen one confirmed case of human scabies in over 20 years and that responded to medication provided by the general practitioner.

Bird fancier's lung

This is a general term for various respiratory conditions experienced by people who keep birds. It has been well known for many years, as its name suggests, particularly in the world of cage bird fanciers and pigeon keepers. Its effect can be severe and can cause keepers to have to stop keeping birds.

As usual prevention is better than cure, so if you are keeping birds try to adhere to the following practices:

(1) Always keep birds in a well-ventilated room or shed
(2) Wear a respiratory mask when cleaning out, particularly when removing dry droppings
(3) At the first sign of your own respiratory problems, go to your general practitioner and tell him/her that you work with birds

Other zoonoses

There are other zoonoses that can be contracted from animals. Most of them, including rabies, come under standard veterinary practice codes of conduct. In general, working cleanly and hygienically should prevent infection. Talk to the veterinary surgeon about the following diseases and learn to be aware of them:

- Rabies
- Salmonellosis
- Toxocariasis
- Pasteurellosis
- Campylobacteriosis

(9) THE ANIMALS

Wild animals are obviously different to companion animals – they demand individual methods of treatment but generally the nursing and care of casualties differs greatly from the 'hands on', reassuring practices that work with our own pets.

Staring

In the wild an animal feels under threat if another animals stares at it. This is in response to the inevitable predator concentrating and staring before it moves in for the kill.

A wild animal can take our direct gaze as a threat so always try not to stare at a casualty but avert your eyes. However, when you are concentrating on handling a dangerous animal then it will demand your full attention even if this does involve staring.

Viewing

A wild animal feels stress every time a human being is close to it. Coupled with the staring it must be terrified. Imagine if there was a constant stream of humans staring at it. Life would be one long torture.

Also a regularly disturbed patient is going to take longer to heal and worst of all might cause itself further injury in its efforts to avoid being seen.

Wild animals going through a period of care in captivity should *not* be put on public display.

Fussing

With a companion animal, patting on the head with a few soft words of compassion can work wonders. But a wild animal takes any touch as a threat and does not recognise the platitudes so effective for our dogs and cats. No petting, stroking, patting, grooming: no contact whatsoever is the order of the day. However, when approaching a wild animal, talk to it quietly – not to pacify it but just to let it know you are there so as it will not be startled.

Imprinting

Similarly and crucially it is imperative not to talk regularly to or handle any young animals and birds. Obviously in raising orphans there has to be a certain amount of bonding but once that vital weaning stage has been reached the animal must be encouraged to sever any links. If this does not happen the animal becomes permanently imprinted on humans and will never interplay with its own species.

A regime to prevent imprinting is to use different people for different stages in an animals development. A foster mother will provide pre-weaning feeding but then the animal is taken over by a juvenile animals' team who integrate it with others of its own species and never handle it again.

Pets

An imprinted animal will never be suitable for release. Kept in captivity its wild instincts will cause it to be forever restless. It will not settle into domesticity like a dog or a cat. Wild animals, in spite of what some of the pet trade suggests, do not make good pets. You could never trust one not to bite or scratch or attack – you could never relax with it – and the animal, which may even be nocturnal, will never settle to a 'nine-to-five' existence.

From the outset strive only to get the wild casualty released back to the wild, but if it is slightly disabled consider finding a sanctuary where it can live with others of its own kind. If not then euthanasia should be seriously considered.

(10) EUTHANASIA

The subject of euthanasia always raises controversy. For one thing it is a human title just like 'putting it to sleep', 'putting down' or 'putting it out of its misery'. All of these platitudes mean one thing – 'killing' – which should be borne in mind, just in case 'euthanasia' is an easy way out.

The trouble is euthanasia is constantly being abused and animals are killed because somebody does not want to put in the time and effort necessary to treat the animal. Animals do not have much. The one thing they have is 'life' and they will fight tooth and claw to preserve that one thing. If we are caring for the animals then it is our duty to give each patient the chance to keep that 'life'.

This is not to say 'Never resort to euthanasia'. Of course sometimes it is necessary. The attitude should be 'Is there another humane option?' If not then euthanasia is the only course.

A good back-up policy is that at least two senior animal staff have to consult on any proposed euthanasia; the inquest is held before the animal is killed.

Candidates for euthanasia

Most cases are blatantly obvious and seem to follow a similar pattern. Guidelines have been drawn up so that a casualty can be killed without unnecessary delay.

Criteria for euthanasia in clear-cut cases are:

• A severed and displaced vertebral column
• The loss of two or more limbs
• A bird that is blind
• A swan, goose or duck that loses a leg
• Most male deer that cannot be released
• Disabled wood pigeons – wood pigeons never settle to captivity

Methods

Euthanasia is all about stopping unnecessary suffering and that very action of killing an animal should not include suffering. To make sure of this, procedures should be adopted that make it unlikely the animal suffers.

The recommended drug that should be used is pentobarbitone sodium. This is a controlled drug so must be given under the direction of the veterinary surgeon, must be kept in locked cupboard and each use must be recorded in a register. The preferred method of injection is rapidly via an intravenous route. So if an animal is on an intravenous drip the drug can be administered easily.

Many animals and birds are too small to be able to access their veins. An intracardiac or intraperitoneal injection can be very painful so all small animals should be deeply anaesthetised before the injection is given.

Disposal

All sharps and syringes must be disposed of safely as clinical waste. Bodies are also clinical waste and must be sent for incineration.

(11) POST-MORTEM

Often it is fairly obvious why a casualty dies but sometimes the reason is a mystery. People working with casualties often blame themselves, and nurses and rehabilitators have left the profession because they thought they were failing.

A wild animal brought into care is not far from death anyway. Saving its failing life is winning against the odds. Many of them are going to die in spite of everything that is done for them. Mistakes might have been made but how can those mistakes be corrected if the causes of the animal's death are not known other than that the patient died.

Every wild animal that dies should receive a post-mortem examination. The veterinary surgeon may not be able to perform every post-mortem examination but can advise when there is a par-ticularly intricate case. Any person with a knowl-edge of hygiene and anatomy can perform a gross examination which will often give the answers as to why an animal died. In most cases a gross exami-nation proves that the animal often had an irre-versible problem that would never have resolved. Also post-mortem examinations may provide pathological information to increase existing data on British wildlife.

Gross Post-mortem

Species:

NAME: **DATE:**

Teeth	Sex	Age	Weight

EXTERNAL	Normal/Mange/Ringworm/Oedematous
INTESTINES	Normal/Gaseous/Haemorrhage/Parasites
STOMACH	Normal/Gaseous/Haemorrhage/Parasites
SPLEEN	Normal/Damaged/Enlarged
LIVER	Normal/Patchy/Discoloured...................../Enlarged
GALL BLADDER	Normal/Enlarged
KIDNEYS	Normal/Discoloured....................
BLADDER	Normal/Enlarged
LUNGS	Normal/Discoloured/Pussey/Bloody
″ Parasites	Live/Dead
HEART	Normal/Enlarged

Fig. 1.4 A gross post-mortem record provides vital data.

Standard post-mortem procedures can be set up and would include:

- A strict adherence to a health and safety protocol designed specifically for post-mortem procedures (The veterinary surgeon will be able to provide a suitable Code of Practice)
- A separate area away from the clinical centre of any facility
- A set of instruments and disposables kept just for post-mortem examinations
- Sets of surgical gloves, aprons and masks for operatives
- A standard gross post-mortem examination form that follows regular procedures (Fig. 1.4)
- Sample bottles and formol saline for body tissues
- Body bags to take clinical waste

Any information and relevant tissues should be kept and stored for future reference and databases.

Post-mortem examinations provide not only vital information but also help carers over that terrible feeling of 'I did not do enough', and they also expand the knowledge of wildlife.

SUMMARY

All these prime directives have been tried and tested by wildlife rehabilitators over many years. They can be adopted even by the smallest facility. Setting up a facility under the direction and assistance of a veterinary surgeon is essential and that veterinary surgeon will appreciate that these wild animals are receiving the best of care even before he or she becomes involved.

2
First Response

Most wildlife casualties are the victims of some form of trauma. They regularly present with severe, infected injuries and shock not commonly seen in companion or domestic animals. The wild animal, however, appears to demonstrate a greater capability to cope with these injuries and will often recover if given the chance and the necessary supportive treatments.

Yet even the most sophisticated nursing and treatments are of no use if the casualty does not survive long enough to reach the treatment table. The first discipline with any wild casualty is to make sure all the life-supporting processes are sufficiently intact to get the animal to the treatment facility.

Getting the animal to the treatment table may involve simply retrieving it from the cardboard box presented at reception or may involve transporting it some distance from the scene of an incident. Assuming the animal is alive when picked up, it is obviously crucial to keep it that way until more sophisticated first-aid resources can be brought into play.

To assist in any situations that might arise, a first-aid kit for wild animals should be to hand. It should contain items to cover the whole range of contingencies that wild casualties can present (Table 2.1).

THE VITAL SIGNS OF LIFE

Vital signs are the clinical indications of the existence and stability of the life of an animal. A practical knowledge of an animal's vital signs and the physiological processes giving rise to them is essential for anybody rescuing or handling wild animal casualties. These vital signs in a healthy animal will be an indication of its well-being.

A body is made up of cells, all of which depend on a good supply of oxygen and nutrients so that cellular metabolism can be fuelled. The waste products of this metabolism, such as carbon dioxide and lactic acid, must be removed from the cells' immediate environment to avoid them being poisoned.

The circulatory or cardiovascular system, the heart, blood vessels and the blood flowing through them, provides the means by which oxygen and nutrients can be distributed to every cell in the body and the waste products removed. Oxygen, nutrients and the waste products that have to be removed can only be exchanged across the walls of the extensive network of tiny blood capillaries. The normal function of this microcirculation is vital for the life of any tissue or any organ in the body.

Breathing is the mechanism by which oxygen is taken into the lungs, or into the air sac system in a bird or reptile, and delivered to the red bloods cells in the lungs' capillaries for distribution throughout the body. Simultaneously waste carbon dioxide is released from the blood and voided as the animal breathes out. Amphibians have the added ability of being able to absorb air through the skin.

An animal's vital signs provide information about the functional state of the cardiovascular and respiratory (breathing) systems and can reveal the condition of the crucial life-support mechanisms. Any compromise of the cardiovascular or respiratory systems can put life itself at risk.

The vital signs of life include:

(1) Heart rate
(2) Pulse rate and strength

Table 2.1 Components of a first aid kit suitable for wildlife casualties.

Stethoscope
Cuffed endotracheal (ET) tubes
K-Y Lubricating Jelly (Johnson & Johnson)
Laryngoscope
Disposable examination gloves
2″ Cotton weave bandage
Artery forceps 2 × pair
Space blankets
Traumastem haemostatic powder (Millpledge)
First-aid protocol
Ambu bag
Mix small ET tubes for birds
10 ml syringe for inflating ET tubes
Sterile swabs
2″ Cohesive bandage
Intrasite Gel (Smith & Nephew)
Scissors
Giant cotton buds
Thermometer
During hot weather – a cool box for drugs and some
    fluids

(3) Quality, rate and gross sounds of breathing
(4) Colour of mucous membranes
(5) Capillary refill time (<2 seconds is normal)
(6) Core body temperature

It is far safer to monitor these vital signs than it is to try to reverse the often irreversible effect of their failure. These monitoring procedures are directed towards assessing the oxygen carrying ability of the blood and the effectiveness of the circulatory system in distributing this blood to maintain an animal's cellular metabolism.

When handling or transporting an animal, frequent monitoring of these vital signs and taking the appropriate action when changes in them indicate a problem, will prevent a number of unnecessary deaths.

(1) Heart rate

Without a functioning heart none of the vital life-supporting mechanisms can work. Heart failure simply means there is no effective output of blood from the heart. It occurs when either the heart has stopped (cardiac arrest) or is misfunctioning due to uncoordinated beating of different parts of the heart (e.g. ventricular fibrillation).

If the heart is beating the veterinary surgeon may ask for the heart rate. This is not the same as a pulse, although it can be. The heartbeat rate should be counted at the chest wall over the heart using a stethoscope. Using a watch, count the number of heartbeats in 15 seconds and multiply by four. This gives the number of beats per minute (BPM).

On this information the veterinary surgeon may prescribe atropine sulphate and other drugs.

(2) Pulse rate and strength

The pulse is the result of the heart pumping blood around the arteries. It is counted and assessed at points around the body where arteries can be felt just under the skin. If the heart is functioning normally the pulse rate will be the same as the heart rate.

Three common sites to take a pulse rate are:

• The coccygeal artery which can be felt underneath the base of the tail
• The femoral arteries as they pass behind and parallel to the proximal third of the femurs on the inside of the thighs
• The brachial arteries which can be located as they cross the distal third of the humerus

In advance of an emergency it is worth familiarising yourself with these points on a dog or cat.

The pulse rate and its quality give an indication of how effectively the heart is distributing blood around the arteries:

• Its strength provides information on the pressure at which blood is being pumped from the heart.
• A peripheral pulse tells you whether blood is being circulated to the peripheral capillary network.
• The pulse will indicate if its regularity is different from the heart.
• Monitoring the pulse may provide a warning that the heart is weakening allowing remedial measures to be implemented under the direction of the veterinary surgeon. It is one of the most important signs of life.

As with heart rate, the pulse rate can be calculated by using a watch and counting how many pulse beats there are in 15 seconds and multiplying by four to give the number of beats per minute.

(3) Quality, rate and gross sounds of breathing

Even if the heart is beating and the circulation functioning, without breathing there is no exchange of oxygen, or removal of waste carbon dioxide, through the lung capillaries.

The vital sign that an animal is breathing is a steady rise and fall of the chest. This is not always obvious in birds and reptiles; their quality of breathing can be assessed by looking in the mouth and observing the opening and closing of the glottis, the entrance to the trachea (Fig. 2.1).

Sounds of breathing, inhaling and exhaling may also indicate the presence of blood or mucus in the mouth or trachea.

The colour of the mucous membranes in the mouth also give a good indication of the presence of oxygen in the microcirculation (see (4)).

Impending failure of the respiratory system can often be detected by:

- A fall in the rate of breathing to less than 50% of normal
- A progressive fall in the depth of breathing
- A pallor or blue appearance of the mucous membranes

(4) Colour of mucous membranes

The mucous membranes or mucosa are the moist layers of tissue lining many of the structures of the body. They are heavily perfused with the microcapillaries of the circulation and their status can be seen. Their normal healthy colour of bright pink is another vital sign that shows there is a good circulating supply of oxygen and good respiration. Changes in this microcirculation can often be seen by the changes in the colour of the mucosa.

(5) Capillary refill time

The gums are part of the mucosa and as such have a microcirculation of capillary blood vessels that can be seen.

By pressing on the gum, with the thumb, the capillaries will be occluded and the gum become pale. By judging how long it takes for the capillaries to refill and the colour return once the thumb has been removed it is possible to assess the capillary refill time (CRT).

Normally the CRT in animals is between 1 and 2 seconds. Anything over this provides another vital sign that the microcirculation is below par.

(6) Core body temperature

Cellular metabolism in an animal is reliant on a series of highly complex chemical reactions within cells. These can only occur within a limited temperature range. Taking an animal's core temperature, usually with a thermometer passed into the rectum, gives an indication of well-being.

However, many species have different normal core temperatures and that must be taken into account before any remedial action is taken (Table 2.2).

SIGNS OF DEATH

There is no point in attempting to monitor vital signs of life if the animal is already dead.

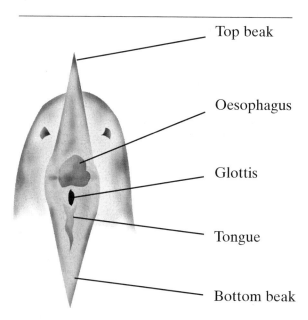

Top beak

Oesophagus

Glottis

Tongue

Bottom beak

Fig. 2.1 The mouth of a bird showing the glottis, the opening to the trachea.

Table 2.2 Some body temperatures of British wild animals.

Animal	Temperature (°C)
Badger	37.8–38.5
Bats	Vary according to ambient temperature
Birds in general	40
Bottle-nosed dolphin	37
Brown rat	37.2–37.8
Cetaceans	36–37.5
Deer	38–39
Ferret	37.8–40.0
Fox	37.8–39
Grey squirrel	37.4–38.5
Hedgehog	34–37 (Hibernation 6°C)
House mouse	36.1–36.7
Mink	37.5
Otter	38
Passerines	40–41
Pigeon	40–41
Rabbit	38–39.6
Seabirds	39–41
Seals	36–38

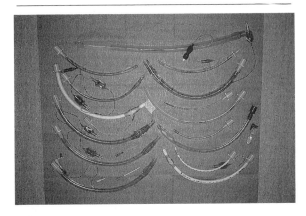

Fig. 2.2 The complete range of endotracheal tubes will be required for emergency procedures.

Just as there are signs of life to watch, there are also signs of death:

(1) Lack of heartbeat
(2) Wide dilation of the pupils
(3) There is agonal gasping
(4) The animal is not breathing
(5) There are no reflexes
(6) Rigor mortis which may or may not be present
(7) And the most positive sign, where the usually smooth, moist fronts of the corneas become glazed and wrinkled

EMERGENCY PROCEDURES

The vital life signs will provide indications as to the well-being of an animal. However, if problems do arise and life signs are not as they should be, it is important to follow the basic principles of first aid – the ABCD of first aid. These are:

A: Airways
B: Breathing
C: Circulation
D: Drugs

Airways

- Check that the passage of air into the lungs is unobstructed
- Remove any blood clots, foreign bodies, mucus or vomit from the mouth
- Make sure the entrance to the trachea is clear of obstruction
- Make sure that the tongue is pulled forward and is not obscuring the tracheal entrance
- Extend the head and neck forward to maintain a clear airway

If there is a problem keeping the airways clear then an endotracheal tube can be passed into the trachea (Fig. 2.2). Make sure the tube itself does not get blocked or become kinked.

Birds, in particular, will find breathing easier if they are maintained in an upright position on their keels.

Breathing

- Check whether the animal is breathing or not

  Signs of respiratory failure can be detected by:

- No signs of breathing for 1 minute
- A pallor or blue appearance of the mucous membranes
- Violent and frequent struggles by the animal to draw in a breath

If there are still no signs of breathing then artificial respiration can be commenced.

Artificial respiration

Chest compressions
Intermittent pressure on the chest wall can be tried to establish an airflow in and out of the lungs but this is extremely inefficient for anything more than a couple of minutes.

Mouth-to-mouth respiration
With an endotracheal tube in place, a form of 'mouth-to-mouth' resuscitation can be effectively accomplished by intermittently blowing into the lungs taking care not to overinflate them. Just enough air to cause the rib cage to lift is sufficient. This is probably the best form of respiratory resuscitation to try with bird casualties.

Mouth-to-nose respiration
Not really recommended because of the danger of zoonotic infection.

The technique, if used, is:

* Check the entrance to the trachea is clear of any obstruction
* Pull the animal's tongue forward so that it is not obstructing the airway
* Holding the animal's nose in the cup of the left hand enables the lower jaw to be held fast closed with the fingers
* This leaves the right hand free to support the weight of the animal's head (Fig. 2.3)
* Then air can be gently blown into the nose and down to the lungs with just enough force to gently lift the rib cage

Ambu bag
One of these should be included in every first-aid kit and animal treatment centre. Quite simply an Ambu bag fits on to the endotracheal tube enabling air to be passed directly into the lungs and waste carbon dioxide removed. Short regular compressions of the Ambu bag, say two breaths a second, will keep the respiration functioning (Plate 3).

The only drawback to Ambu bags is that they should not be used on birds, reptiles or amphibians

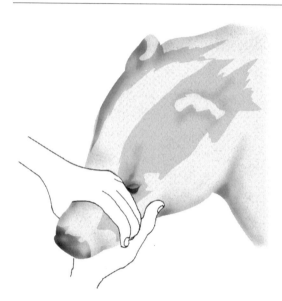

Fig. 2.3 How to hold the nose while applying mouth-to-nose respiration.

who are particularly susceptible to injury by over-inflation of their lungs or air sacs.

Acupuncture
Just below the nares or rhinarium is the nasal philtrum which, when pricked with a sterile needle, can stimulate a breathing response (Fig. 2.4).

Drugs
In an attempt to encourage the animal to breathe while you are performing artificial respiration a few drops of doxapram hydrochloride (Dopram-V – Willow Francis Veterinary), a respiratory stimulant, should be placed under the tongue. Its effect is comparatively short-lived and should be repeated every 10 minutes or to effect.

Injectable doxapram can be given intravenously at 1–2 mg/kg.

Circulation

* Listen to the chest with a stethoscope or feel for a pulse

If neither are present or are not normal then various conditions could be present.

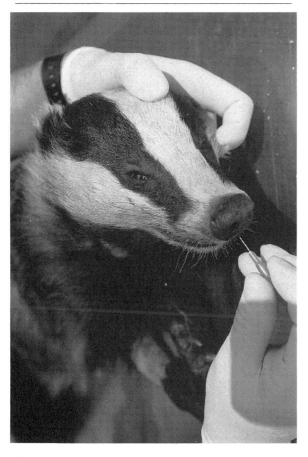

Fig. 2.4 Using a hypodermic needle (25 g) to stimulate the acupuncture point at the nasal philtrum can encourage an animal to take a breath.

sions for cardiac resuscitation it must be borne in mind that the animal may have some chest damage, e.g. broken ribs, and it is possible to cause further injury. Coupled with this should be some attempt to support and reinstate the respiratory system with artificial respiration and oxygen, if it is available.

Under the strict direction of a veterinary surgeon adrenaline can be administered and may stimulate the heart to start beating again. Adrenaline is administered intravenously at 0.01 mg/kg every 3–4 minutes or as a last resort may be injected into the heart. Simplified this would be 1 ml 1/10000 adrenaline per 10 kg.

Even if the heart does respond the effect may be only temporary so the patient must be monitored closely and any sign of the heart slowing taken into account and reported to the veterinary surgeon.

With cardiac arrest there will be respiratory failure. Attempts at resuscitation should combine both cardiac stimulation and artificial respiration. Respiratory failure usually precedes cardiac failure giving little opportunity to be prepared for cardiac arrest.

Where there has been failure of both systems there is very little likelihood that your attempts at resuscitation will be successful. However, if there is just respiratory failure, and the attempts to restart the breathing are successful, then the patient must still be closely monitored for any signs that the respiratory system might fail again.

Cardiac arrest

Feeling the side of the chest of a normal animal you should be able to detect a heartbeat even if it is very slow. Listening with a stethoscope helps in tracing even the faintest heartbeat and, of course, the lack of a heartbeat. Therefore, it is crucial that the heart is monitored constantly.

If the heart fails, within 3 minutes the lack of oxygen to the brain results in irreversible brain damage. Time is of the essence so external cardiac massage, intermittent pressure on the chest wall over the heart, may help to keep the blood circulating to the brain and other organs. Placing the head down will assist the blood flow to the brain. However, with any compres-

Ventricular fibrillation or rapid heartbeat

Ventricular fibrillation (VF) is disorganised electrical activity in the ventricles of the heart which, in fact, will have stopped pumping blood.

In some birds, particularly wood pigeons, pheasants and some passerines, the heart will be felt to start racing. The rapid vibrations can easily be described as fibrillation although technically this is not the case. As a bird's heart rate accelerates it will lead to cardiac arrest. The only hope of saving the bird is quickly and urgently to place the bird in a dark, warm environment, i.e. in a cardboard box or under a towel, and leave well alone. It is, however, unlikely that the bird will recover.

Table 2.3 Crash procedures and dosages notice for instant reference.

St Tiggywinkles
The Wildlife Hospital Trust

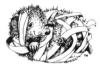

Crash Procedures

Follow A, B, C and D

> # A – Airway
> # B – Breathing
> # C – Circulation
> # D – Drugs

Adrenaline
Use only 1:10000

Supplied as 1:1000 mix with 10 parts water for injection e.g. 2 ml syringes = 0.2 ml adrenaline plus 2 ml water

Dose: 1 ml/10 kg

Use only in cases of cardiac arrest unless directed by veterinary surgeon.

Dopram V Injection (Fort Dodge Animal Health)
Intravenous injection 0.1 ml/kg repeat after 15 minutes.

Dopram V Drops (Fort Dodge Animal Health)
Orally 2–3 drops per animal under tongue. Repeat after 15 minutes.

Use in cases of respiratory arrest, unless directed by veterinary surgeon.

Atropine Sulphate
Intravenous 0.1 mg/kg

Drugs

Various specific drugs can be useful in life-threatening situations. They should always be to hand both for routine emergencies and for prescription by the veterinary surgeon (see also Table 4.3). Preferably they should be kept together and separate from other drugs in an emergency container, 'a crash box' or 'a crash trolley', where they will be immediately accessible in the event of an emergency (Table 2.3).

SHOCK

All wildlife casualties will show some degree of dehydration and can be assumed to be suffering from some degree of shock. Generally brought on by trauma, it can also be precipitated by severe dehydration, haemorrhage, diarrhoea or vomiting.

Shock is not a mental condition. It is a failure of the microcirculation (basically the capillary network) to provide adequate perfusion of the tissues with blood. Cells are deprived of oxygen and nutrients, and waste products like carbon dioxide and lactic acid are not removed. Local cellular death will occur followed by the death of the animal. Various categories of shock can be diagnosed by the veterinary surgeon but of most practical importance is hypovolaemic shock, due to the loss of blood, plasma, or just water and electrolytes. Without the input of a veterinary surgeon it is safe to assume that any animal suffering from shock is suffering from this 'low volume shock'.

The clinical signs of shock include:

(1) Pale mucous membranes
(2) Capillary refill time (CRT) longer than 2 seconds
(3) Hypothermia and cold extremities
(4) Lower level of consciousness
(5) Weak rapid pulse
(6) Increased heart rate
(7) Increased breathing
(8) Weakness in the muscles

Shock is a complicated medical condition that needs countering in different ways. In particular the use of fluid therapy is essential. Its effect and uses are more fully discussed in Chapter 3.

HYPOTHERMIA

This is where the animal's core body temperature falls below normal. The ambient temperature can have an effect on whether an animal becomes hypothermic or not. Animals that are wet and in a cold environment are particularly susceptible to hypothermia as are animals that are debilitated in some way.

Treatment could entail warm fluid infusion (see Chapter 3) or warming by fanning heat from a car heater, hair dryer or a closely monitored infra-red lamp over the animal. Immersion in a bath of water at normal body temperature is particularly effective as long as the animal is dried thoroughly afterwards.

Contact heat with a heat pad will only heat one part of the animal and may cause burning or other tissue damage. To counter hypothermia the animal's total environment has to be warmed.

HYPERTHERMIA

Hyperthermia is the exact opposite of hypothermia and can also be exacerbated by the ambient temperature. It is caused by an excessive rise in body temperature either through exposure to too much heat or else is the result of an abnormal production of body heat. Clinical signs include: rapid pulse, breathing and panting; extreme weakness, trembling and collapse. Unless urgent measures are taken to reduce the body temperature, convulsions and death will follow.

Treatment could entail putting the animal in the shade, immersing it in cold water, wrapping it in wet towels or even packing it with ice bags. Increased ventilation will enable the animal to disperse some of its own heat by increased respiration and panting. Cold water lavaged into the rectum will greatly assist the reduction of body heat, e.g. from a sports bottle with a spout.

HAEMORRHAGE

Even with a good heartbeat and a regular breathing pattern, any casualty's life could still be in danger from haemorrhage. Most wildlife casualties will be suffering from some form of bleeding, whether it be a minor scratch or a life-threatening major wound. It may be external bleeding that is obvious or it may be internal bleeding that is undetectable without sophisticated diagnostic techniques or surgery.

External bleeding is where blood appears on the surface of the body. This may be from open wounds or may be blood, lost internally, escaping from the mouth, ears, nose or intestinal or urinary tract. Internal bleeding cannot be readily seen and may be the result of severe bruising or damage to internal organs like the spleen, liver and lungs.

At the scene of an incident or when you first see the animal casualty, take note of any signs of blood and where it may have come from. Also try to assess how much blood has been lost. Any animal's body has its own defences against blood loss and any bleeding may well have stopped before you attend the animal.

There are four natural defences that may stop an animal bleeding although they may not be sufficient to save its life:

(1) *Clotting.* All natural ways of stemming haemorrhage involve clotting at the point of injury – the bleeding point. If the flow of blood is not too great, e.g. from the capillaries, then it will probably clot without any assistance. It is only when the blood vessel is large or under the enormous pressure of an artery that clotting cannot take place without a first aider's assistance.

(2) *Constriction of the blood vessels.* Arteries by nature have elastic walls that when torn across will constrict and try to close the vessel promoting clot formation. A tear has more chance of closing than a straight cut caused by something sharp.

(3) *Low blood pressure.* As an animal bleeds its blood pressure becomes lower until there may not be enough pressure to expel any further blood. At this point clots will be able to form at the bleeding points in the damaged blood vessels.

(4) *Back pressure.* Where an animal is bleeding internally into a body cavity, when the cavity is full and the pressure of the blood in it equals that escaping from the blood vessel(s) no more blood can escape and once again clots will form.

An animal that has ingested warfarin, or other types of anticoagulant rodent poison, will have its blood clotting mechanism impaired. There may be so many small haemorrhages that it may be nigh on impossible to save an affected animal. However, injections of vitamin K (Konakion – Roche) at 1–2 mg/kg repeated after 6 hours, may aid clot formation.

Health and safety

Through any of these natural processes any bleeding may have stopped before you approach the animal to move it. At this point it is worth considering whether the blood stains noted are from the animal's blood or did it bite someone who was trying to help it. An experienced handler of wildlife, especially of badgers, foxes, otters, seals or even squirrels, should not get bitten. The good samaritan, however, is very likely to get bitten and bleed profusely. There is a danger of infectious disease being transmitted between humans so surgical gloves are essential if the situation arises.

The experienced handler should not get bitten but be aware that infection can be carried in a bite or in an animal's body fluids. Notably animals' urine is the usual medium for transmitting leptospirosis, which causes the potentially fatal Weil's disease in humans.

Reactionary haemorrhage

Hopefully the natural processes have taken effect with an animal's blood clotting to stop any further bleeding. Unfortunately, the efforts of first aiders may well dislodge the clots and start the bleeding again.

There are three ways this reactionary haemorrhage can be provoked and all are unavoidable:

(1) Just moving an animal by picking it up or taking it out of a container can dislodge a blood clot and start the bleeding all over again.

(2) As you pick an animal up it may struggle and its heart rate may increase enough to raise its blood pressure enough to dislodge any blood clots.

(3) The introduction of intravenous fluids to increase the circulating blood volume may also dislodge any clots that have formed. But as will be seen in the next chapter, on fluid therapy, shock is the most likely cause of a casualty's death and must be given priority over other likely conditions.

External haemorrhage

From these examples it is easy to see how the first aider can do little to cope with internal haemorrhages. External haemorrhages emanating from wounds are much more accessible giving the first aider an opportunity to control life-threatening haemorrhages until the animal can be delivered to, or be seen by, the veterinary surgeon.

Far more birds are found as wildlife casualties than mammals; to be effective their blood pressure tends to be higher than mammals and in small birds even the loss of little more than 10% of their blood volume could be fatal. This could be just the equivalent of one or two drops spilt by the neighbourhood cat.

There are three classes of external haemorrhage:

Class I Where haemorrhage is mild, for example 10–15%, there will be few if any changes in the animal's vital life signs.
Clinical signs: Animal alert
   Mucous membranes pink
   Capillary refill time: <2 seconds
   Pulse pressure appears normal

Class II With a moderate degree of haemorrhage any changes in the animal's vital life signs will be appreciable.
Clinical signs: Animal alert but nervous
   Mucous membranes pale pink
   Capillary refill time: 2 seconds
   Pulse pressure slightly weak

Class III With severe or life-threatening haemorrhage, for example with 30% of the circulatory volume lost.
Clinical signs will be obvious and will include:
   Animal depressed or comatose
   Mucous membranes very pale or
     white
   Capillary refill time: >2 seconds
   Pulse pressure weak or absent

The first aider may feel helpless with an animal bleeding internally; fluid therapy and speed to the operating table are the only ways to possibly save the animal's life. Yet the first aider can be very effective in controlling bleeding from exterior wounds.

The point of bleeding needs to be located and the type of blood loss noted. Blood from wounds will either be arterial, venous, capillary or more usually a mixture of all three:

- *Arterial bleeding – bleeding from a major artery.* Arterial bleeding will usually be seen being pumped under great pressure in pulses which coincide with the heartbeat. It will be bright red and may be pumped out over considerable distances. This is the most serious form of haemorrhage which will result in copious blood loss unless it is controlled immediately.
- *Venous bleeding.* This is a much darker red and tends to pour out of a wound with a little low pressure. Occasionally, however, there may be a slight pulsing but nothing near the force shown by arterial bleeding. In large wounds the blood can be seen coming from the side of the wound furthest from the heart. Even though it is not under great pressure, extensive venous bleeding can result in major blood loss.
- *Capillary bleeding.* The whole body is packed with small capillary blood vessels, the microcirculation, which will rupture with the slightest wound. Any bleeding will be of small amounts, as capillaries are fine vessels, allowing clots to form more easily.
- *Mixed bleeding.* The trouble with mixed bleeding from more than one type of blood vessel is that it is difficult to identify the source and decide on which first-aid measures to use. Unfortunately virtually all wounds will show a mix of bleeding from any of these sources.

Controlling haemorrhage

As a general measure it is a good idea to dress each wound with Intrasite Gel (Smith & Nephew) before any procedures are started. This helps control the inevitable bacteria in all wounds and keeps further debris out.

Direct digital pressure

Not requiring any instruments or materials, the use of clean or surgical gloved fingers can control the haemorrhage from many wounds especially those of venous or capillary blood vessels. A finger and thumb is placed on the intact skin on each side of the wound. The intact skin is then pinched, effectively closing the blood vessels at the same time. The sides of the wound, if there are no foreign objects in it, are then pushed together and held.

This direct digital pressure needs to be held for 5 minutes giving the blood in the veins time to clot. The pressure must not be relaxed until the 5 minutes is up or else any clots that have formed will be dislodged and you will have to start all over again.

Once the bleeding has ceased apply a pressure pad and bandage to prevent reactionary bleeding. Direct digital pressure can be effective but in practice the use of pressure pads and bandage are more practical and even more effective.

Pressure pad and bandage

A bleeding wound that you cannot control with direct digital pressure may be stemmed with a pressure pad or pads and bandages. In this procedure a pad of sterile gauze swabs is used to completely pack the wound. Then a non-adhesive cohesive bandage (Co-Flex – Millpledge Pharmaceuticals) is used to tightly wrap the pad into the wound (Fig. 2.5). If the wound is still bleeding add another pad over the top of the old one and re-wrap. The old pad should not be removed because this will probably dislodge any clots that have formed. The pad and bandage should be left in place until the animal is seen by the veterinary surgeon.

Ring pad

A wound will often have foreign bodies embedded in it. In these circumstances the use of a straight pressure pad would only serve to push this debris deeper into the damaged tissue. A ring pad uses the same principle as the pressure pad but is a rolled towel or bandage laid around the intact skin at the edge of the wound, completely encircling it. The pressure bandage is then applied over the ring with just enough pressure to stem the flow of blood.

Artery forceps and ligatures

Where a major blood vessel, an artery or vein, is damaged it may be possible to isolate it and it is crucial to identify the vessel that is damaged. It is dangerous to just grope around the wound with artery forceps as irreparable damage can be inflicted on the many nerves present in the skin area.

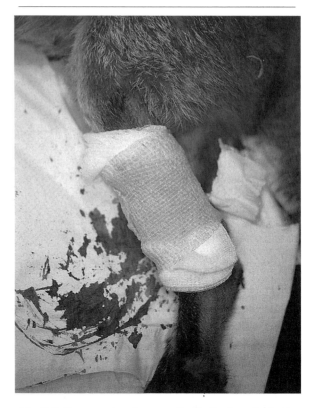

Fig. 2.5 Pressure bandage applied to the leg of a fox to stem haemorrhage.

If it is definitely located the vessel can be clamped closed, but do not be overconcerned about closing a major artery. Once a blood vessel has been effectively closed off, surrounding vessels will slowly expand and re-route the blood supply to areas beyond the defect. Eventually even new blood vessels may form to cope with the change. The clamped vessels can be ligatured with suitable suture material or the forceps can be left in place until the animal can be seen by the veterinary surgeon.

Pressure points

Sometimes the flow of blood at a wound makes it impossible to identify the offending blood vessels, usually arteries. With wounds to the limbs and tail it is possible to apply digital pressure to the arteries at the pressure points between the defect and the heart.

The pressure points are the same on all animals and can be located by feeling for the pulse on a dog or cat.

(1) The *brachial artery* runs down the inside of the humerus with its pulse being clearly felt over the distal humerus. Pressure on this point will slow any arterial bleeding below the elbow.
(2) The *femoral artery* pulse can be felt as it runs down the inside of the thigh behind and parallel to the femur. Pressure here will slow any arterial bleeding below the stifle.
(3) The *coccygeal artery* passes along the underside of the tail. Pressure under the base of tail will slow any arterial bleeding in the rest of the tail.

Tourniquets

Tourniquets are very dangerous in that they occlude all blood vessels, damage underlying tissue and, if left in place for longer than 15 minutes, can cause tissues beyond them to effectively die off. They can, however, be used if a limb has sustained major injury which may necessitate amputation. Only flat material or a belt should be used. String or any other thin material will cut into the animal causing even more damage.

The tourniquet can be applied on the intact skin above a wound. It must be released every 15 minutes and moved closer to the wound allowing the tissues under its original position to recover.

Wherever possible tourniquets should be avoided, a pressure pad and bandage can be just as effective and are far safer.

Haemostats

A product from Millpledge Pharmaceuticals called Traumastem may be used to control small arteriolar or venous bleeding in combination with the application of short-time digital pressure or pressure packing.

Other bleeding points

The nose

Epistaxis, or nose bleed, is often seen where an animal has suffered a head injury. There may well be damage to the bones of the nose. No real remedy is available to stop the bleeding although cold compresses may help.

With epistaxis it is crucial to make sure the animal can breathe by keeping its nostrils clear or, if that is not possible, its mouth clear.

Toe nails

Both birds and mammals bleed copiously from nails or claws damaged in accidents. Usually it is not too serious and can be stemmed with the use of Traumastem (Millpledge).

Pin or blood feathers

When a bird is growing new feathers, at each moult, these feathers have a major blood supply. If one of these pin feathers is broken there could be a massive loss of blood which could be life-threatening especially to small birds. Clamping the feathers with artery forceps or plucking them should stop the bleeding.

Taking all these measures on board should make sure that any wildlife casualty stands a good chance of staying alive to receive the next crucial stage of its first-aid treatment, that is the introduction of fluid therapy, either at the scene of the incident or at the medical facility.

3
Fluid Therapy
Part I: Building Blocks

TRIAGE

The vast majority of wildlife casualties taken into care are the victims of some kind of trauma. Only too often their obvious injuries attract attention while the real life-threatening conditions are unseen but already in progress, taking the animal to a point of no return. These less obvious results of trauma, shock or dehydration, are often overlooked whereas they must be countered before any attempt should be made to deal with other injuries.

The first procedure is to provide a quick and accurate assessment of the needs of the casualty. This is known as 'Triage'. The principle of triage is to sort casualties into categories of priority for treatment. With wildlife casualties there is usually only one animal presented at any time but a variation on triage can be applied specifically tailored to suit the available resources and, in particular, not to call on the veterinary surgeon to each admitted case. An experienced nurse or rehabilitator can provide instant triage and only call the veterinary surgeon for life-threatening conditions, whereas other cases can be fitted into a planned programme.

All casualties will require some treatments and examination at some stage but initially they can be categorised as, in order of ascending priority:

(3) Not in a life-threatening condition and only requiring routine first-aid treatments. An example would be an orphaned baby bird.
(2) Injured, not in a life-threatening condition but requiring first aid, stabilisation, pain relief and probably radiographs to enable the veterinary

surgeon to fully assess the animal. Candidates for euthanasia fall into this category.
(1) In a life-threatening condition demanding emergency life-saving measures and the immediate summoning of the veterinary surgeon.

These guidelines on triage can also be applied when there is more than one casualty at a time, for instance during an oil spill (see Chapter 18).

Unfortunately shock, especially, is not often encountered with companion animals but it is safe to assume that every wildlife casualty is suffering from some degree of shock or dehydration which should be addressed if there is to be any degree of successful rehabilitation.

DISTRIBUTION OF WATER IN THE BODY

An animal's body is made up of a great deal of fluid which in an adult can mean that 50–60% of the body is water (Fig. 3.1). Younger animals will have a higher water content, about 70–80%, whereas older animals have reduced body water, about 50–55%. Also, fat contains less water than other types of tissue so consequently fat animals might have proportionally less water.

Two-thirds of a body's water (equivalent to 40% of bodyweight) will be inside the cells of the body tissues. This is known as intracellular fluid (ICF). The remaining one-third (equivalent to 20% of bodyweight) will be outside the cells and is called extracellular fluid (ECF).

The ECF is further divided into:

- 5% plasma water which is contained within the blood vessels

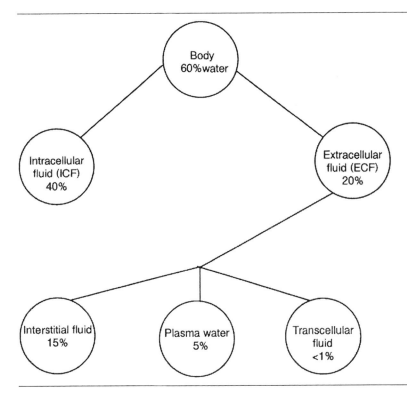

Fig. 3.1 The breakdown of a body's water content.

- 15% interstitial fluid which is contained in the spaces between the cells
- Less than 1% transcellular fluid for the processes like gastrointestinal secretions and cerebrospinal fluid

The body constantly loses water unconsciously from the ECF. This inevitable water loss is essential to support the four functions where the loss emanates from:

(1) *Respiration.* From the respiratory tract during breathing since expired air is moistened as it passes through the nasal passages and the respiratory system.
(2) *Urination.* From the kidneys during urination, although the body's metabolism will adjust for changes in hydration and water availability for excretion.
(3) *Gastrointestinal processes.* From the gastrointestinal tract in the faeces or serious fluid losses through diarrhoea or vomiting.
(4) *Skin losses.* Reliant on ambient conditions, fluids are lost through the skin or from pores in the feet during perspiration. Birds will open their mouths to disperse heat by vibrating the gular region in their throats.

To replace this lost water an animal, on average, must ingest the equivalent of about 50 ml/kg of water per day. Smaller animals, especially birds, may have a greater water requirement than this, e.g. a range of 66–132 ml/kg per day, the smallest needing the most pro rata to body size.

Inevitable water loss needing replacement in mammals also varies according to the size of the animal:

Weight of animal	Approximate daily fluid intake
1 kg	100 ml/kg
10 kg	50 ml/kg
100 kg	30 ml/kg

Drinking is obviously the best way of getting water but some birds and other animals very rarely drink. Their water intake is gained from their food whether it be meat, vegetable matter, or as some finches manage, the metabolism of dried seeds and nuts for their water content.

DEHYDRATION

An animal that does not manage to eat or drink for any length of time will still be losing fluid at the rate of about 50 ml/kg per day for a 10 kg animal. Although as dehydration sets in the kidneys will concentrate the urine to reduce water loss, losses from respiration, the skin and gastrointestinal tract cannot be reduced. Therefore a reduced water intake can easily become life-threatening to the animal, as can an increased fluid loss such as may be incurred by having serious diarrhoea or vomiting. Described simply as a fluid deficit percentage of bodyweight, a 15–25% deficit can generally be taken as fatally irretrievable (Tables 3.1 and 3.2 and Plate 4).

Commensurate with its size any animal will survive going without food for far longer than it will survive without fluid intake.

Many wildlife casualties, especially orphans, will be showing some degree of dehydration. This is just because they will not have eaten or drunk for a period of time and may have been lying unprotected from hot summer weather. In fact any wild bird taken into care can be assumed to be 5% dehydrated. Unless the dehydration is very pronounced, 10–15%, the condition may not be life-threatening. However, the added stress of being brought into captivity and handled may well push the casualty to its limits.

Whatever the degree of dehydration it is absolutely crucial that the casualty is given the right amount of fluids without any delay. Too much fluid, especially parenterally, can cause pulmonary oedema in some species while too little will not remedy the situation. Coupled with the animal's weight (every casualty should be weighed as it arrives) (Fig. 3.2), and an assessment of its degree of dehydration, using the guide in Tables 3.1 and 3.2, it is possible to estimate its fluid requirements without the need for laboratory tests such as packed cell volume (PCV) which, anyway, may be misleading unless interpreted by the veterinary surgeon.

Calculate the likely fluid deficit as a percentage of bodyweight. Added to this would be the animal's daily maintenance requirements at an average of 50 ml/kg per day or 60–132 ml/kg per day for birds depending on their size. The protocol is to try to replace the deficit over 2–3 days while still providing daily maintenance for those days (Example 3.1). If there is any doubt about calculating the fluid

Table 3.1 Estimate of dehydration in birds.

Clinical signs	Estimated percentage of dehydration
No obvious changes but assume all injured birds have some fluid deficit	≤5%
Skin appears tight, especially over the keel (breast bone). The skin forms temporary tents if pulled up. The eyes look dull. The inside of the mouth is dry, not moist as is usual	5–10%
The mouth is very dry. The feet and wing tips are cold. The skin stays tented if it's pulled up (Plate 4). The heartbeat is rapid and the bird looks ill, listless and depressed. The bird is near death. Not moving. It feels cold as shock sets in	10–15%

Table 3.2 Estimate of dehydration in mammals.

Clinical signs	Estimated percentage of dehydration
No obvious signs of dehydration but a history of fluid loss and assume all casualties have some deficit	≤4%
The skin appears tight. Mouth is dry, eyes starting to dry. Mucous membranes in mouth are dry and red. The skin appears even tighter. Eyes beginning to sink. Urine is concentrated and reduced in volume	5–7%
Pulse very weak. Animal very cold. Eyes shrunken. Animal almost comatose. Skin remains tented (Plate 4). Mucous membranes pale. Life-threatening	8–10%

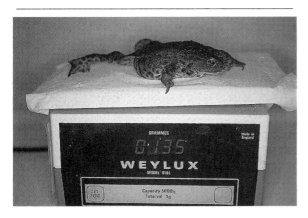

Fig. 3.2 Every casualty should be weighed on admittance.

A tawny owl weighing 400 g is presented in a dehydrated condition. Its dehydration is estimated at 10% of its bodyweight.

Assume its pre-trauma weight would have been 420 g

Fluid deficit: 10% × 420 = 42 ml

Protocol adopted is to replace deficit over 3 days giving the owl an extra 60 ml/kg per day over and above its deficit.

The owl would receive

Day 1:	$\frac{1}{2}$ deficit	21 ml
	Maintenance	25 ml
		46 ml
Day 2:	$\frac{1}{4}$ deficit	11 ml
	Maintenance	25 ml
		36 ml
Day 3:	$\frac{1}{4}$ deficit	10 ml
	Maintenance	25 ml
		35 ml
Day 4:	Maintenance only	25 ml

These amounts are further divided into smaller doses given throughout the days.

Example 3.1 The calculation of the fluid requirements of a tawny owl (*Strix aluco*) admitted in a dehydrated and shocked condition.

deficit then just provide fluids for maintenance until the veterinary surgeon advises further.

Animals suffering from lesser degrees of fluid or blood loss may not actually be in shock as various adjustments in the body's fluid distribution will have been made to compensate for these losses. This, initially, maintains the microcirculation. However, they will be heading towards shock and such losses should be replaced to prevent shock occurring.

Therefore assume that every casualty is suffering from some degree of shock. Dehydration is tantamount to shock and its assessment gives some idea of the depth of shock the patient is suffering from. Fluid therapy will counter this as will the use of corticosteroids which are generally considered to aid recovery (Fig. 3.3).

X-rays for fractures and other internal injuries can wait 24 hours for the animal to stabilise. An urgent x-ray such as for a suspected fractured spine may be one of the exceptions, whereby a short anaesthetic with isoflurane may be the only way to get a satisfactory radiograph. Otherwise the prudent use of sedatives like diazepam can safely quieten the animal to permit x-rays and the putting up of an infusion line.

TONICITY

The administration of particular fluids will assist many animals in overcoming the life-threatening perils of shock. True, an animal that starts drinking will be able to maintain its own body water content but it will benefit from assistance in replacing any deficit.

In the water content of the body, divided into the intracellular and extracellular compartments, are dissolved various electrolytes. The concentration of these solutes in both compartments is kept on an equal footing by the osmotic pressures of the solutions. A process called osmosis allows water to flow from one compartment to the other in order to maintain equilibrium.

Different fluids exert different osmotic pressures but using plasma as a yardstick those fluids exerting the same osmotic pressure as plasma are said to be *isotonic*. Those fluids that exert a higher osmotic pressure are said to be *hypertonic* and those exerting a lower osmotic pressure are *hypotonic*.

When we provide fluids to an animal we must make sure they are not hypertonic or else existing life-supporting fluids may be drawn out of the extracellular fluid. Usually isotonic or hypotonic

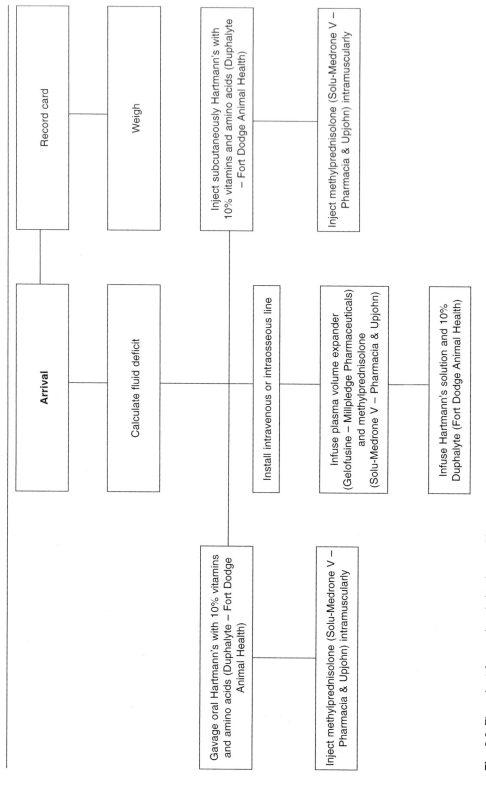

Fig. 3.3 Flow chart for newly admitted casualties.

fluids should be given to a dehydrated or shocked animal, unless a different approach is prescribed by the veterinary surgeon. They may need hypertonic fluids like glucose but advice on their use should also be left to the veterinary surgeon.

FLUID REPLACEMENT

Fluid replacement can be provided through a number of routes including orally, intravenously, subcutaneously, intraperitoneally or intraosseously, the latter being the route suitable for most small birds and other animals.

Various proprietary fluids are available to suit any situation. However, wildlife first aid will only ever need a few of these just to overcome dehydration and possible starvation. All of these are either hypotonic for oral use or isotonic for parenteral use.

International rehydration fluid (IRF)

This is very much a 'stopgap' measure if nothing else is readily available. It can usually be made up from ingredients found in any kitchen cupboard. It is hypotonic and can only be given orally. International rehydration fluid (IRF) is made up by mixing:

A dessertspoonful of sugar
A teaspoonful of salt
1 litre of warm water

It should be discarded after 24 hours.

ORAL REHYDRATING SALTS

There are many brands of oral rehydrating salts manufactured for human consumption available at chemists. They are perfectly adequate for use in animals and may even taste better than the veterinary equivalent. Similarly there are various brands manufactured for animal consumption. Usually obtainable through veterinary practices, Lectade (Pfizer) is available in packets to make 1 pint thus saving a lot of waste as it also has to be discarded 24 hours after mixing.

It is possible to mix your own equivalent oral rehydrating salts by using the following ingredients:

7 g	sodium chloride
5 g	sodium bicarbonate
3 g	potassium chloride
40 g	glucose
2 litres	water

The solution must be mixed thoroughly and discarded after 24 hours.

Oral fluids can be effective if nothing else is available and if an animal is not severely dehydrated. They are useful as maintenance fluids after an animal is stabilised and before it is drinking or feeding itself. They are probably not very effective in replacing major fluid deficit especially in a shocked animal where its gastrointestinal processes may be compromised. They are, in the main, more readily absorbed than subcutaneous fluids.

SYSTEMIC FLUIDS

Apart from the oral fluids, all other fluid preparations are prescription-only medicines which should be used under the direction, but not necessarily in the presence, of a veterinary surgeon. They are given by injection or via intravenous cannulae from a drip bag (Plate 5). In all cases they must be used in aseptic practice as their entry point offers a perfect ingress for bacteria and infection.

With wildlife casualties only a few preparations are needed to cope with all first-aid situations. These are: compound sodium lactate, amino acids and vitamins, dextrose saline and plasma volume expanders. Their use is either subcutaneous, intravenous, intraosseous or intraperitoneal. The intraperitoneal route involves entry into the body cavity, this is unnecessary in a first-aid situation and should be strictly the province of the veterinary surgeon, as a practice controlled by the Veterinary Surgeons Act 1966.

Plasma volume expanders

The main purpose of any fluid replacement is to increase the circulating blood volume. Fluid preparations are either colloid or crystalloid. Colloids, which are the plasma volume expanders, stay in the bloodstream a little longer than crystalloids and are important to maintain any initial expansion in the circulating blood volume.

In cases of shock the plasma volume expanders are the first fluids added once an intravenous catheter has been installed. They are not to be used for subcutaneous infusion. As a first administration they replace about one-twelfth of the fluid deficit. A standard rate could be 10ml/kg which could be doubled if there are signs that there has been severe haemorrhage. Like all fluids they should be warmed to about 39°C before infusion at a rate of 20–30 ml/kg per hour.

A proprietary brand of plasma volume expander is Gelofusine (Millpledge Pharmaceuticals).

Corticosteroids

To combat shock, coupled with the plasma volume expanders, massive doses of corticosteroids are recommended. They can be infused directly in an intravenous line or if that is not available given by intramuscular injection.

The intramuscular route, however, may be slow or pointless if the animal is in profound shock where its peripheral circulation has closed down and the absorption will be impaired. The drug of choice in this situation is methylprednisolone sodium succinate (Solu-Medrone V – Pharmacia & Upjohn) at a dose rate of 20–50mg/kg. It can be repeated 4–6 times daily.

Compound sodium lactate

This is a crystalloid solution to be used once the plasma volume expander has run in. It is usually known as Hartmann's solution and its smaller molecular structure allows it to pass more freely from the extracellular fluid (where it is added) to the interstitial fluid. It replaces lost water and electrolytes especially after diarrhoea.

The other benefit in a wildlife casualty situation is that Hartmann's contains bicarbonate of soda which is a buffer in countering metabolic acidosis which is another after effect of shock. In metabolic acidosis the pH value of the blood is disturbed. Large changes in pH may result in the animal becoming depressed and ultimately dying. Diagnosis of metabolic acidosis, or its opposite – metabolic alkalosis, is not easy and is strictly the province of the veterinary surgeon. A prescription to counter the more likely of the two, acidosis, would be bicarbonate of soda. The amount of bicarbonate of soda in Hartmann's solution offers some buffering in possible cases of acidosis even before the condition is diagnosed.

Amino acids and vitamins

Hartmann's solution, although full of essential salts like sodium chloride and bicarbonate of soda, does not contain the amino acids and B vitamins contained in Duphalyte (Fort Dodge Animal Health). When added to the Hartmann's at a rate of 10% it provides these extras as well as sodium acetate trihydrate which requires less metabolism to be utilised than the lactate in Hartmann's. The fluid replacement can now be utilised by tissues other than the liver, for example by the muscles. In severe cases of dehydration and starvation it can be used undiluted with seriously compromised birds or reptiles.

Dextrose and saline

Dextrose/saline is another isotonic parental infusion like Hartmann's. It contains 0.18% sodium chloride in a 4% dextrose solution.

With 10% Duphalyte (Fort Dodge Animal Health) added, dextrose/saline is useful to replace primary water loss and to provide maintenance once an animal is stabilised.

Other systemic fluids

Once an animal is stable, clear of its dehydration and recovered from shock its recovery will be slow and may not even happen if it does not get some nutrition. Wild animals are understandably nervous when in captivity. Even if they are on the point of starvation many of them will refuse to eat, and although fluids will keep them alive their condition will deteriorate. With animals like deer, who have complicated nutritional processes, their gastrointestinal mechanism may cease to function.

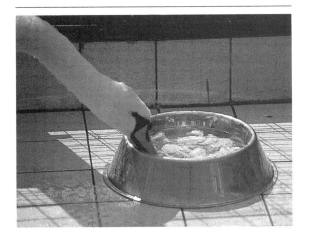

Fig. 3.4 Swans will often only take white bread floating on water.

Before any attempt to provide liquid nutrition it is important to try to offer the animal the type of food it normally sees. For instance, many mute swans (*Cygnus olor*) have grown up on lakes and ponds on a diet of bread given to them by passers-by. Often a swan in care seems to ignore other more nourishing diets but will polish off bowl after bowl of white bread floating on water (Fig. 3.4).

Think about nutrition carefully. Identify the animal and look up in books what its natural diet would consist of. Try to copy that diet if you can and hope that the animal starts to feed on its own. Sometimes a non-aggressive member of the same species that is eating while in care will encourage the reluctant feeder. If all this fails liquid nutrition or force feeding are the inevitable answers.

ORAL NUTRITION FOR BIRDS

Birds are classic animals that may not feed once they are in care. Many of them arrive in a severely emaciated state. Once their hydration is returning to normal, say after 24 hours, then it is important to provide artificial nutrition by mouth. Birds in particular are ideal candidates for a therapy called gavage, wherein a stomach tube is passed into the oesophagus or crop and liquidised foods are syringed directly into the bird. Many products are available for use in gavage for birds especially Complan (Crookes Healthcare) and Ensure

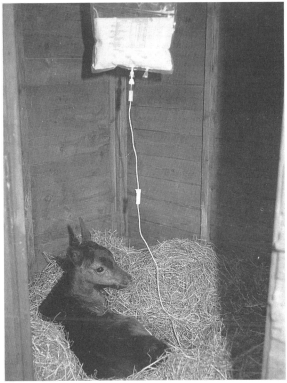

Fig. 3.5 Larger animals can benefit from nutrition given by intravenous infusion.

(Abbott Laboratories) both liquid nutrition available from chemists for human consumption.

There are, however, products specifically formulated for gavaging to birds. Manufactured by Vetafarm Europe, Poly-Aid provides all the nutrients a bird needs until it starts to feed for itself.

PARENTERAL NUTRITION

Gavage is not really an option with mammals.

For many years humans have received the benefit of being able to be fed by intravenous infusion. It has always been a complex process involving intensive nursing and monitoring as well as a constant replacement of the fluid reservoir and giving sets in major veins. B Braun Medical has now perfected an intravenous nutrition system, Nutriflex Lipid Peri, which is more flexible and versatile than previous systems.

Self-contained in a three-compartment sterile container, Nutriflex Lipid Peri (B Braun Medical) provides all the constituents of a complete building diet simply administered through peripheral veins like the cephalic and lateral saphenous veins. At The Wildlife Hospital Trust (St Tiggywinkles) we have been using it successfully to rally deer, who seem to lose condition rapidly, and other animals, especially those with mouth and jaw problems (Fig. 3.5).

All of these liquid preparations are available to benefit wildlife casualties and all have a place in the arsenal of anybody dealing with wildlife. Wild animals are quite different to companion animals and often demand innovative measures to assist them. Over the years many wildlife rehabilitators have worked perfecting techniques of administering the fluid products at their disposal. The next chapter seeks to highlight the systems evolved to provide fluid therapy to wildlife casualties.

4
Fluid Therapy
Part II: Administration

FLUID ADMINISTRATION IN BIRDS

Oral rehydration (gavage)

This is a comparatively non-invasive method of administering fluids and liquid nutrition to birds of all sizes. In many parts of the world it is the preferred way of rehydrating birds, primarily because it can be carried out without any veterinary facilities.

Using two people, one holds the bird with its head erect while the other inserts a lubricated soft rubber blunt-ended tube attached to a syringe down the bird's throat. Using a water-based lubricant will not effect the bird (K-Y Lubricating Jelly – Johnson & Johnson). The tube is passed by the glottis, the entrance to the bird's trachea and respiratory system, and allowed to slide, no pressure should be used, into the bird's oesophagus (Fig. 4.1). In the crop, not all birds have crops, it may well meet resistance. Without pushing, the tube should be twisted towards a point just to the left of the top of the bird's keel (Stocker, 1991b). Then the oesophagus continues down to the proventriculus and the bird's gizzard. This point should be estimated and marked on the tube before it is inserted. The gizzard, in fact, lies just to the bird's left, just below the sternum or breast bone (Fig. 4.2). Having the syringe (which can range from 1 ml to 50 ml) attached to the tube and both filled will ensure that the first compression of the syringe does not push just air into the bird.

Quantity of oral fluids

A bird's alimentary system is capable of taking 25 ml per kg of bodyweight. This yardstick will calculate how much fluid to gavage into the bird at any one time. This method of infusion poses no threat of over-perfusion like intravenous or intraosseous fluids.

The liquid should be warmed to 39°C and drawn up into a syringe which is attached to the end of the rubber tube. As the liquid is passed down the tube into the oesophagus it is absolutely vital to watch down the bird's throat for any liquid backing up. This would show that too much liquid is being offered so a pull back on the syringe would then be necessary to draw up any excess.

Do not separate the syringe and the tube when removing them. Still attached to each other they will be holding any excess liquid. Separate them and this will flow back into the bird and possibly into the glottis and trachea.

This method of gavage can be used for first-aid fluid administration, maintenance fluids and liquid nutrition. However, its progress is not as efficient as providing intravenous fluids. To provide intravenous therapy a managed range of fluids and disposables allows for instant fluid infusion via parenteral routes (Table 4.1).

Intravenous fluids

More effective than oral fluids but only really suitable for larger birds, intravenous infusion does allow the first aider to provide instant plasma volume expansion and effective access for emergency drugs. Smaller birds receive the same benefit through intraosseous infusion which is more practical as the veins of small birds are too small for the insertion of cannulae.

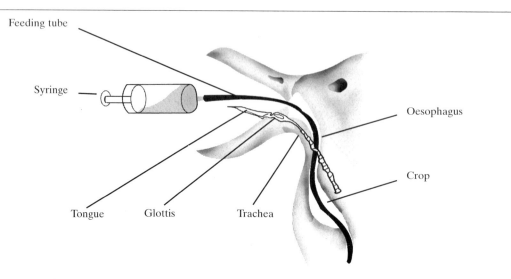

Fig. 4.1 A gavage tube should pass the glottis.

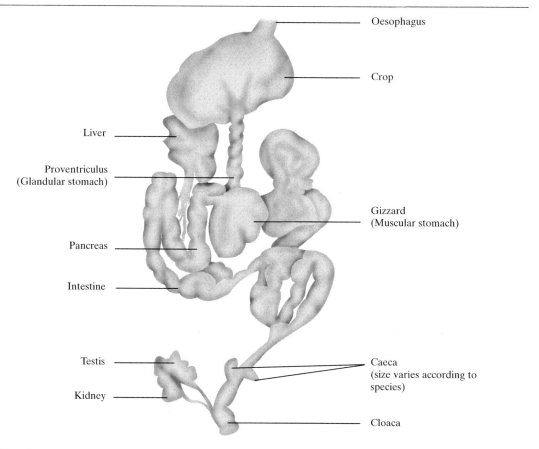

Fig. 4.2 The alimetary canal in a bird possessing a crop.

Table 4.1 Fluids and disposables instantly accessible for emergency fluid administration.

Bags of sterile fluids:
    Hartmann's solution
    Dextrose/saline
    Plasma volume expander
    Duphalyte (Fort Dodge Animal Health)
Giving sets to fit infusion pumps
Giving sets for gravity feed
Over-the-needle intravenous catheters:
    $20\,g \times 32\,mm$
    $22\,g \times 25\,mm$
    $18\,g \times 51\,mm$
$23\,g$, $25\,g$, $27\,g$ butterfly catheters
Heparinised water for injection (5000 units in $100\,ml$
    sterile water, $1:50\,000$)
Vetbond (3M) tissue glue
$2.5\,cm$ adhesive plaster
Alcohol or surgical swabs
Sterile swabs
Solu-Medrone V (Pharmacia & Upjohn), $500\,mg$ and
    $125\,mg$
Diazepam, $10\,mg$ vials
No. 11 scalpel blades (for use with muntjac)
Artery forceps and elastic bands to use as tourniquets
$20\,g$ and $18\,g$ Cookes intraosseous cannula introducers
$20\,g \times 40\,mm$ spinal needles and smaller if they are
    available
$25\,g \times 16\,mm$ hypodermic needles

Intravenous therapy for, in particular, swans, geese, herons and any large bird of prey or corvid can be provided where a vein can be accessed. The veins of choice are the medial tibia veins which run up the inside of both legs (Plate 6). These veins have more support around them than the large cutaneous ulna veins, in the wings, and are less likely to be damaged by cannulation. Butterfly infusion sets are ideal as they are simple to insert and can be held in place by a small drop of instant tissue glue (Vetbond – 3M). The size of butterfly catheter depends on the size of the bird but a range of $23\,g$, $25\,g$ or $27\,g$ will suit swans to herons, respectively. They will, however, need flushing with a heparinised solution before insertion as a bird's blood will instantly clot and clog them.

Most intravenous infusions rely on gravity to operate. Because of the minute size of some of these catheters a much surer and more accurate infusion can be guaranteed using either an infusion pump or a syringe pump.

Larger over-the-needle type intravenous catheters can be used to infuse into the cutaneous ulna vein where it crosses underneath the humerus. It is a larger vein capable of accommodating a $22\,g$ over-the-needle catheter but it has been found to be very mobile and fragile without the stability of a leg to fix it too.

Like all intrusive procedures the area around the catheter and all the components must be sterile.

Intravenous infusion via intraosseous cannulation

Although it may be possible to introduce a catheter into the veins of small birds, the practice is particularly difficult which invariably results in torn or ruptured veins. A much more stable, rigid and accessible route for fluid infusion is via the cavities in some of the limb bones.

A bird's bones are heavily vascularised and as receptive as a vein to fluid infusion (Ritchie *et al.*, 1990). The bones of choice are easily accessible; the ulna in each wing or the tibiotarsus in each leg.

Entry is obtained by gently pushing either a spinal needle or a small hypodermic needle through the centre of the proximal end of each bone until it reaches the bone's intramedullary cavity. The site must be prepared aseptically after one or two feathers have been plucked out.

While steadying the proximal end of the bone in one hand and gently pushing and rotating the needle into the centre of the bone, a sudden lack of resistance shows that it has entered the cavity. If the needle misses or exits the bone it can be detected by the hand steadying the bone and re-sited. There may be some bleeding back into the needle which may clot unless a small drop of heparinised solution is passed through it.

Small hypodermic needles such as $30\,g$, $27\,g$, $25\,g$, $23\,g$ may become clogged with bone as they are inserted. Using a syringe to aspirate the clogging allows a small amount of sterile fluid or heparinised solution to be syringed through to clear the needle completely.

With slightly larger birds, from the size of a pigeon and upwards, it is possible to cannulate the bones with spinal needles. These have an indwelling stylet that prevents the needle being clogged during placement. The stylet can be removed to facilitate infusion and can be replaced to keep the site viable.

20g or 22g × 40mm spinal needles serve to suit many species (Plate 7). The hypodermic needles in smaller birds can be closed with a luer stopper to keep them viable. They can all be held in place by Vetbond (3M) instant glue but should be removed after 48 hours. A coating of antiseptic ointment or cream around the insertion site and a cover made from a 5cm sterile swab with a slit cut in it will assist in preventing infection at these very sensitive sites.

The advantages of using the ulna in the wing rather than the tibiotarsus in the leg seems to be that the indwelling cannula there causes less interference with the bird's mobility.

Quantity of intravenous fluids for birds

Wild birds seem to fare better on intermittent boluses of sterile fluids than on the continuous infusion so suitable for mammals. As with mammals it is absolutely crucial that the correct amount of fluid is provided. With too much fluid circulatory overload can easily occur and cause major problems. Any bird must be weighed accurately, its fluid deficit and maintenance calculated and divided into as many doses (boluses), not exceeding 10ml/kg, as it takes to rehydrate it (Example 4.1).

The use of infusion or syringe pumps facilitates precise administration of the amount of fluid and a precise time, say 2 or 3 minutes, over which the infusion is given (Plate 8). Before infusion all fluids should be warmed to 39°C and kept at that temperature. Fluids running through a giving set will cool rapidly. Running the set through a bowl of warm water will keep it nearer the desired temperature. To allow more precise control there is a new piece of equipment due to come on the market called 'Thermal Angel' (Estill Enterprises Inc. in manufacture). This will attach to the giving line and be adjustable to provide the precise temperature required for infusion.

Subcutaneous infusion for birds

While intravenous or intraosseous fluids are the therapy of choice for birds, injecting fluids subcutaneously (under the skin) can be effective in providing maintenance for birds that are stable or not seriously dehydrated. It is doubtful whether, because of the shutdown of the peripheral blood vessels, it is of much benefit to a deeply shocked bird. It is, however, suitable for birds that appear to be less than 5–7% dehydrated and can be very useful in encouraging orphan birds to feed.

Only crystalloid fluids, like Hartmann's solution laced with 10% Duphalyte (Fort Dodge Animal Health), should be given subcutaneously. A bird's skin is not very elastic so the maximum bolus at any one time should be restricted to 10ml/kg, but it can be inserted into more than one site.

Tawny owl (*Strix aluco*) estimate 10% dehydrated
Estimated pre-trauma bodyweight 420g
Calculated to receive on its first day in care (see Example 3.1)

50% fluid deficit	21 ml
Maintenance	25 ml
Amount of fluids to be given in first 24 hours	46 ml
With a maximum bolus of 10 ml/kg	= 4.2 ml

Therefore:
(a) 11 boluses of 4.2 ml to be given in 24 hours	= 46.2 ml
or	
(b) Six boluses of 4.2 ml every hour	= 25.2 ml
Six boluses of 3.5 ml every two hours	= 21.0 ml
	46.2 ml

These provisions are also applicable to intraosseous infusion in birds.

Example 4.1 Calculating the amount of each bolus of fluids given to a dehydrated tawny owl.

As with all intrusive fluid administration, the sites must be aseptically prepared and only sterile equipment and fluids used for the actual infusion. They should be warmed to 39°C. The wing, web or the area of the sternum can be used as infusion sites but the capacity is somewhat restricted. A far better site is found inguinally on the inside of each thigh where the loose area of skin adjoins the leg to the body (Plate 9). Another site often used is over the back, the pelvis and the synasacrum. Fluids should never be infused in any other areas on a bird for there is a danger of putting fluid into the bird's extensive air sac system which could prove fatal. Do not try to put too much fluid into any one site as over-stretching the skin may cause necrotic areas. After the fluids have been injected in, and the needle withdrawn, pinching the skin over the site will prevent fluids leaking back out.

FLUID ADMINISTRATION IN MAMMALS

Oral rehydration

Oral rehydration by gavage is not really an option in mammals. For one thing they have teeth and sometimes it is very difficult to see the opening to the trachea where fluids could inadvertently kill an animal by drowning.

The only oral support really available to wild mammal casualties is to bottle feed infants or to slowly dribble oral rehydration salts into a co-operative mammal's mouth. In both cases it is imperative to make sure that the animal swallows properly.

Animals that will drink for themselves, provided they have the right kind of drinking dispenser, will not need any further assistance other than the provision of rehydration fluids for their consumption.

The incapacitated adult mammal may also benefit from liquid food given to it by mouth (Plate 10). Notably Ensure (Abbott Laboratories) or Complan (Crookes Healthcare) will provide nutrients even if the animal drinks them from a bowl rather than a syringe.

Do not on any account give any mammal, or bird for that matter, any of the following liquids:

- Brandy ⎫
- Whisky ⎭ a depressive

- Bread and milk ⎫ some animals cannot
- Milk on its own ⎭ digest the lactose
- Blood   bats do not drink blood

Their use should be condemned as 'old wives' tales'.

Intravenous infusion

Intravenous infusion is the route of choice for therapy to mammals. Most British mammals presented for rescue are of a size where the venous system is reasonably easily accessible. Of the animals not suitable for intravenous therapy the hedgehog is just about borderline, so anything smaller is reliant on subcutaneous fluids. The hedgehog itself is one of the few mammals that is suitable for intraosseous fluids.

Other animals – badgers, foxes, deer, otters, wildcats and larger mustelids – can all be given intravenous first-aid therapy. The problem with all these animals is that they are wild and unless comatose they will not cooperate and will bite or kick. Sedatives like diazepam are safe for use in these animals. A dose rate of 1 mg/kg should quieten an animal enough to allow an intravenous line to be set up and maintained.

All the carnivorous species are potentially dangerous whether they look lively or not. It is safer to muzzle the animal while it is being handled but be aware that if it is bleeding into the nose or mouth or seems to vomit then the muzzle must come off. These animals are much better at biting than humans are at avoiding a bite. Concentrate at all times and never put anybody in a situation where they may get bitten.

The cephalic veins are the veins of choice for intravenous infusion, but just as accessible are the lateral saphenous veins on the back legs. Of course there is the choice of the jugular veins if there is difficulty accessing the others. In general do not attach an intravenous line to a leg that is injured.

The line is fitted to an over-the-needle catheter and strapped to the leg with adhesive plaster. They generally will not last long before a lively casualty will either twist them beyond recognition or chew through the lines. 'Buster' collars do not seem to suit wild animals who seem very adept at destroying them.

A badger (*Meles meles*) is presented having been caught in a snare. It weighs 7.6 kg and appears to be between 7 and 10% dehydrated.
An intravenous line is set up using a 20 g × 32 mm over-the-needle catheter in a cephalic vein.

Its fluid deficit is calculated at 10% of an estimated weight of 8.5 kg   = 850 ml

Its maintenance requirements for 24 hours   = 425 ml

It is decided to replace deficit over 2 days

Therefore in the first 24 hours the badger is to receive 50% deficit plus maintenance   = 850 ml

On an infusion pump drip rate of 3 drips per second in a infusion set giving 15 drips per ml

In the first half hour the badger can be given 40 × maintenance rate which is 360 ml leaving the rest of the day to be infused with only 490 ml in 23.5 hours

However, as there is still 50% of the deficit to recover on the second day, it is an advantage to infuse, for the rest of the first 24 hours, at maintenance rates

For the rest of the first day the badger would receive via an infusion pump say 425 ml at 18 ml per hour   = 423 ml

With no infusion pump and a giving set giving 15 drips per ml the setting would be 4 drips per minute   = 384 ml
The shortfall with the remaining fluids on the first day is to prevent over-perfusion

---

Example 4.2 Calculating the quantity of fluids necessary to stabilise a badger casualty.

Quantity of intravenous infusion for mammals

Mammals, especially the livelier ones, do not allow intravenous lines to stay viable for long. For this reason it is often advantageous to run quite a lot of fluids in, say, the first hour and let the animal call a halt to the infusion when it is only relying on maintenance fluids. In fact in cases of profound shock the infusion at 40 times the maintenance rate can be given in that first hour.

All larger wild mammal casualties should receive the full treatment to counter shock. This means using plasma volume expanders, corticosteriods and crystalloid infusions. Maintenance fluids can be at an average of 50 ml/kg per day with all the calculations worked on that basis (Example 4.2).

Infusion of too much fluid could lead to over-perfusion of the circulation and result in pulmonary oedema. So with all intravenous infusion it is vital to closely monitor the animal and its condition (Table 4.2).

Intraosseous cannulation

Similar to the procedure seen with bird therapy, intraosseous cannulation can be the most suitable means of infusing some of the smaller mammals

(Otto *et al.*, 1989). Hedgehogs (*Erinaceuseuropaeus*), for instance, are the most frequently presented wild mammal requiring first aid and many of them are in a dehydrated, emaciated or shocked condition. The hedgehog's femur is easily accessible under it spiny pelage and is an ideal site for intraosseous cannulation.

Mammalian bones, however, are much more resistant to needles, than avian bones. For this reason inserting any form of needle requires mechanical assistance. Cook Veterinary Products now market an intraosseous cannula introducer. Basically an intraosseous cannula fits over a stylet attached to a small handle. The handle gives the added purchase to wind the catheter into the bone. The stylet prevents clogging with bone particles. Once inserted the handle and the stylet merely unclip.

To place a catheter into the proximal end of the femur the site is first clipped and cleaned. Local anaesthetic such as lidocaine or amethocaine should be applied to anaesthetise the site. The intraosseous cannula introducer is aimed at the trochanteric fossa of the femur in order to avoid involvement of the sciatic nerve. Slowly at first, rotate the introducer by the handle and once it has established a seating on the bone slightly more pressure and rotation drives the needle through. As the needle passes through the bone and into the

Table 4.2 Maintenance rates of fluid infusion wall chart.

	Fluid therapy – maintenance rate Standard giving set at 50 ml/kg per day, 15 drops per ml			
Body weight (kg)	Daily intake (ml)	Hourly rate (ml)	Drops per minute (no. drops)	Time per drop (seconds)
0.5	25	1	—	240
1	50	2	—	120
2	100	4	1	60
3	150	6	2	40
4	200	8	2	30
5	250	10	3	24
6	300	12	3	20
7	350	14	4	18
8	400	16	4	15
9	450	19	5	13
10	500	21	6	12
11	550	23	6	11
12	600	25	7	10
13	650	27	7	9
14	700	29	8	8
15	750	31	8	8
16	800	33	9	7
17	850	35	9	7
18	900	37	10	7
19	950	39	10	6
20	1000	42	11	6
21	1050	44	11	6
22	1100	46	12	5
23	1150	48	12	5
24	1200	50	13	5
25	1250	52	13	5
26	1300	54	14	5
27	1350	56	14	5
28	1400	58	15	5
29	1450	60	15	4
30	1500	62	16	4
31	1550	65	17	4
32	1600	67	17	4
33	1650	69	18	4
34	1700	71	18	4
35	1750	73	19	4
36	1800	75	19	4
37	1850	77	20	4
38	1900	79	20	3
39	1950	81	21	3
40	2000	83	21	3
45	2250	94	24	3
50	2500	104	26	3

Add deficit	3–5 × maintenance over 2 days
Shock	40 × maintenance for 30–60 minutes (Gelofusine (Millpledge Pharmaceuticals) as a plasma expander)

medullary cavity a loss of resistance is felt. Flicking the needle with a finger will show that it is properly inserted – it will be steady, if not it will wobble. Once in place gentle suction with a syringe should be applied to the needle which should then be flushed with a heparinised solution. The needle can be held in place by suturing or the use of a tissue glue (Vetbond – 3M).

Fluid infusion is at the same rate as birds, a maximum of 10 ml/kg per hour, although an infusion or syringe pump would facilitate a continuous feed infusion at standard rates per kg.

Subcutaneous fluids

Although intravenous fluid infusion is the most direct way of overcoming dehydration or shock, the facilities for cannulation especially of the smaller mammals are not always available. In these situations and with very small mammals, mice, shrews, voles, dormice and bats, subcutaneous fluids are the only answer. Hartmann's solution laced with 10% Duphalyte (Fort Dodge Animal Health) is warmed and injected under the skin over the back of the animal. Too much in one place may cause the skin to stretch and slough so subcutaneous fluids can be spread over more than one injection site.

The amount to give is about equivalent to 10% of bodyweight, i.e.:

a 400 g hedgehog should receive 40 ml fluid.

The smaller the hypodermic needle the better it is for the animal. A guide to which needle to use is:

Needle size	Animal
22 g	Squirrels, rabbits
23 g	Hedgehogs, moles, weasels
25 g	Water voles
27 g	Mice, voles, bats, shrews and dormice

FLUID THERAPY FOR REPTILES AND AMPHIBIANS

People are becoming aware of the importance of protecting Britain's reptile and amphibian populations. Consequently more are being picked up whereas in the past it was assumed that an injured snake or toad had to be killed.

As more of these cold blooded animals are presented for treatment so more techniques are being developed to help them. Fluid therapy is just as important to these animals as it is to their warm blooded neighbours.

Fluid administration for reptiles

Snakes

Snakes are now being found injured especially grass snakes (*Natrix natrix*). When presented they demonstrate the classic signs of dehydration, especially skin tenting.

Rehydration, at about 10% of bodyweight, can be orally via a stomach tube passed to a point about one-third of the way along a snake's body. Hartmann's solution laced with 10% Duphalyte (Fort Dodge Animal Health) should be used even though this is an oral procedure.

Subcutaneous fluids at 10% of bodyweight can be given into the lateral sinuses about halfway along the snake (Plate 11).

Care must be taken with adders (*Vipera berus*) which are the other common British snake. They are poisonous quite unlike the superficially similar, but now very rare, constricting smooth snake (*Coronella austriaca*) which is very unlikely to turn up injured.

Lizards

The other native British reptiles are lizards including the slow worm (*Anguis fragilis*). These are often caught by cats and benefit from subcutaneous fluids at 10% of bodyweight.

Terrapins and tortoises

Terrapins and tortoises are not native British reptiles. Escaped from captivity they should be referred to the veterinary surgeon for treatment.

Fluid administration for amphibians

Common native amphibians are frogs (*Rana temporaria*), toads (*Bufo bufo*) and newts (*Triturus* sp.). Frogs and toads especially get injured regularly in gardens or on the roads. Subcutaneous fluids at 10% of bodyweight are the best way to counter dehydration and shock.

Table 4.3 Check list notice of components of intravenous therapy.

St Tiggywinkles
The Wildlife Hospital Trust

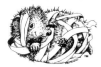

Emergency Intravenous Therapy

All intravenous (i/v) infusions should be warmed to body heat

Catheters
Swans, herons	24 g × 16 mm
Foxes, badgers, small deer	20 g × 32 mm
Large deer	20 g × 32 mm, 18 g × 51 mm
Muntjac	20 g × 32 mm

Plasma expander
Gelofusine (Millpledge Pharmaceuticals)   10 ml/kg (for severe haemorrhage use 20 ml/kg)

Severe shock and cardiovascular collapse
Methylprednisolone (Solu-Medrone V – Pharmacia   50 mg/kg
& Upjohn) *or*
Dexamethasone – slow infusion   0.1 mg/kg

Fluids
Primary loss, vomiting, diarrhoea: Hartmann's solution
Long-term loss, dehydration: dextrose 4% with sodium chloride 0.18%
[Both with 10% Duphalyte (Fort Dodge Animal Health) added]

For drip rate – see separate chart (e.g. Table 4.2)

Sedative
Diazepam   1 mg/kg (can go intramuscularly)

Antibiotics
I/V:	Enrofloxacin	5 mg/kg
	Metronidazole	40 mg/kg
Subcutaneous:	Amoxycillin	40 mg/kg (varies with species)

Analgesic
Buprenorphine (Temgesic – Schering-Plough Animal Health)	0.012 mg/kg
Flunixin (Finadyne Injection for Dogs – Schering-Plough Animal Health)	1 mg/kg
Carprafen (Rimadyl – Pfizer)	4 mg/kg

Anti-toxaemic (established infection)
Flunixin (Finadyne Injection for Dogs – Schering-Plough   1 mg/kg
     Animal Health)

Pulmonary oedema
Frusemide (Lasix – Hoechst Roussel Vet)   2.5 mg/kg

PROCEDURES RELATED TO FLUID ADMINISTRATION

Antibiotics

When an animal is in shock the microcirculation of the gut mucosa may be compromised. This means that bacteria could cross from the gut lumen into the circulation. For this reason all animals that are being treated for dehydration or shock must receive a broad-spectrum antibiotic. The antibiotic we use is long-acting amoxycillin at standard dose rates. Injection is subcutaneous. The veterinary surgeon may prescribe other antibiotics or even those that can be given intravenously such as enrofloxacin.

Analgesics

Pain killers are available for animals if required. They can be given intravenously through the intravenous infusion. Carprofen and flunixin are longer acting than buprenorphine but all should be prescribed for individual cases by the veterinary surgeon.

Diuretic

On listening to the chest with a stethoscope if there are signs of pulmonary oedema from either over-perfusion of the circulatory system or even from the trauma then the veterinary surgeon must be advised immediately in order for remedial action to be taken.

Oxygen (O$_2$)

It has been found that animals with head injuries or concussion fare better if provided with 100% oxygen therapy by face mask.

SUMMARY

Fluid therapy is recommended for all wildlife casualties. Carried out properly it will save many lives. The golden rules are:

(1) Maintain a check list of components of intravenous therapy (Table 4.3)
(2) Always use the correct fluids and none of the 'old wives' tales' remedies
(3) Only use sterile products for intravenous, intraosseous or subcutaneous administration
(4) Keep all areas of insertion aseptically clean
(5) Monitor all animals in case problems arise at the insertion site
(6) Monitor respiratory response in case pulmonary oedema is apparent
(7) Discard all disposables after use

5
Wound Management
Part I: The Biology of Wounds

In dealing with wildlife casualties, the large number and variety of wounds seen means that any type of wound in any condition should be expected. Many of these wounds would rarely be seen in normal veterinary practice, but in spite of the severity of some of them a good wound management protocol will ensure that most of the casualties will recover enough to be released back into the wild.

Basically all external wounds go through similar stages of healing, so it is important that any treatments complement the natural processes and do no further harm.

A wound may be defined as a break or division in any tissue caused by injury or surgical operation. It is obvious that wildlife care and treatment only initially needs to cope with wounds from injury. Surgical wounds are part of a surgical nursing programme instituted by the veterinary surgeon and are outside the scope of this book.

The majority of wounds that wildlife care is concerned with are open wounds where there is a break in the skin or accessible mucous membranes. Closed wounds are within the body covering and, although some may benefit from the use of compression bandages, they really are the domain of the veterinary surgeon.

The differences between the two types of wound are:

Open wounds
- Can usually be seen
- Blood loss can be evaluated
- Blood loss can be controlled
- Can usually be treated without surgery

Closed wounds
- Cannot always be detected by superficial examination
- Contusions and haematomas may be seen as swelling or bruising under the skin
- May include wounds to internal organs, e.g. ruptured liver
- Hard to access or control blood loss
- Only accessible by surgery

At the time of injury natural processes will immediately try to start the healing processes. It is very important to understand these processes so that proper management can assist and speed them, culminating in a much stronger scar site. On healing, all wounds except the finest surgical or incised wounds will leave a scar. Scarring can lead to problems which should be taken into consideration before an animal is released.

Typical scarring problems are:

- The loss of protective or insulating plumage or pelage
- The distortion of structures such as the eyelid
- Actual scarring of the cornea
- Scarring around small orifices, e.g. the tip of the penis or prepuce

All open wounds can be further categorised into:

- Clean
- Clean contaminated
- Contaminated
- Infected (dirty)

A clean wound can only occur where the surgeon aseptically cuts the skin covering during surgery.

Even this clean wound is likely to become contaminated if the surgery invades unclean body tissues or products. These two types of clean wounds will never be encountered other than in the surgery.

Contaminated wounds are those which to all intents and purposes are inflicted with a clean object. Puncture wounds and wounds of compound fractures may appear clean but already debris and bacteria will have invaded the unprotected wound. It is said that it can take bacteria 4–6 hours to gain a foothold in a wound. If the circumstances are right, this 'golden period' allows for the wound to be cleaned and closed with less risk of infection.

Infected or dirty wounds are the type most commonly seen with wildlife casualties. Often it will have been several days since the injuries occurred with the bacteria firmly entrenched and in a battle with the body's natural defence mechanisms. This natural defence may be able to cope with minor wounds but the infection seen in some major wounds will inevitably lead to the death of the animal.

Infection or dirt in a wound will inhibit healing for the following reasons:

- Debris in the wound can inhibit the function of the defending white blood cells and antibodies
- Infection can damage the vascular supply preventing systemically administered antibiotics from reaching the wound
- Infection prolongs the inflammatory phase of wound healing
- Infection produces enzymes that digest the collagen needed to close a wound
- Infection reduces the vascular supply
- Exudate, containing white blood cells, bacteria and necrotic tissue, separates the wound edges

The main purpose of all wound management, whether natural or artificial, is to get the wound cleaned so that it can eventually be closed and prevent any further invasion by infection. Closing a fresh wound that has not been cleaned properly will only provide a safe haven for bacteria to multiply. A wound cannot heal with all the cumulative exudate of dead leucocytes (white blood cells) and ingested debris and bacteria. This type of closed-up dirty wound will then become an abscess

which will need to be cleaned out before healing can start to begin.

TYPES OF HEALING

There are two types of healing classified as (Fig. 5.1):

- First intention
- Second intention (granulation)

First intention healing

This type of healing occurs when two damaged but clean, uninfected tissues are brought together. Blood capillaries will migrate from one side to the other forming a vital union. This type of healing is usually seen in surgical incisions that are sutured. Occasionally a wild casualty will have clean but contaminated incised wounds which respond well to cleaning and suturing, and with the wound edges in apposition will heal by first intention (Fig. 5.1a).

Second intention – healing by granulation

Most wounds seen in wildlife casualties have too much soft tissue damage and with the edges not in apposition they cannot heal by first intention (Fig. 5.1b). These wounds, infected or not, have to heal from the inside out by the processes of granulation. All wounds precipitate natural processes in the body from the moment that the body tissue is damaged. The processes have evolved to clean and eventually close a wound and involve four stages:

(1) Inflammatory phase
(2) Granulation
(3) Re-epithelialisation
(4) Maturation

(1) Inflammatory phase

Immediately on wounding, an increase in blood flow to the damaged area will cause extra bleeding while delivering fluids rich in protein and white blood cells (leucocytes) to the damaged tissues.

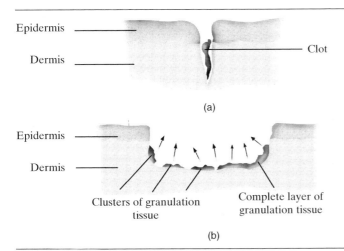

Epidermis ————

Dermis ————

———— Clot

(a)

Epidermis ————

Dermis ————

Clusters of granulation
tissue

Complete layer of
granulation tissue

(b)

Fig. 5.1 The process of wound healing. (a) First
intention; (b) granulation.

The initial bleeding serves to flush debris from
the wound. Inflammation caused by the initial
insult and the release of chemical agents from
the cells serves to close off damaged blood vessels
to assist the clotting of the blood. An increase in
the permeability of the blood vessels allows a
concentrating of antimicrobials and leucocytes into
the wound site.

Inflammation is characterised by the redness,
heat and swelling caused by the increased blood
flow and by fluid released from the interstitial fluid
through increased permeability of the capillaries.
With major inflammatory reactions the diversion of
the blood to the wound area can lead to further
decreases in circulating blood volume so crucial to
shocked animals.

At this stage various leucocytes (neutrophils
and macrophages) start to ingest (phagocytose)
bacteria, foreign matter and necrotic tissue in a
debridement phase. The resulting exudate of
dead leucocytes and ingested debris and bacteria
is the pus so commonly seen in the wounds of
wild mammals. Pus may appear repulsive but its
production is essential as the leucocytes destroy
infective material and bacteria, and in mammals
its liquidity can flow away from the wound.

Unfortunately the exudate itself is an irritation
to the healing process. Its presence continually
incites more dead leucocytes which in turn prohibits the next phase of healing, the granulation,
from beginning. Also at this time an increased
blood supply is brought in for defence so the

inflammation will not recede. This is also a deterrent to the process of granulation commencing.

(2) Granulation

Once the wound is cleared of infection tissue and
exudate, probably after 3–4 days treatment, fibroblasts, which are cells of corrective tissue, migrate
into the wound and form a matrix which will fill the
wound. Capillaries in the surrounding tissues then
proceed into the matrix and provide the copious
blood supply that is necessary for the healing
process. Then the fibroblasts start to contract and
pull the edges of the wound together.

This 'granulation' tissue with a copious blood
supply appears bright pink and is very resistant to
infection. Comprising a matrix of fibroblasts and
blood capillaries, this tissue then forms a healthy,
secure foundation over which the delicate epithelium can form to create a base for the eventual
closure of the wound.

Granulation tissue is so well supplied with blood
that it will bleed profusely if it is damaged. This is
why when it comes to cleaning wounds the author
would recommend that lavage is the method of
choice (Chapter 6).

(3) Re-epithelialisation

On the bed of granulation tissue the delicate
epithelial cells migrate inwards from the edges of
the wound to form a one-cell thick layer. Obviously

this is very fragile and should be protected. However, at this stage of healing there is little danger of further infection as long as a protective dressing prevents damage to the epithelial layer.

(4) Maturation

Once the first layer of epithelium is in place more cells will be added to, very gradually, thicken the layer. This process is very slow and may take some weeks to provide a reasonable cover for the wound. While this is taking place the majority of the capillaries supplying the granulation tissue will recede. Eventually the new epithelium will show as a scar but this will not be quite as strong nor as flexible as the original skin layers before the wound damaged them.

By managing these four stages of wound healing the ideal conditions for each process can be achieved. This will accelerate the healing period allowing a much earlier release of the animal.

TYPES OF WOUND

All open wounds, not healing by first intention, have to go through the processes mentioned above before they can heal. All the different types of wound encountered in wildlife casualties benefit from being identified and managed accordingly.

All open wounds can be identified as falling into one of the following categories (Fig. 5.2):

- Simple incised wounds
- Avulsed incised wounds
- Simple lacerated wounds
- Avulsed lacerated wounds
- Puncture wounds
- Abrasions
- Burns

Simple incised wounds

Simple incised wounds are caused by sharp object matter like a surgeon's incision with a scalpel. In the wild they can be caused by glass, cans, barbed wire and, in the case of deer, other animals. Muntjac (*Muntiacus reevesi*) and Chinese water deer (*Hydropotes inermis*) have razor sharp tusks which are specialised canine teeth. In rutting fights

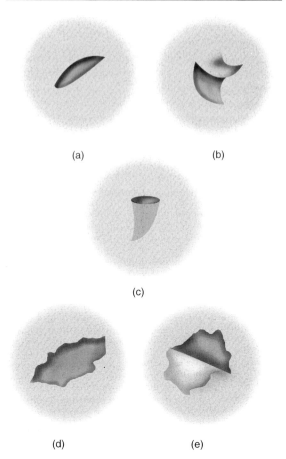

Fig. 5.2 The types of wound. (a) simple incised; (b) avulsed incised; (c) puncture; (d) simple lacerated; (e) avulsed lacerated.

the males attempt to slash their opponents and although deer skin is very tough the occasional slash will inflict a simple incised wound.

Because the wound is caused by a sharp object any injured blood vessels will be cut cleanly and will bleed profusely. However, small incised wounds may stay closed and restrict blood flow allowing clotting to take place. Large incised wounds may gape open demanding the first-aid measure of holding them closed until a more permanent remedy can be arranged.

Apart from contamination carried in by the object inflicting the injury, these incised wounds remain reasonably free of environmental debris like soil or sand.

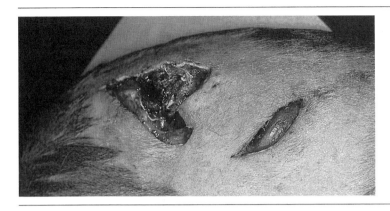

Fig. 5.3 Muntjac casualty showing simple incised wound and avulsed lacerated wound.

These are the wounds that can only be seen in a recent casualty picked up immediately after sustaining its injuries (Fig. 5.3). Within the 'golden period' of 4–6 hours the wound can be cleaned, closed and should heal by first intention.

Avulsed incised wounds

An avulsed wound is where a flap of skin has been torn away from the underlying tissue but one end of the flap is still attached. They are often triangular shape and will fit back into the defect from whence they came.

If the wound is fresh and uninfected the flap can be thoroughly cleaned and sutured back into position in the defect which has also been cleaned. In most cases the edges of the wound will heal by first intention but sometimes some of the flap will die back and have to be removed. When the remainder is in place in the defect, the remaining cavity will have to be treated as a lacerated wound.

Simple lacerated wounds

Simple lacerated wounds are anything but simple and are the wounds most regularly seen in wildlife casualties. They are usually extensive and have ragged, torn edges making closure difficult. They are usually not very deep and being exposed attract environmental debris and bacteria which stick to the exposed surfaces. There is not much bleeding as contraction of the blood vessels will in itself stop bleeding. They can cover a wide area and are characteristically accompanied by heavy bruising and pain (Fig. 5.4).

There are many causes of this type of injury with the commonest being road traffic accidents, attacks by other animals, collisions and being trapped on wire or fencing.

Sometimes the casualty is presented shortly after it has received its injury but even then there will normally be too much debris and bacteria to allow early closure and healing. First intention healing is out of the question but thorough cleaning of the wound and the use of systemic antibiotics may facilitate an early attempt at closure. However, usually it is impossible to remove all the debris and bacteria, so infection will set in and cause the wound to break down, necessitating removal of any suturing.

Most wildlife casualties will persevere with their lacerated wounds until finally the infection gains a major foothold, spreads throughout the animal and it can persevere no longer. This is when the animal drops its defences, is found and brought into care. By then any wounds will be grossly infected, demonstrating prolific exudate (quantities of pus), much necrotic tissue or, more often than not, maggots devouring not just the pus and dead tissue but often the animal itself. These wounds look appalling and often smell horribly but with proper cleaning and management they can be treated successfully. As most wounds in wild animals are of this nature it is essential that any care facility is geared up to cope with them.

Avulsed lacerated wounds

Just like avulsed incised wounds, these avulsed lacerated wounds consist of flaps of skin torn away

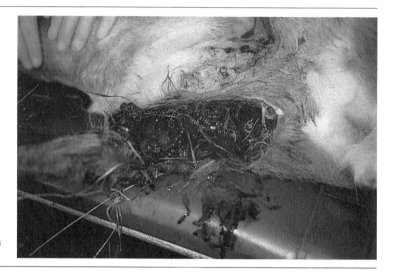

Fig. 5.4 A typical lacerated wound on a muntjac.

from the underlying tissues. Attempts can be made to clean the wounds and suture the flaps back in place (Fig. 5.5).

However, just like most lacerated wounds, they will be dirty and even already infected. In most cases the flap will be necrotic beyond redemption and should be cut back to healthy tissue. The underlying wound would then be treated like a simple lacerated wound encouraged to heal by granulation.

Puncture wounds

Wildlife casualties have often suffered puncture wounds that may be difficult to see. They are usually small in diameter but are often deep. Shot wounds often course right through the body, exiting from the other side.

The circumstances of an animal's injuries may give a clue that there are unseen puncture wounds. For instance any of the following incidents will probably have left puncture wounds which need to be found:

- *Shot wounds.* If the animal has, reportedly, been shot then searching through the fur or feathers may reveal shot wounds. X-rays will determine whether there is shot still in the body.

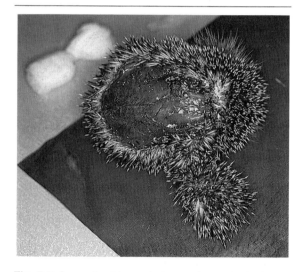

Fig. 5.5 An avulsed lacerated wound on a hedgehog.

If not then there will be exit wounds opposing the entry wounds.

- *Bite wounds.* Sometimes animal attacks are reported but often the casualty is just presented with bloody patches on its fur or feathers. Bite wounds are usually in pairs where the canine teeth of the attacker have penetrated the skin. Opposing these two puncture wounds will usually be two more puncture wounds from the attackers other two canine teeth.

- *Talon wounds.* Similarly, mammals or birds attacked by birds of prey will have talon wounds where they have been captured. Usually the back talon penetrates the deepest but the opposing three talons will have also punctured the skin. This is the case for both feet so an animal attacked by a bird of prey will have at least eight puncture wounds.

- *Impaling wounds.* These are easily located as the unfortunate casualty is usually firmly impaled on the sharp object causing the puncture wound. In wildlife this could be fishing hooks, wire from fencing or litter.

Whatever their cause puncture wounds are usually comparatively small, but deep. They are contaminated but if found early enough can be cleaned and will heal very quickly. One problem that does arise is because of the smallness of the entry into the wound, any exudate cannot escape and an abscess can form.

Abrasions

An abrasion is a wound wherein the skin is not completely punctured but the outer layers have been torn away. They are usually caused during road traffic accidents when the animal is dragged along the carriageway. Due to the traumatic way in which they are inflicted they are usually accompanied by bruising and pain.

Abrasions are normally heavily contaminated but after cleaning will heal very rapidly as epithelial layers are already intact.

Burns

The final category of wounds are those caused by burns. These are usually serious and can account for a massive loss of fluids and the ensuing shock. Burns that affect wildlife can be caused by a number of incidents including:

- Dry heat from the fire of a bonfire
- Excessive cold in the form of frostbite
- Chemical burns from a variety of sources
- Sunburn where an animal lies exposed to the sun and is unable to move

Burns may be classified as:

- *Superficial burns (1st and 2nd degree burns)* that do not penetrate the skin or underlying tissue. They are extremely painful.
- *3rd, 4th, 5th and 6th degree burns* that occur where the skin has been penetrated or destroyed and the underlying tissue involved. As most of the nerve endings in the skin will have been destroyed this degree of burning may not always be painful.

The classification of burns also requires the assessment of the amount of body surface affected. For instance 40% burning would mean the whole of one side of the animal was affected and pro rata.

Unless there is a reported history of burning, any burns may not be immediately recognised. It may even take a few days for the tell-tale signs to materialise. Good indications of possible burns are:

- Redness and heat radiating from the area as the blood vessels dilate in the inflammatory phase of wound healing.
- The tissues in the affected area will swell with the inflammation but may also have a moist appearance where tissue fluid is allowed to percolate from the capillaries on to the damaged surface.
- Pain may be apparent with superficial burns but many wild animals will mask any discomfort.
- Singed hair, feathers or spines (Plate 12).
- Sometimes if the fur was not burnt away at the time of injury it will fall out after a few days. This is due to damage incurred by the hair follicles.
- Often burns destroy the vitality of the surface tissues and after some days the affected skin will dry, become black and eventually peel away exposing a granulating wound underneath.

Chemical burns

Normally chemical burns are known to exist because the animal was found in contact with the hazardous substance. It is important when accepting a casualty to learn the identity of the chemical in case the animal has ingested some in trying to clean itself. In these cases the animal will need treatment for poisoning as well as for its burns.

It is also crucial that Health and Safety guidelines are followed in case any chemicals involved are toxic to handlers. Gloves should always be worn. The Veterinary Poisons Information Service (see Appendix 7) can give advice on treatment for chemical burns and ingestion.

6
Wound Management
Part II: The Treatment of Wounds

The treatment or management of any wound should start the moment the wild animal is picked up. First of all, wounds should be covered with clean gauze or lint to stop any further contamination. Under this cover a layer of Intrasite Gel (Smith & Nephew) or K-Y Lubricating Jelly (Johnson & Johnson) will give extra protection against further contamination which can easily be removed with water once the animal reaches the treatment facility. In fact if Intrasite Gel (Smith & Nephew) is left in the wound for 24 hours or even 12 hours there is a considerable decrease in bacterial contamination (N. Mills, pers. comm.).

Compound fractures may be obvious as the animal is picked up or there may be a small hole pierced by a bone fragment that is covered with fur or feather. These are common in wildlife casualties but can usually be treated if the exposed bone remains vital. Covering a compound fracture with a wound dressing, like the paraffin-tulle dressings (Grassolind – Millpledge Pharmaceuticals) now available, will keep the exposed area moist until further treatment can be considered. The paraffin-tulle is covered by a non-adherent dressing and held in place with non-adhesive cohesive bandage (Co-Flex – Millpledge Pharmaceuticals).

At the treatment facility a routine protocol for the treatment of wildlife casualty wounds should follow a regular pattern and have available the various products and dressings necessary to cope with any type of wound. The routine should be to treat, in a set order, the following:

- *Shock* – all casualties must, as a priority, be treated for shock and dehydration before any other procedure is attempted.

- *Fractures* – any fractures must be temporarily stabilised to ease the animal's discomfort and prevent further injury if the animal moves.
- *Burns* – these are painful, cause a lot of fluid loss and are ideal for invasion by bacteria. Treatment at this stage will help overcome shock and pain leaving a more stable animal to be treated.
- *Clean or contaminated wounds* – the cleaning of these should only be considered once the animal is stabilised, comfortable and free of pain.
- *Fly-stricken wounds* – at this stage removal of the maggots or fly eggs will prevent further damage to healthy tissues.
- *Infected wounds* – although often unsightly and smelly, infected wounds have been on the animal for some time. Leaving the cleaning of them may not make any difference to their pathogenicity and will give the animal that much longer to recover from its shock and admission. However, over 24 hours bacteria can spread into the blood stream and also toxaemia can set in so each casualty should be cleaned as soon as it is stable.

TREATMENT OF BURNS

The first response procedures to cope with shock or fractures are dealt with in more depth elsewhere in other chapters. Burns need to be addressed just as urgently at a first-aid stage whereas further treatment will require the input of the veterinary surgeon.

Dry heat burns

The protocol once the burns have been identified is to:

- Cool the affected area as quickly as possible. Running cold water over the wound will bring pain relief and in cooling the tissues prevent more cells from dying. It will also counter the risk of hyperthermia. Running water over the wound is better than cold packs as there is less pressure on painful areas.

  Wrapping the areas in cold wet towels will also relieve pain and swelling.
- At the same time the rest of the animal must be kept warm not by direct heat but by wrapping in blankets or space blankets.
- Burns are initially sterile in that the heat will have killed any bacteria on the skin surface. Covering the wounds with sterile non-stick dressings or paraffin-tulle held in place by a small amount of sterile absorbent dressing secured with a bandage will prevent further contamination. Cold wet towels can be wrapped around the dressing sites to cool the area. Finally wrapping the whole area in polythene will keep the wound moist until the veterinary surgeon can be summoned.

  Normally any ointments should be avoided but a cream, silver sulphadiazine (Flamazine – Smith & Nephew) does provide some relief from pain and infection.

Frostbite

In very severe weather conditions some animals may be exposed to frostbite and severe freezing burns. This has been seen in water birds and some birds of prey.

Frostbite is a rare occurrence in the milder parts of Britain. However, if it does occur the use of Preparation H (Whitehall Laboratories) may be beneficial as well as a suggested protocol (Plunkett, 1993). Preparation H (Whitehall Laboratories) is a haemorrhoidal preparation for humans containing shark liver oil and yeast cell extract. Its use, rubbed into an area, seems to increase the flow of blood and assists the revitalisation of constricted tissue.

Also:

(1) Apply warm compresses to the affected areas
or
(2) Immerse the affected areas into *warm* water
(3) Do not rub the affected areas but dry them gently and apply cotton bandages
(4) Do not apply pressure bandages
(5) Do not administer corticosteroids but do provide broad-spectrum antibiotics and analgesia
(6) Do not initially amputate as many apparently non-viable tissues will recover

Chemical burns

Whereas in handling all wildlife casualties you should wear latex surgical gloves, where there has been chemical pollution a pair of industrial rubber gloves will protect you from burning.

Preferably, before handling, reference should be made to the Control of Substances Hazardous to Health (COSHH) paperwork of the chemical involved. The Veterinary Poisons Information Service (see Appendix 7) will be able to advise on previous animal incidences involving that particular chemical.

If an animal has chemical burns, the affected area should be vigorously washed with copious amounts of water. The chemical should be identified and if it is a known:

- *Alkali*, like caustic soda, it should be washed off with a solution of equal parts household vinegar and water
- *Acid*, it can be washed with a concentrated solution of bicarbonate of soda or washing soda

Also check inside the mouth for burns and ingestion.

Chemical burns are not usually very deep but their severity is because they are usually caused by substances that are highly toxic.

Sunburn

Seen especially where cetaceans are stranded on beaches, there are now recommended protocols to deal with these situations. Guidelines can be found in Appendix 2.

Other incidences of sunburn have been where young unfurred or unfeathered orphans have been found lying in full sunlight. Apart from the standard treatment for burns, Flamazine (Smith & Nephew) and a homeopathic ointment (Ointment for Burns – Nelsons) have proved effective in sunburnt casualties (A.C. Creswell, pers. comm.).

TREATMENT OF CLEAN OR CONTAMINATED WOUNDS

Just as there should be protocol procedures for any practices at a treatment centre, so there should be an order of approach to wound management and treatment. In order of practise these should be:

(1) The removal of any dressings put in place before the admission of the animal
(2) Any haemorrhage resulting from this procedure should be controlled
(3) At this point a bacteriology swab should be taken for the purposes of bacteriological culture and sensitivity test to establish the most appropriate course of antibiotics
(4) Any causative agents like wire, glass or pellets should be removed
(5) The wound should be packed with Intrasite Gel (Smith & Nephew) or K-Y Lubricating Jelly (Johnson & Johnson) to prevent the ingress of more debris especially when the animal is clipped or prepared for cleaning
(6) The area around the wound is clipped; or in the case of birds, the feathers plucked
(7) The surrounding area is cleaned with a skin cleaner or antiseptic
(8) The wound itself is cleaned
(9) The wound is dressed   *or*
(10) The wound is closed.

Removal of dressings

Hopefully any dressings put on to wounds, before the animal is brought in, are on a base of Intrasite Gel (Smith & Nephew) or K-Y Lubricating Jelly (Johnson & Johnson). These should simply lift without causing further damage. If the dressings have dried in situ then they will need soaking off with warmed water or saline solution.

Haemorrhage

Removing dressings may dislodge any blood clots that have formed. Any ensuing bleeding can be controlled with sterile pads of preferably a haemostatic dressing like Kaltostat (Conva Tec) that can be left in position for 24 hours if necessary. Cut to fit inside the wound, this type of calcium alginate dressing will assist the debridement and can be soaked or pulled away bringing much of the wound debris with it.

Sensitivity

Before any of the wound is properly cleaned it is useful to arrange a bacteriology culture and sensitivity test to establish the most suitable course of antibiotics.

Gross debris removal

Any large amounts of debris in the wound can now be lifted free with a pair of clean forceps. Where there is a large object like a stake or a long thorn piercing deep into the underlying tissue it should be cut short for convenience but left in place for the veterinary surgeon to remove. This is in case removal releases haemorrhage, in the deep body tissues, that might need surgery.

In a shot-wounded animal it is not always possible to retrieve any shot. When the shot entered the body it will have dragged either hair, or feathers in a bird, into the wound. Left in place it is going to be a constant source of irritation and infection but is not always easy to access, especially in the abdominal cavity or chest. In these situations the shot can be left in situ as long as the veterinary surgeon is happy that it will not interfere with life processes or locomotion.

Protecting the wound

Packing the wound with Intrasite Gel (Smith & Nephew) or K-Y Lubricating Jelly (Johnson & Johnson) not only provides a barrier to fur or feathers further contaminating the wound as the surrounding area is prepared, but also stops antiseptics or cleansing agents, used on the skin, running into the wound.

This practice also continues keeping the wound moist, an essential for good, rapid healing.

Preparation of the wound site

All areas surrounding *all* wounds should be thoroughly prepared before any attempt is made to deal with the wound itself.

The skin surrounding the wound needs to be clipped in a mammal, plucked of feathers in a bird, and cut back with curved scissors in a hedgehog. Shaving mammals should not be considered as it can cause irritation and further complications.

Plucking a bird's feathers is the accepted way of preparing bird wounds. Once plucked the feather will be replaced by fresh growth. However, if they are cut, feathers will not be replaced until the next moult which may be months away. Just a word of warning, the plucking of feathers seems to be one of the few practices that can cause pain to a bird. Take this into account, be quick and precise and only remove the minimum number of feathers. Plucking primary feathers in a large bird can be very difficult as they are firmly anchored to the periosteum.

Cleaning of the wound environment

Once it is cleaned of fur or feathers, the skin surrounding the wound should be cleaned with dilute proprietary skin cleaners, see Table 6.1.

It is preferable but not essential to avoid getting any of these cleaning products into the wound itself. Some antiseptic or disinfectants may be cytotoxic to the cells still intact inside the wound.

Wound cleaning

The wound at this stage is still full of gel and the original small debris and bacteria. At the base of the wound exudate is forming as the leucocytes phagocytose the debris and bacteria. Underneath all this is a wound base of original tissue now profusely supplied with a blood supply and an army of blood cells. It is important when cleaning all the foreign material out that any sound material and healthy cells are not damaged.

Mechanical cleaning of the wounds with swabs or cotton wool will damage sound tissue and will force debris further into the wound. Also loose strands from the swabs or the cotton wool will themselves be deposited as further debris.

The safest way to remove all the offending matter and used gel is to flush all the wound, lavage, with sterile saline. No antiseptics or disinfectants are necessary and anyway some of these may be cytotoxic and destroy healthy cells around the wound although chlorhexidine gluconate in a less than 0.05% solution is apparently not cytotoxic.

Plain water can be used for initially flushing out the bulk of the foreign matter in really dirty wounds. However, it is not isotonic and may prompt changes in osmolarity and damage to fragile healthy cells.

As mentioned above, by far the safest fluid to use in lavaging wounds is sterile saline solution but any sterile isotonic fluids, like Hartmann's or dextrose/saline, that are left over from infusing a patient are suitable. A mix of one teaspoonful of salt to one litre of cooled, boiled water can be made up if none of the others is available.

Pumping any of these fluids into the wound at between 9 and 25 lb per square inch should

Table 6.1 Recommended dilution factors for skin cleaners.

Generic name	Trade name (manufacturer)	Recommended dilution for cleaning skin
Chlorhexidine gluconate	Hibiscrub (Coopers Pitman-Moore)	1:1000
Cetrimide solution	Savlon (Coopers Pitman-Moore)	1:1
Triclosan	MediScrub (Medichem International)	1:1

dislodge all the gel, debris and bacteria. This pressure can be attained by linking an 18 g hypodermic needle to either a 60 ml or a 35 ml syringe. Similarly a 30 ml syringe with a 19 g needle will produce the same effect.

To make lavage even simpler there is a wound lavage system available from Kruuse that fits on to any standard bag of fluid and provides up to a litre of lavage at the right pressure (Plate 13). Also on the market, and especially useful for lavaging wounds where there are maggots, are little electric pumps with nozzles sold for dental hygiene purposes. These have a little tank that is filled with the fluid and the pump pulses jets of it out through a nozzle into the wound.

An additional support to lavage is the availability of a chemical debriding agent. A mixture of malic, benzoic and salicylic acids (Dermisol Multicleanse Solution – Pfizer) will enhance removal of necrotic tissue from the wound without damage to the underlying healthy tissue. Its use is particularly helpful on animals where it is not possible to dress any wounds and which are dangerous to handle. Dermisol has been successfully used to treat wounds in badgers, otters and deer, all of which are unapproachable to treat in any other way.

Dressing the wound

The aim of all wound dressing is to keep the wound in a moist condition so that any necrotic material can be easily removed either by the body's natural processes or by further sessions of lavage.

Primary dressing

The first few days of treatment are a period of debridement and cleaning of debris. Any dressing during this period can be positive because the sooner the wound is clean the sooner it will start healing.

Types of suitable dressings for use during this debridement phase are:

- *Hydrogels*:
  - Intrasite Gel (Smith & Nephew) – a convenient hydrogel in a re-sealable tube
  - Vigilon (Seton Healthcare) – semi-permeable sheets of gel on a polyurethane mesh support

- Bio Dress Wound Dressing (BK Veterinary) – a hydrogel on a supportive sheet

- *Hydrocolloids*:
  - Comfeel (Coloplast) – an impregnated soft elastic pad or paste for application directly into the wound
  - Lyofoam (Seton Healthcare) – a polyurethane foam dressing to fill the wound

- *Tulle dressings*: Grassolind (Millpledge Pharmaceuticals) – a cotton or viscose fibre network impregnated with soft paraffin

These primary dressings will cover and keep the wound moist to aid debridement. They should be changed daily or every second day and will clean the wound without damaging healthy tissue.

Wet packs are the alternative dressing where lint swabs are soaked in saline solution and allowed to dry in the wound. Necrotic and tissue material become attached and as the packs are pulled free much of this material comes with them. Unfortunately the use of wet packs constantly damages the healthy tissue underlying the exudate.

Much is written about adding antibiotics directly to the wound. Generally, topical antibiotics may be effective during the first few hours but after that their use is pointless. Targeted systemic antibiotics are the only treatment that will be effective.

There should be strict guidelines with any wound management protocol. In particular, these are some practices which are contraindicated in wound treatment:

- Powders of any sort should not be used in wounds except where maggots are present in large animals
- Antiseptics and disinfectants, unless proven, can be cytotoxic to healthy cells in a wound
- Povidine-iodine for cleaning is ineffective as it is de-activated by any debris
- Wounds should not be mechanically scrubbed with swabs or cotton wool

Second-phase dressing

These are applied once the wound is clean, free of infection and starting to granulate. Pink granulation tissue will be seen forming around the edges and across the floor of the wound. The fibroblasts may already be causing the wound to shrink.

The continued use of hydrogel or hydrocolloid dressings will protect the granulation tissue while providing the right environment for tissue growth. Remember when changing these dressings that although the wound is now free from infection the granulation tissue is still extremely fragile and should be treated carefully.

Final dressing phase

The second-phase dressings are changed regularly until the thin, fragile layer of cells, the epithelium, starts to form across the granulation tissue. Then any dressing is just to protect the fragile re-epithelialisation.

Suitable dressings include:

- Allevyn (Smith & Nephew) – a hydrocellular polyurethane dressing
- Tegaderm (3M) – a semi-permeable polyurethane film
- Opsite Flexi-grid (Smith & Nephew) – a semi-permeable polyurethane film
- Melolin (Smith & Nephew) – a low adherence dressing
- Rondo-Pad (Millpledge Pharmaceuticals) – a low adherence dressing
- Co-Flex (Millpledge Pharmaceuticals) – a non-adhesive cohesive bandage to keep dressings in place

Generally all wounds benefit from a moist environment. However, dressings must not be allowed to get wet from external sources or else bacteria can pass through them into the wound. Change dressings regularly.

Artificial closing of wounds

A clean incised wound should be cleaned and closed as soon as possible, preferably on admittance. To heal it must be held with both sides of the wound touching. After the sound edges of the wound have been clipped, or plucked in a bird, the wound can be held closed with an adhesive dressing or butterfly strips. If practical a non-adhesive bandage can be applied to also assist in keeping the wound edges together. The aim is for the wound to

heal quickly by first intention. It may not be possible to hold the wound closed in this way especially if the animal will not tolerate dressings. In these incidences suturing or stapling are the only solutions.

Stapling is becoming more popular as it is reasonably quick and effective in forming good adjacent healing surfaces (Plate 14). Surgical staples are available in ready-to-use staplers or else have to be fitted into a stapling machine. They have to be removed, say after 10 days, with a special surgical staple remover. It is important to record how many staples were inserted to make sure the same number are removed.

Suturing is a procedure that is best learnt under the auspices of a veterinary surgeon or on one of the veterinary nurse suturing courses. It may be the only way of closing some wounds and is the only method of repairing damaged underlying tissues like muscles or prolapses (Fig. 6.1). It is preferable to use sutures with swaged-on needles as they cause less traumatic damage especially with the fragile skin of some birds.

It is important:

- To only place sutures in viable tissue
- Not to tie sutures too tightly or tissue necrosis may be the outcome – the interfaces should just about be touching

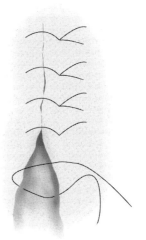

Fig. 6.1 How to tie a simple interrupted suture.

- To allow a fairly large margin between the suture and the wound edge
- To place the sutures at a suitable distance apart, say 1 cm for small wounds
- To use mattress sutures in order to get the most suitable interface for healing (Fig. 6.2)

Incised wounds and any clean avulsed wounds that are artificially closed should heal by first intention. Apart from these incised wounds, and the occasional 'suitable for suturing' granulation wound, all other wounds will need to run the full course until granulation and re-epithelialisation brings about closure.

TREATMENT OF EXCEPTIONAL WOUNDS SEEN IN WILDLIFE CASUALTIES

As well as the usual wounds already mentioned, wildlife casualties do suffer other types of wounds which, because of their idiosyncrasies and regularity, ought to be highlighted here.

Fly-stricken wounds

Any wild casualty injured during the warmer months of the year is in danger of attracting

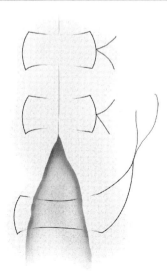

Fig. 6.2 How to tie a mattress suture.

flies that will invade any wound. Also, contrary to popular opinion, flies will attack healthy animals that have some kind of contamination on them. In particular flies will be attracted to flea faeces on any hedgehog that ventures out during the day. Similarly rabbits may be attacked around the anal and genital area. Animals with diarrhoea or faecal contamination around the hindquarters are typically at risk. In fact every casualty brought in during the warmer months, especially hedgehogs, should be thoroughly examined for fly strike.

The fly eggs themselves are like tiny grains of white rice (Plate 15). They will hatch quickly into tiny maggots that immediately start attacking necrotic or healthy tissue. Fly eggs can be brushed off with a stiff washing-up brush or picked off in clumps with forceps. Particular attention should be taken of all potentially damp areas; around the anus and genitalia, in the ears, in the eyes, in the mouth and under each leg.

In order to cover any missed eggs that might hatch it is worth starting any affected animals on a course of ivermectin (Ivomec Injection for Cattle – Merial Animal Health) or doramectin (Dectomax Injectable Solution for Cattle and Sheep – Pfizer), (Stocker, 1992). Do not use on chelonia.

If the animal is presented with actual maggots in a wound, or around its body in any orifice available, then it is imperative that these are removed or else they will kill the animal.

Sterile maggots in small quantities are being used in human medicine to clean wounds but in wild casualties there are too many maggots to restrict their consumption to necrotic tissue. When necrotic tissue is not available they will quite happily consume healthy tissue. At the same time the sheer numbers of them produce masses of toxic waste products and even toxins that can percolate through the tissues.

Maggots can be picked off with forceps but if there is a massive infestation then an electric pump like a Water Pik (Teledyne) will flush them out while also lavaging the wounds.

There is one larvicidal product on the market that effectively kills maggots. Containing coumaphos, propoxur and sulphanilamide, Negasunt (Bayer) can be effective for large animals but may not be suitable for small animals like hedgehogs and birds.

A topical larvicide that kills maggots can be made, as it is required, by mixing a solution of one part ivermectin to nine parts ordinary tap water. Only small amounts should be used and as it is unstable it should be applied immediately it is mixed.

Once again to cover any straggling maggots missed in the clean-up, the animal should be started on a course of ivermectin or doramectin. Also, as maggots do seem to produce toxins, a non-steroidal anti-inflammatory like flunixin (Finadyne Injection for Dogs – Schering-Plough Animal Health) will help counter any endotoxic shock.

Ligature wounds

In wildlife casualties ligature wounds are very common. They are caused by: pieces of string, fishing line or netting lying in the environment; snares, which are unfortunately still legal; fences particularly with fallow deer (Fig. 6.3) and muntjac (Fig. 6.4); and somehow minute pieces of hair around the legs and feet of feral pigeons, starlings (*Sturnus vulgaris*) and sparrows (*Passer domesticus*).

An animal that becomes caught up in such a hazard will, in its struggle to free itself, cause the ligature to become tighter and tighter. Sometimes the ligature gets so tight that the limb below the stricture falls off leaving a nice clean amputation site. The animal can then usually cope very well with a leg or toe missing. Where the ligature does not actually cut through the skin and tissue it will put pressure on tissues underneath it causing skin and cells to die through pressure necrosis.

Once you remove every trace of the ligature you will be left with a necrotic, infected wound following the line of the stricture. Where the wound is on a leg it is possible to treat it as any other infected wound with a course of dressings. However, if the wound is around the neck or body then dressings are not practical. Then the wound has to be treated with regular dressings of Intrasite Gel (Smith & Nephew) or Dermisol Multicleanse Solution (Pfizer).

The insidious nature of ligatures causing these wounds is only the tip of the iceberg. Many animals are freed from ligatures, especially snare victims, with apparently no injuries. However, the ligature would have already caused serious damage to the cellular structures beneath the skin surface. After a few days the pressure necrosis affecting these tissues will be seen as an open infected wound along the line of the ligature. A badger was released from a snare with apparently no injuries and within a week pressure necrosis had cut that badger in

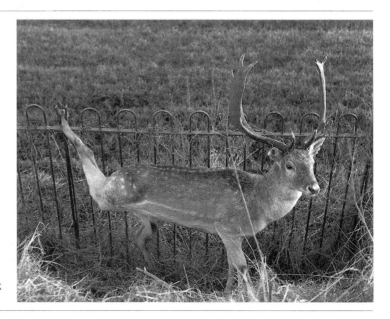

Fig. 6.3 Fallow deer trapped by the back leg.

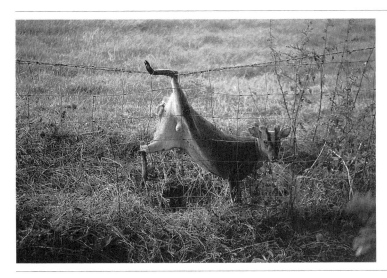

Fig. 6.4 Muntjac buck trapped in a fence.

half and killed it. This is why any animal released from a ligature or snare should be held in captivity for at least a week in order to monitor the stricture line.

Prolapses

Often seen in garden birds caught by cats, not very common in mammals but life-threatening for any animal is an intestinal prolapse where the body wall has been punctured and the abdominal organs exposed. If there is a veterinary surgeon available refer the animal immediately. If not, and if there is to be any delay in treatment, first aid is essential to save the animal's life (Table 6.2).

This is one of those major procedures that is both first aid and life saving. The animal might still die but it definitely will if no action is taken.

Eye wounds

Wild animals do suffer damage to their eyes, usually during collision incidents. The assessment of eye damage and treatment is a specialised veterinary procedure which should not be attempted except by a veterinary surgeon.

If the eye is prolapsed covering it with paraffin-tulle will keep it moist until the veterinary surgeon can take over.

Abscesses

External abscesses are formed when a wound is closed before any debris or bacteria have been evacuated. They are noticeable as they fill with pus, the exudate of phagocytosis. They are probably painful and can grow huge. Some will burst spontaneously, while closed abscesses will need opening by lancing with a No. 11 scalpel blade. At this stage it is beneficial to expand the exit hole by blunt dissection with dressing scissors.

The wound will never heal while there is still exudate present so this must be expressed and any remainder cleaned out by lavage with saline solution or Dermisol Multicleanse Solution (Pfizer). It needs to heal by granulation so the veterinary surgeon may decide to cut away some of the skin covering to allow the wound to drain more freely.

Bacteriology cultures and sensitivity tests can be done on the exudate but sometimes pus will be sterile and not register the need for antibiotics. However, antibiotic cover should be instigated with the addition of an antibiotic effective against anaerobic bacteria. Metronidazole (Torgyl Forte – Merial Animal Health) by injection will control all anaerobic bacteria present.

Wounds caused by compound fractures are very common in wildlife casualties and can lead to

Table 6.2 Emergency procedures to deal with prolapsed abdominal organs.

St Tiggywinkles
The Wildlife Hospital Trust

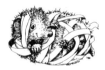

Intestinal Prolapse First Aid Procedures

The procedures which do not have to be expert are:

(1) Put the animal on an intravenous drip

(2) Wash exposed abdominal organs in warmed sterile saline

(3) Any tears in the intestines should be cleaned and sutured the best you can with 4/0 Vicryl (Ethicon), all the time bathing the exposed organs with the warm saline

(4) Gently push all exposed tissue back into the body cavity

(5) Then locate the tear in the abdominal muscle wall and suture it closed with Vicryl (Ethicon)

(6) Next treat the skin tear as a lacerated wound, clip and clean the defect and then suture or staple closed

(7) Provide broad-spectrum antibiotic cover, e.g enrofloxacin in adults

(8) Pass the animal, as soon as possible, to the veterinary surgeon

---

abscesses. The wounds themselves can be treated as any other wound whereas there is a whole range of measures to deal with any fractures (Chapter 7).

WOUNDS IN BIRDS

Wounds in wild bird casualties behave differently to those in mammals. Initially they bleed, bruise and get dirty but avian blood clots much more quickly than that of mammals and their higher body temperature makes them more resistant to infection.

There is also a theory that birds have a distribution of pain receptors different to that of mammals. Consequently even with fractured wings or legs they continue to try to fly or walk and cause far more soft tissue damage than that inflicted by their initial accident.

Being more resistant to infection, after wounds have been cleaned, and possibly sutured, birds put down granulation tissue rapidly underneath any debris or contamination. The battle of leucocytes

and bacteria does not often produce the exudate seen in mammal wounds, in fact pus in birds is usually solid or semi-solid.

When a wound in a bird starts to granulate a process called dry necrosis conglomerates dead tissue and debris into a solid mass that can be picked away, often intact, with forceps. Underneath, the granulation tissue will have apparently sealed off the wound and needs no further cleaning. Every 2 or 3 days this dry necrosis is picked away until re-epithelialisation reduces the amount and fills the wound cavity.

There are, however, bacteria that are occasionally seen in the wounds of birds and are particularly foul smelling – bird wounds very seldom smell. It seems to be particularly virulent and rapidly destroys all the soft tissues leaving a typical smelly, liquid residue. At present it seems that once the infection has taken hold it advances so rapidly that no treatments seem to be effective. Cleaning off the residue only leaves necrotic tissue prompting amputation if the infection is in a wing.

7
Biology and First Aid of Fractures

A fracture is defined as a complete or incomplete break in the continuity of a bone. Displacement of the bone fragments is not always evident.

Wild casualties are particularly prone to bone fractures. These are usually as a result of collision, trauma, predator damage or gunshot wounds. There are also fractures that have no apparent cause.

In most wildlife cases, if it is possible to catch a normally elusive adult wild bird, or mammal, then it is often a fractured limb or limbs that disables the animal enough so that it can be caught. In fact all wildlife casualties should be thoroughly examined especially looking for fractures of the limb bones, pelvis, spine and jaw.

The veterinary nurse or wildlife rehabilitator are often the first to see an animal and suspect any skeletal damage. It is then their responsibility to institute management of any fractures until the veterinary surgeon can examine the animal, obtain radiographs and prescribe a course of treatment.

Before any animal with suspect fractures is moved, those fractures must be immobilised, albeit temporarily, until the animal can receive further treatment. Any immobilisation ensures that there is:

- No further displacement at the fracture site
- Some pain relief
- No further soft tissue damage
- No further contamination of an open wound

To be able to immobilise even the simplest fracture, it is crucial to have some understanding of the skeletal structure of mammals, birds and to some degree reptiles and amphibians (Fig. 7.1). Noticeable fractures usually involve the limb 'long bones'

or the jaw. The long bones include the humerus, radius and ulna, femur, tibia and fibula (tibiotarsus in birds). There may well be fractures of bones set in deep tissue and not easily recognised. Because of these all wildlife casualties should be handled carefully until radiographs rule out fractures of the pelvis and spine.

A very useful adjunct is a range of mounted skeletons of the species normally encountered (Fig. 7.2).

In describing any suspect fractures of a long bone an indication of their site on a particular bone can be provided by these terms:

- *Proximal* – that part of the bone nearest to the body
- *Distal* – that part of the bone farthest from the body
- *Mid shaft* – a fracture more or less in the centre of a long bone

Further location detail can often be provided after radiographs have been taken. These are:

- *Physeal* – a fracture through the growth plate of an immature animal
- *Diaphyseal* – a fracture of the diaphysis or mid shaft of the bone
- *Epiphyseal* – a fracture of the epiphysis
- *Condylar* – a fracture of the epiphysis when condyles are involved

Radiographs will also provide evidence of fractures to the spine, pelvis, shoulders, ribs and skull, and in birds will highlight fractures of the coracoid and other bones.

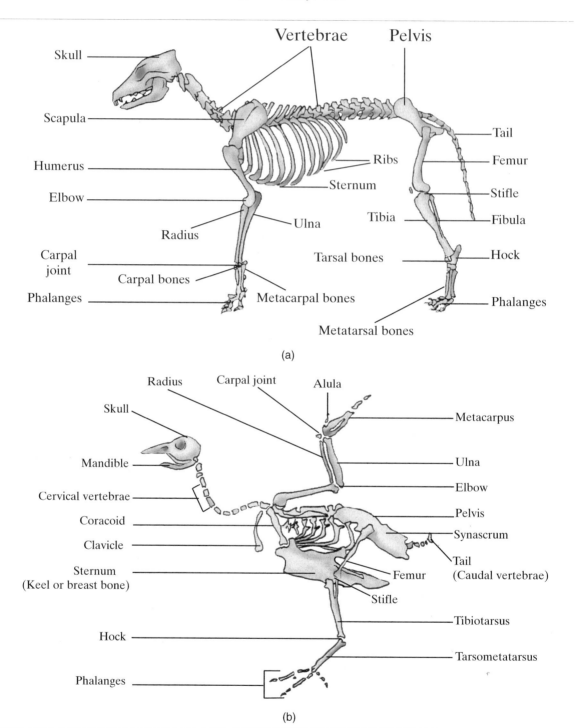

Skull

Vertebrae

Pelvis

Scapula

Tail

Humerus

Femur

Ribs

Elbow

Sternum

Stifle

Ulna

Tibia

Fibula

Radius

Carpal
joint

Tarsal bones

Hock

Carpal bones

Phalanges

Metacarpal bones

Phalanges

Metatarsal bones

(a)

Radius

Carpal joint

Alula

Skull

Metacarpus

Mandible

Ulna

Cervical vertebrae

Elbow

Coracoid

Pelvis

Clavicle

Synascrum

Sternum
(Keel or breast bone)

Femur

Tail
(Caudal vertebrae)

Stifle

Tibiotarsus

Hock

Tarsometatarsus

Phalanges

(b)

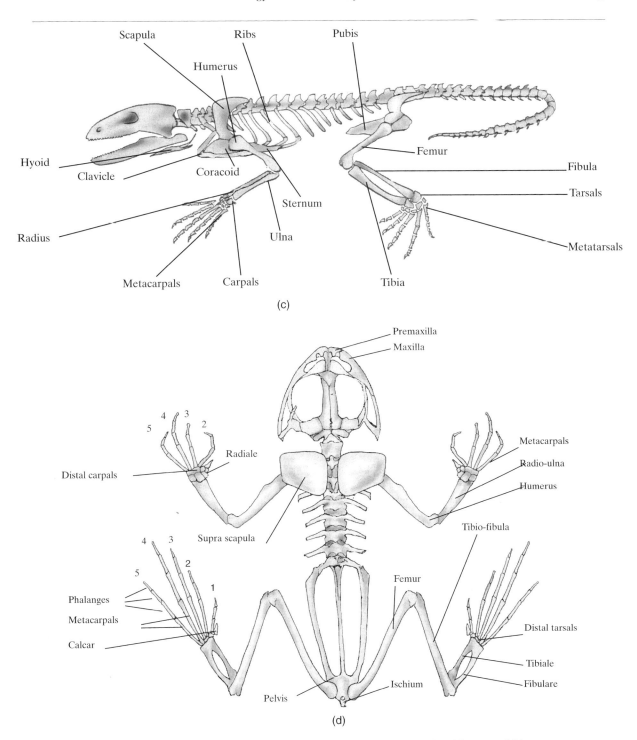

Fig. 7.1 Diagrams of the skeletal frames of: (a) a mammal; (b) a bird; (c) a reptile; (d) an amphibian.

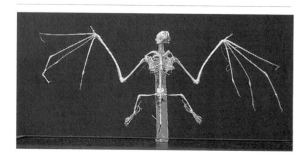

Fig. 7.2 A mounted skeleton, this a noctule bat, is a useful reference for orthopaedic injuries.

The fracture itself is further classified as:

- *Simple fracture* – where there is only a single fracture line through the bone.
- *Comminuted fracture* – where there are three or more bone fragments.
- *Open* or *compound fracture* – where there is a break in the skin above the fracture site.
- *Closed fracture* – where there is no break in the skin.
- *Greenstick fracture* – often seen in immature animals where the fracture does not pass right through the bone.
- *Pathological fracture* – usually means where disease has damaged a bone. This can be seen, for example, in young animals reared on an inappropriate diet (see metabolic bone disease in Chapters 9 and 10).

SIGNS OF A FRACTURE

Although some fractures cannot be confirmed without the use of radiography there are often detectable signs of the most common fractures, those in the limb bones. Signs to look out for include:

- *Open or compound fracture.* Quite often there will be fragments of bone emerging from skin wounds. Even without obvious fragments of bone, any bleeding or skin damage around a suspect fracture site could signify a compound fracture.

- *Deformity.* Often the first suspicion of a possible fracture is where an animal's leg or wing appears to be at an unusual angle.
- *Immobility.* Usually any limb carrying a fracture will hang loosely and uselessly.
- *Lameness.* An animal with a fractured limb will be unable to walk or fly properly. Although wildlife casualties will continue to try to use an injured limb their lameness points to a fracture.
- *Paralysis.* Fractures of the spine or pelvis may prevent an animal from using its hind legs. Occasionally a fracture of the neck vertebrae will also paralyse the front legs. Suspicion of this type of fracture needs radiography to provide a complete assessment. The animal's bladder will probably need expressing.

These are signs for observation but when the animal is contained it may be possible to identify further indications of fracture injury:

- *Heat.* The tissues around a fracture site will feel hot.
- *Swelling.* Most of the swelling at a fracture site is cased by haemorrhage, i.e. a haematoma.
- *Pain.* The animal will be in some degree of pain but wild animals, except perhaps badgers, will give no indication of the discomfort.
- *Crepitus.* As a fracture site is moved a grating may be felt, and even heard, as bone fragments grate against each other. Moving the fragments will be very painful and should be resisted until the animal is anaesthetised at the treatment facility.

FIELD FIRST AID FOR SUSPECT FRACTURES

A wild animal with fracture trauma will obviously be in some distress and may appear motionless and easy to catch. But even with more than one fractured limb a wild animal's innate flight response will enable it to move away from any would-be rescuer at an amazing turn of speed. So before any fractures can be immobilised the animal has to be caught and unfortunately handled forcefully until it is under control. Sometimes further damage during the capture is unavoidable but once the animal is under control any fractures can be temporarily immobilised in order to transport the casualty to the treatment facility. It is important to get to a treatment facility as soon as possible but simple precautions can be taken to maintain the animal's condition without causing any unnecessary delay.

First aid for fracture wounds

Any compound or open fractures should be covered with a sterile dressing or a piece of clean cloth. A pressure ring pad held in place with cohesive bandage will protect any wound site, control any further haemorrhage and restrict excess inflammation. Once these are covered any fractured limbs can be quickly and simply splinted.

First aid for mammal fractures

Possible fractures of the spine, pelvis, neck, femur or humerus cannot be immobilised by simple splinting. Animals suspected of sustaining any of these injuries should be strapped to a stretcher or laid out on the bottom of a suitable carrying basket. With larger animals like deer it is important that more than one person lifts or rolls the casualty on to the stretcher. If a stretcher is not available then any flat piece of wood will provide the requisite stability.

Paralysed deer should not be moved without a stretcher even if euthanasia is to be used. There are probably fractures present and these will cause extreme pain if the animal is moved carelessly.

Suspected fractures of the radius, ulna, tibia, fibula, carpal or tarsal bones can be temporarily immobilised by binding the injured limb to a splint or piece of wood. A few layers of padding (cotton wool) should be wrapped around the limb. No attempt should be made at this time to reduce the fracture. It is sufficient that the bones are approximately aligned.

The splint is then applied to the caudal surface of the limb and held in place with three or four strips of cohesive bandage. Where possible joints above and below the fracture should be included in the splint.

Various types of splinting material can be carried for just this purpose:

- *Zimmer splint* – is a malleable aluminium strip up to 30 mm wide with foam padding on one side.

- *Gutter splints* – come in various sizes and are plastic gutter-shaped lined again with foam padding.
- *Half casts* – saved from treatments of similar animals these are just leg casts cut in half to be used like a gutter splint.
- *Wooden splints* – any pieces of flat rigid wood can be cut roughly to the shape of a leg.
- *Inflatable splints* – these are used for human casualties and can be used for some animals but there are hazards commensurate with their use, including them getting bitten and deflated.
- *Newspapers or Magazines* – if nothing else is available then a thick whole newspaper or magazine can be wrapped around a broken leg and held in place with cohesive bandage.

With any splinting it is necessary to leave toes exposed to detect any swelling.

First aid for bird fractures

Apart from swans, geese, herons and the large birds of prey, most bird casualties are smaller than most mammal casualties. The concept of first aid to temporarily immobilise any fracture is the same. However, birds seem to have little sensation of pain from a fracture and, especially with wing fractures, will continue trying to fly with the bone fragments increasingly shredding the soft tissues of the wing. The potential for irreparable damage makes it paramount that fractures in birds are rendered harmless until more sophisticated immobilisation can be put in place at the treatment facility.

Fractures of the legs are not as common as wing fractures and can be quickly and simply immobilised with a splint and cohesive bandage.

By far the most common injury a bird will suffer is a fracture of one or more of the brittle wing bones. A fractured wing will hang uselessly beyond the fracture site although the proximal wing may still be used to flap. To simply immobilise the whole wing for a short period the bird, with both wings held folded against the body, can be slipped into a length of tubular bandage or an old sock or stocking with the end cut out. This will also contain the legs.

Large birds should have the damaged wing strapped in a folded position to the side of the body (Plate 16). Cohesive non-adhesive bandage (e.g.

Co-Flex – Millpledge Pharmaceuticals) should be crossed over the injured wing in its folded position. Then it is taken under the bird to behind its legs and then up under the other wing passing in front of the shoulder. The bandage is then taken across the back of the bird, down over the injured wing and back under, this time in front of the legs. It is then brought up under, but behind, the other wing and over the back to be secured over the injured wing.

Birds will tend to sit if they are transported in an aerated dark box with a towel on the bottom for their feet to grip. Larger birds that cannot fit into a carrying box will benefit from having their heads covered with a towel or cloth.

TRIAGE AND TREATMENT OF FRACTURE PATIENTS

Once the casualty is at a treatment facility and has received its life-saving first aid and fluid therapy, then any fractures can be evaluated and receive more sophisticated fixation or treatment.

A fracture heals in a similar way to any other wound. The body's first response is to divert blood to the fracture site where a haematoma will form as the blood vessels are damaged. In a clean and stable fracture site granulation tissue will form and stem cells migrate into it to form a callus. The callus will provide some stability but it is only formed with fibrous tissue, cartilage and immature bone. As time passes the fibrous tissue is replaced with more cartilage and bone until the fracture is stable. Then in a period of remodelling the callus is gradually replaced with new bone to bring about the original shape of the bone. Any initial misalignment of the original fragments may result in a distorted callus leading to a somewhat mis-shaped bone which in most cases will be acceptable but a deviation in any of the bones of a bird's wings can lead to problems with flying. For this reason the first attempts at definitive fracture stabilisation, at the triage stage, should take into account that any fracture has four criteria without which it will not heal satisfactorily. These are:

- *Reduction* – the fracture fragments must be aligned in their original positions.
- *Fixation* – the fracture fragments must be held rigidly until a substantial callus has formed. Even

the slightest movement may impede capillary buds trying to migrate across the fracture gap and will encourage a large callus.
- *Blood supply* – there must be a viable unimpeded blood supply to the fracture area.
- *Soft tissue* – soft tissue surrounding the fracture site must remain relatively undamaged with all tendons, ligaments and nerves intact.

Failure at any stage of a fracture's treatment can result in complications that may or may not be able to be resolved:

- *Non-union* – is where the bone fragments do not join.
- *Delayed union* – is where a considerable length of time is taken for the connective tissue to provide a stable callus.
- *Malunion* – the fragments will have healed together but not in their original line. There is a danger of entrapment of the tendons and other soft tissues.

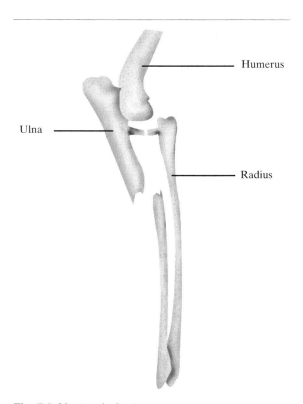

Fig. 7.3 Monteggia fracture.

- *Osteomyelitis* – is where infection is in the bone preventing final healing and callus formation.
- *Short limb* – is where the bone fragments are overridden, shortening the limb and causing contraction of the tendons.
- *Fracture disease* – particularly applicable to birds, is where the callus and healing of a fracture expands and involves nearby joints, causing them to ankylose.

Assessing the severity of any fractures will give some lead as how to initially treat them. Fractures can be classified in one of three categories:

(1) *The critical fracture* requires immediate intervention by the veterinary surgeon. They are generally life-threatening or non-sustainable requiring definitive treatments or drug application.

These emergencies include skull fractures, spinal fractures, jaw fractures and joint dislocations. One condition we see regularly in deer casualties is the Monteggia fracture where a fracture of the ulna is accompanied by a dislocation of the radial head (Fig. 7.3). The veterinary surgeon may want to operate as soon as possible. Any delay may make the fracture harder to treat or even inoperable.

These fractures, together with fresh open or compound fractures, should be dealt with immediately on admission. Failure to do so could be inflicting unnecessary pain on the casualty and may jeopardise the chance of satisfactory healing.

(2) *The semi-critical fracture* may lead to complications if it is not handled appropriately from the outset. Initially at triage the semi-critical fracture can be immobilised for future assessment by the veterinary surgeon within 24 hours.

Semi-critical fractures include old open fractures, closed fractures of the long bones, joint surfaces and epiphyseal growth plates as well as fractures of the pelvis.

(3) *The non-critical fracture* is still important but can often be immobilised with coaptation splints requiring no further intervention. These include closed fractures of the lower limb bones, greenstick fractures and tail fractures.

This chapter has dealt with the general biology and first aid of fractures. The management of fractures will be dealt with in the next chapter (Chapter 8).

8
Fracture Management

Part I: Fractures in Mammals

Fractures in mammals may be classified according to the three categories detailed in Chapter 7, namely critical, semi-critical or non-critical.

THE CRITICAL FRACTURE

Any suspicion of a critical fracture must be referred to the veterinary surgeon for immediate intervention.

Spinal fractures

Any sign of paralysis may involve a spinal fracture. A casualty must be kept strapped to a stretcher or medical trolley until the veterinary surgeon has been able to obtain radiographs and make a prognosis.

Although euthanasia is usually the only option available sometimes the veterinary surgeon may decide there is a chance of surgery or recovery. Keeping the animal completely immobile will assist if there is a chance of recovery.

Paralysed animals have usually lost bladder function so to ease this life-threatening condition the bladder can be expressed at least twice daily. There may also be loss of anal tone and reflexes leading to constipation and/or contamination of the area.

Skull fractures

Animals with suspect skull fractures should, like all casualties with head injuries, be provided with 100% oxygen by face mask or nebuliser. The veterinary surgeon may require radiographs but the animal should be kept immobile until this time.

Muntjac deer have two stems of the skull that provide bases for the pedicles and antlers. Being skull tissue they are much more fragile than the antlers and often get fractured in collision injuries. They can usually be immobilised by wrapping them together with 2.5 cm fibre-glass casting tape (Vet Glas – Millpledge Pharmaceuticals). These skull fractures usually heal with no complications in about 6 weeks (Fig. 8.1).

Jaw fractures

Until a jaw fracture is stabilised an animal is not going to be able to eat or drink. Nasogastric or oesophageal feeding tubes are not really appropriate for wild mammal nutritional therapy as any handling or approach to the animal only succeeds in creating extra stress.

At triage a fractured jaw of any mammal with a well-defined muzzle can be supported by a tape muzzle (Welsh, 1981). This consists of two rings of tape, one around the animal's muzzle just below the eyes with the other around the neck just behind the ears (Fig. 8.2). The rings are made of two lengths, each of 2.5 cm zinc oxide tape, placed adhesive sides together as rings around the muzzle and neck. They are joined by similar double straps of zinc oxide plaster to keep them in position. The nose ring should be loose enough so that the mouth can open slightly in case the animal vomits. This will keep the jaw secure until the veterinary surgeon decides on treatment.

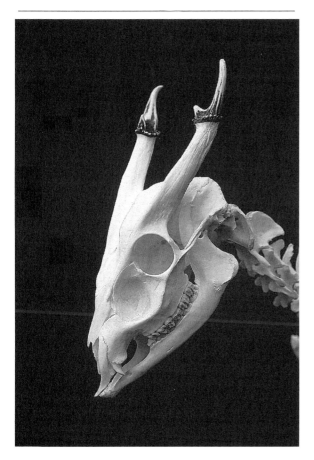

Fig. 8.1 Muntjac skull showing, below the pedicles, the skull stems that are often fractured.

Fresh open or compound fractures

Although not often seen in veterinary practices, open or compound fractures are very common in wildlife casualties. They add the hazard of infection to a fracture site and the possibility of osteomyelitis affecting the bone itself. There is also the threat of damage to soft tissues like blood vessels, nerves, ligaments and tendons. Treating the fracture site, just as with any other wound, it is easy to see that if advantage could be taken of the so-called 'golden period' then infection may be kept at bay so reducing the period the bone takes to heal.

In spite of an attempt to obviate any infection, a bacteriological swab for sensitivity testing should be taken before any attempt is made to clean the wound. This is to provide guidance as to which antibiotic therapy is most suitable.

The fracture site should then be treated along the lines of any other clean but contaminated wound (see Chapters 5 and 6). This involves covering the wound, clipping and cleaning the surrounding intact skin and lavaging the wound and bone fragments with sterile saline solution.

Any exposed bone should be manipulated to beneath the skin covering. This does not mean a reduction of the fracture but the skin covering will keep the bone moist, vital and clear of further infection. Temporary sutures or skin staples covered with a non-adhesive dressing will hold the covering skin until the veterinary surgeon operates.

The veterinary surgeon may well decide on a system of internal or internal/external fixation of any fracture. Before this takes places any fractured limbs should be immobilised especially those with open fractures that are temporarily covered.

Without either internal or internal/external fixation, fractured limbs can be reasonably well immobilised with a series of coaptation devices that at least diminish the opportunity for the animal to cause itself any more trauma by trying to use a fractured limb. These devices consist of three recognised bandaging techniques:

- The Robert Jones bandage
- The Velpeau sling
- The Ehmer sling

or a mixture of innovative splints and casts.

Robert Jones bandage

A Robert Jones bandage can be applied to provide stability to fractures of the lower limb bones, namely the radius, ulna, metacarpals and the tibia, fibula and metatarsus. When it is applied to include the joints proximal and distal to the fracture it provides sturdy support without applying too much pressure to the soft tissue involved. Yet as with any immobilisation method two toes should be left exposed just in case any swelling develops. If it does the bandage must be immediately removed.

Application of the Robert Jones bandage (Fig. 8.3)
(1) Cut two strips of 2.5 cm adhesive tape long enough to cover the metacarpal or metatarsal

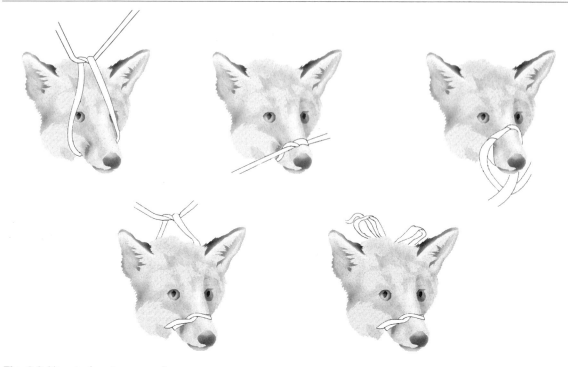

Fig. 8.2 How to tie a tape muzzle.

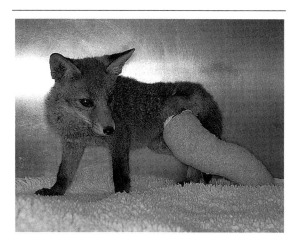

Fig. 8.3 A fox coping with a Robert Jones bandage immobilising a fracture.

(2) The leg is held extended by these two tapes while four or five layers of a complete roll of cotton wool is wrapped around the leg covering the fracture site and the joints above and below it. It is stopped short on the foot so that two toes are left exposed.

(3) Then bandage over the top of the cotton wool with white open-weave bandage starting distally and working up the leg.

(4) 'Flick' the bandage with a finger. It should make a resonant sound that lets you know there is sufficient tension on the cotton wool.

(5) Pull apart and reflect back along the bandage the two strips of adhesive tape to provide stirrups to stop the bandage slipping.

(6) Now cover the whole bandage with either adhesive tape or cohesive bandage.

Velpeau sling

It is not possible to externally splint either a fractured humerus or scapula. As a temporary support

bones plus about 10 cm. These are then applied to the front and back of the foot with the extra 10 cm of tape overhanging the foot and being stuck to each other.

a Velpeau sling will prevent the animal from using the front leg that is injured.

Application of the Velpeau sling (Fig. 8.4)
(1) The shoulder area and forearm should be lightly padded with cotton wool.
(2) The elbow is then placed in flexion at an angle of about 90°.
(3) Conforming (Knit-Fix – Millpledge Pharmaceuticals), open-weave, or self-adhesive cohesive bandage is then wrapped around the forearm, passed up the side of the chest and over the shoulder.
(4) It is then taken down the side of the other shoulder, across the chest and back under the original forearm.
(5) This is repeated several times, each time progressing the bandage on the forearm towards the foot and all the time keeping the elbow below the carpus.
(6) The Velpeau sling is secured with adhesive tape.

Not an ideal solution to injury of the upper front leg but as a temporary measure the Velpeau sling should not impede the animal's movement and can provide stability until surgery is arranged.

Ehmer sling

The femur and hip area of an animal are usually so well covered in muscle that it is impossible to successfully immobilise fractures or dislocations without surgical intervention. However, the Ehmer sling will support that area of the leg and reduce the opportunity for further trauma or dislocation.

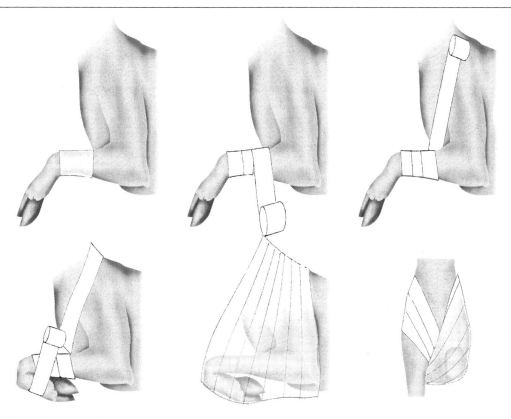

Fig. 8.4 How to apply a Velpeau sling.

Application of the Ehmer sling (Fig. 8.5)

(1) The animal is laid on its side with its injured leg uppermost.
(2) Cotton wool is wrapped around the metatarsus to prevent rubbing and swelling.
(3) The hock and stifle should be slightly flexed – full flexion could impair circulation to the region.
(4) Using cohesive self-adhesive bandage (Co-Flex – Millpledge Pharmaceuticals) wrap it a few times around the metatarsus.
(5) Flex the whole leg and turn the foot inwards bringing the bandage up over the inside of the stifle.
(6) Bring the bandage down and once more pass under the metatarsus and back over the stifle.
(7) This time bring the bandage down over the stifle but behind the hock.
(8) Bring the bandage back under the metatarsus, back over it and up over the inside of the stifle once more.
(9) Repeat this figure-of-eight bandaging until the hip and leg feel secure.
(10) Secure with adhesive tape.

Splints

Splints are much easier to apply than a Robert Jones bandage to fractures of the lower limb bones. However, they are not as effective and if fitted incorrectly can cause restriction or damage to the soft tissues or conversely can be too loose to be effective.

Splints are available to buy or can be made quite easily:

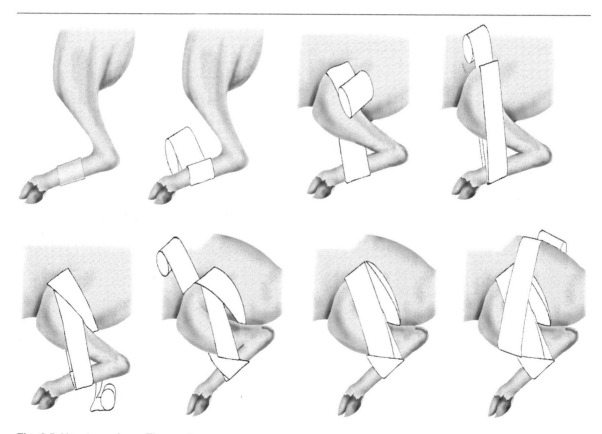

Fig. 8.5 How to apply an Ehmer sling.

- *Zimmer or finger splints* (Alumfoam – Millpledge Pharmaceuticals) are made of aluminium, of different widths, padded on one side with foam rubber. They can easily be moulded to fit the leg but are not very strong and would be easily bent by larger animals.
- *Gutter splints* are plastic padded inside the gutter groove. They can be bought in different sizes and can be cut to fit. They are stronger than aluminium splints and can be used even for deer.
- *Wooden splints* can be cut from any piece of flat wood. Marine plywood of 10 mm thickness is ideal for cutting to the shape of an animal's hind leg.
- *Split casts* are the remains of a cast that has been used on another animal of similar shape and size. When a cast is removed it should be cut on both sides of the leg with an oscillating saw. The half from the back of the leg can then be used for other animals.

Application of splints

All splints should be fitted as follows:

(1) A layer of padding is wrapped around the limb to include joints above and below the fracture site.
(2) The splint is placed on the back of the leg.
(3) Several more layers of padding are wrapped around the leg and the splint.
(4) This is all covered with conforming or white open-weave bandage starting distally and leaving the toes exposed.
(5) Adhesive or cohesive bandage is then used to cover the whole splint.

Stirrups like those used on Robert Jones bandages may help to keep splint bandages in place.

All open fractures still require immobilisation or else any bone fragments can jeopardise any healing. Bandaging techniques offer stability while still being simple to remove and replace at each dressing change.

THE SEMI-CRITICAL FRACTURE

Although semi-critical fractures may not be immediately life-threatening, it is still crucial that they are managed correctly before the veterinary surgeon decides on a course of treatment.

Chronic open fractures

It is not uncommon to receive animals with long-standing open fractures. These will be grossly infected and contaminated with obvious necrosis and often necrotic bone. They need to be treated as infected wounds but the veterinary surgeon will need to debride the area and possibly remove non-vital bone. However, as the lesion has been festering for some time this procedure need not be classed as urgent. A course of broad-spectrum antibiotics should be instituted and standard wound management dressings applied until the surgeon prescribes otherwise.

Immobilising the fracture may be of benefit in the long term and initially it will give some pain relief and prevent further damage.

Wound dressings (see Chapter 6) under standard fracture bandaging techniques will start the debridement process. These bandages and dressings will need changing each day.

Sometimes, especially with hedgehogs, a chronic infected open fracture wound will not heal until the fracture is immobilised. Usually, as a last resort to save a leg, the veterinary surgeon can fit external fixation which will hold the bones rigid while leaving the wound uncovered to be treated topically with hydrogels like Intrasite Gel (Smith & Nephew).

Basically, four hypodermic needles are placed traversely through the uninfected skin and through the unaffected bones – two proximal to the fracture and two distal to it. With small pliers bend the tips of the four needles at right angles. Next a moulding of Hydroplastic (TAK Systems) is formed around the ends of the pins. This is carried out on both sides of the fracture so that each set of four points is firmly held. The wound can then be treated like any other infected wound with bone fractures held rigid and not impeding the healing process. The wound will then have a chance to heal and if any necrotic bone was removed before the extracutaneous fixation was attached, the fracture will also heal. External fixator kits using stainless steel nuts, bolts and rods are available for use with larger animals.

Closed fractures of the limb bones

These are not life-threatening like open fractures but unless they are properly managed they may well become compound and develop complications to healing. They can be initially stabilised with bandaging techniques which may even be adopted by the veterinary surgeon as the long-term treatment of choice. The surgeon may, however, opt for internal or internal/external fixation but the bandaging will provide temporary stability

Casts

Some animals, particularly deer, make it impractical to try to maintain a Robert Jones bandage or a simple splint on a fractured leg. In these instances the temporary splinting can be with synthetic casting material that is easily removed with an oscillating saw.

Application of a cast
(1) Two pieces of adhesive tape are attached as stirrups.
(2) The whole leg is wrapped in one or two layers of cotton wool or fibre bandage with extra padding over it.
(3) The casting material is activated and wrapped on, working distal to proximal overlapping by one-half to two-thirds at each turn.
(4) Pull apart and reflect back along the cast the two strips of adhesive tape to provide stirrups to stop the bandage slipping.
(5) The whole is covered with cohesive bandage leaving the usual toes exposed.

Once again the veterinary surgeon may opt for casting to provide the long-term treatment of some closed fractures, especially comminuted fractures with many fragments.

Pelvic fractures

These will often cause an animal to temporarily loose the use of its back legs. But once confirmed by radiograph the veterinary surgeon may prescribe 'cage rest' as the long-term treatment of choice.

However, if the animal is a female an assessment should be made of any distortion to the pelvis that may prevent her giving birth. Sometimes a female brought in with a fractured pelvis is seen on radiograph to already be pregnant. The veterinary surgeon may decide to operate to remove the fetus and spay the animal. Similarly a female with a pelvic distortion which could lead to dystocia should be spayed before she is released.

Nobody is quite sure how spaying would affect a female's interchanges with others of her species. Certainly in pack species like coyotes (*Canis latrans*) a change in a female's scent may make her subject to harassment by other pack members. We do not have major pack animals in this country although foxes and badgers do maintain small colonies but not with the fierce hierarchical system seen in coyote and wolf (*Canis lupus*) colonies.

Just as more research is needed on the fate of released rehabilitated animals so more research is needed on the outcome of spaying a wild animal.

THE NON-CRITICAL FRACTURE

This description encompasses fractures that would probably heal even if left alone. Included could be foot fractures, greenstick fractures and tail fractures. All these would probably heal but would benefit from immobilisation by one of the bandage, splint or casting methods.

This first part of the chapter has covered the triage and treatment procedures that would benefit mammals with fractures. However, by far the greatest number of fractures in wildlife are suffered by birds. Their bones and the treatment of them is a vast subject which will be addressed in the next part of this chapter.

Part II: Fractures in Birds

By far the greatest number of wildlife casualties in this country are birds. Basically the skeletal structure of a bird is both light yet strong (Fig. 8.6). However, because the bones are very thin and supported by a network of internal braces, they are also very brittle. Consequently the slightest impact or

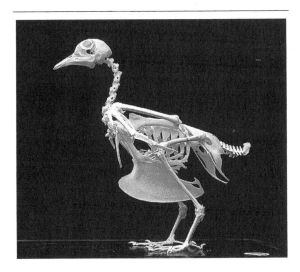

Fig. 8.6 A mounted skeleton of a pigeon will assist orthopaedic treatments to this commonly injured bird.

stress will shatter bird bones, often into many pieces.

On the plus side, apart from apparently not causing much pain for the bird, a bird's bones, given the right circumstances, will heal much more quickly than will those of a mammal. In fact within 5 days of a fracture, fibrous tissue will already be stabilising the fracture. In 9 days cancellous bone is being laid down in the callus until at 3 weeks a bony union is in place and the bird can use the limb again. Another 3 weeks sees the remodelling of a simple fracture callus back to the original shape of the bone (Coles, 1997).

However, things can easily go wrong and, because of the speed of healing in a bird, unless remedial action is taken quickly this healing could be less than perfect, jeopardising the functional use of a limb and possible release. Complications not often seen with mammal fractures must be taken into account from the moment a bird arrives at the treatment table. These complications would be:

- *Mis-alignment.* Bird fractures are usually grossly displaced due to the pull of the muscle masses. Even when grossly displaced, within days fibrous tissue and callus will be forming, linking the fragments together. Once in place this fibrous tissue will be hard to remove in order to get a decent reduction. This is why it is essential to strive for a perfect reduction from the outset.
- *Entrapment.* The build-up of fibrous tissue can be exceptional and it can entrap vital soft tissue mechanisms like tendons. Once again good reduction from the outset is crucial.
- *Deviation.* A bird's bones have evolved to provide strength yet be flexible enough to withstand the ever-shifting aerodynamic forces involved in flying. Even a slight rotation of a fracture in the wing will alter the air flow over the wings causing a less than efficient flight capability. This may be acceptable for a duck that does not need to fly perfectly but, for instance, a hunting bird like a kestrel (*Falco tinnunculus*) must have perfect aerodynamics. Any deviation could cause it to fail to catch its prey with the resultant starvation.
- *Ankylosis.* The condition most often forgotten about until it is too late is ankylosis in a bird's joints, particularly in the wing. Its onset is surprisingly rapid, often within 5 days.

A fracture near to or in the joint will cause fibrous or scar tissue to be laid down in or around the joint in a process that is not always avoidable. However, it seems that just not using a joint will cause that joint to ankylose preventing the bird from regaining normal flight.

For this reason any long-term immobilisation of a fracture in a bird, over 5 days, should not involve the joints distal and proximal to the fracture, the practice in mammals. Even where a fracture is near to a joint, leaving the joint free and mobile from any fixation may prevent the build-up of fibrous and scar tissue on the moving surfaces.

Of course, not immobilising the joint predisposes to rotation or moving the fragmented bone. So any treatment of fractures in birds, particularly in the wings, has to involve stabilising the fracture and somehow preventing the fragments twisting as the joints proximal and distal are still functioning.

Time is of the essence in dealing with fractures in bird casualties. Since a bird with even a slight disability is a doubtful candidate for release, the author feels that all fractures should be treated as critical fractures.

TYPES OF FRACTURE

Spinal fractures

Many bird casualties are presented with a noticeable flaccid paralysis of both legs. On examination the legs may not be fractured pointing either to damage of the nervous system by a spinal fracture or a head injury. A radiograph of the spine or pelvis may provide an answer but these x-rays are notoriously difficult to interpret (see later in Fig. 12.5).

If there is definitely damage to the spine of the bird then euthanasia is recommended. Where no damage is discernible then the bird should be treated as a head injury case being given initially 100% oxygen therapy followed by a course of dexamethasone coupled with antibiotic cover. There should be some improvement in the tone of the legs after a few days. However, if there is no improvement over a period of 1–2 weeks then euthanasia should be applied.

It is worth noting that a bird that is recumbent for any length of time will not be able to evacuate its cloaca. These birds will need assistance to keep their cloacae and surrounding feathers clean.

Skull fractures

The common occurrence of a bird flying into a window and knocking itself unconscious could result in a skull fracture. In fact Klem (1989) revealed that of 500 birds examined after being killed hitting windows, all died of head injuries and not of broken necks as was widely supposed. From this information all window collision casualties should be treated for head injuries on the assumption these may involve fractured skulls.

Generally these cases either respond to oxygen and dexamethasone therapy or rapidly die (see 'Head trauma' in Chapter 9).

Coracoid fracture

According to Coles (1997) this is a massive bone counteracting the compressive forces of the pectoralis muscle. Fractures of the coracoid render a bird unable to fly. Remedial surgery is possible with birds weighing over 500 g but in smaller birds the bone may heal by itself and the bird be able to fly again.

Any fractures of the coracoid are only discernable by radiograph and must be immediately referred to the veterinary surgeon.

Beak and jaw fractures

Broken beaks are not uncommon but are not always suitable for repair. The beak is made up of the maxilla (top jaw bone) and the mandible (bottom jaw bone). The front of these is overlaid with keratin giving the maxillary rhamphotheca and the mandibular rhamphotheca.

Fractures of the bone of one side of the maxilla and mandible can be stabilised by the veterinary surgeon with stainless steel wire sutures. However, damage to the keratin will not resolve by healing. Coles (1997) suggested using epoxy resin, super glue or bone cement (cyanomethylmethacrylate) but even that will eventually break down and have to be renewed. The bird will need to be kept in captivity, it would not survive in the wild.

With more serious fractures which involve breaks on both sides of the beak then simple sutures will not be strong enough. Many attempts have been made by various operatives to pin or wire the fractures but none have been truly successful. However, the author knows of a Canada goose (*Branta canadensis*) that survived in captivity with a pin through the whole length of each side of the bottom jaw.

Similarly, where the beak is missing, various prostheses have been tried but none have been truly successful. The leverage forces employed in a bird's beak are very powerful. To overcome these powerful forces a prosthesis would have to be securely anchored. Unfortunately the lightweight nature of the bird's skull means that there is no firm solid bone in which to fix and secure prostheses for a top beak.

Birds in captivity can cope without a top beak, although their preening would be impaired, but they cannot survive without a bottom beak because for one thing there is no support for the tongue.

With any broken or missing beak it really is worth persevering to find a solution. In particular the modern dental acrylics and glues may provide an answer for just one bird. But whatever happens the bird must never be released (Plate 17).

Open or compound fractures

Although the bones of birds are very light but strong, the bone cortex is very thin and brittle. Coupled with a bird's apparent scant recognition of pain, a fractured bone has sharp jagged edges still being used as if it were whole. Consequently any soft tissue in the area of a fracture can be quickly torn to shreds and the covering skin punctured. Most bird casualties with wing bone fractures have succeeded in making them compound.

Even though a compound fracture can be serious in birds, a planned course of treatment can quickly bring about healing. Apart from the complications in the healing surfaces that can occur and prevent healing, osteomyelitis in birds does not seem to cause the same systemic infection seen in mammals with open fractures (Coles, 1997). However, it is responsible for the failure of a great many open fractures so management from the admission and triage process should include a bacteriological swab for sensitivity testing. The institution of a broad-spectrum antibiotic, like enrofloxacin (Baytril 5% – Bayer) at 10 mg/kg b.i.d., may provide a better spectrum of activity than either amoxycillin or gentamicin (Bennet & Kuzma, 1992).

At this stage, before any cleaning or stabilisation is considered, notice should be taken of open fractures of the humerus. In a bird the thoracic air sacs extend into the pneumatic cavity of the humerus. If the humerus is exposed to contamination it is worth the veterinary surgeon considering prophylactically treating the bird for aspergillosis, especially as trauma can exacerbate this fungal disease.

Aspergillosis is not particularly sensitive to antifungal drugs but itraconazole (Sporanox – Janssen-Cilag) has been effective at 20 mg/kg b.i.d. for up to 30 days. Sporanox (Janssen-Cilag) comes in 100 mg capsules, far too large for most birds but it can be diluted in Diet Coca-Cola® (Coca-Cola Co.) to make it easier to divide. The method used is: dilute one capsule of 100 mg Sporanox in 4 ml of cola making a suspension of 25 mg per ml, this suspension should be left for 24 hours before using.

The wound should be prepared and cleaned using the same principles applicable to open fractures in mammals. The major difference is that rather than clipping hair around the wound site any surrounding small feathers are very carefully plucked out. Where a feather is plucked a new one will grow to replace it but if the feather is cut it would not regrow and would only be replaced at the next annual moult which could be months away.

Larger primary or secondary feathers should, preferably, be left in place. Plucking them may cause damage to the feather follicles and may lead to problems as new feathers grow without the support of a mature neighbouring feather. In moulting, most birds naturally moult one primary feather at a time so that any soft new feather has support from neighbouring feathers as it grows.

At first-aid treatment, after the wounds are cleaned and any fragments replaced under the skin, any fractures should be dressed and stabilised until the veterinary surgeon decides on a course of management. Wounds should be temporarily sutured and covered with a non-adhesive dressing. Adhesive tapes should never be used on birds because they could damage the intricate structure of the feathers as they are removed. A non-adhesive cohesive bandage such as Co-Flex (Millpledge Pharmaceuticals) is much more suitable but many birds will be attracted to coloured bandages, especially birds of prey who will tear at red bandages. For this reason only white bandages should be used on bird casualties.

STABILISATION OF FRACTURES

Until the veterinary surgeon operates to provide internal or internal/external fixation to a fracture in a bird, the fractures, which are usually in the wing structure, need to be immobilised by external co-aptation which may even be adopted as the long-term treatment of choice. In birds both closed and open fractures require the same methods of immobilisation, the criteria being to immobilise any fractures but avoid ankylosis of the joints.

Various methods of immobilisation, including surgical techniques, have varying degrees of success. Whatever the fracture of a wing bone and whatever the expertise available 'There are options. There are always options' (Ness, 1997). The protocol is to adopt the option most likely to succeed and, of course, to be available (Table 8.1).

Table 8.1 Comparison of the likely success rates of fracture treatments of the long bones of wild birds.

Method	Suitable for which bones	Surgery or triage	Likely outcome	Release potential
No treatment at all, only cage rest	All	N/A	Misalignment and fracture disease	Doubtful
External coaptation (splints)	All	Triage	Some misalignment	Possible
Intramedullary pinning	Humerus Radius/ulna Femur Tibiotarsus	Surgery	Ankylosis	Possible
Intramedullary shuttle pin	All	Surgery	Good	Probable
External fixations	All	Surgery	Good	Probable

No treatment

Should there be no facilities at all, a bird with a fracture can be kept confined and its fracture will probably heal. The healing will not be very suitable and there may well be misalignment, entrapment, shortening and even ankylosis. This, of course, should never be considered, as there are many groups and practices, with veterinary back-up, that will take on any casualty.

However, with very tiny birds like wrens (*Troglodytes troglodytes*), goldcrests (*Regulus regulus*), redpolls (*Carduelis* sp.), warblers and some finches any form of immobilisation will probably fail because these small birds do not seem to tolerate treatment of any sort. Often these birds will recover sufficiently if they are kept confined in a cage for a week or two and then exercised in an aviary. Sometimes even a distorted wing will be counteracted at the next moult when new feathers are somehow adjusted to cope with the disability.

External coaptation

Ever since wild bird rescue and rehabilitation first started, soon after World War II, external coaptation with cardboard and lolly sticks has often been the only treatment available. Gradually over the years these external splints have been modified to try to overcome the problems of, primarily, fracture disease or ankylosis.

Only recently have more sophisticated surgical techniques become more widely acknowledged. But even now these are not available in many situations so the tried and trusted splint still has a place in wildlife care. It is also the treatment of choice to stabilise fractures until surgery can be performed. Each bone, particularly in the wings, requires a different form of external coaptation and in many cases these techniques have produced birds that are able to be released.

TREATMENT OF FRACTURES

Fractures of the humerus

This is probably the most important bone in a bird's wing. Apart from being involved in the respiratory system it transfers the power from the massive pectoral muscles into flight. Consequently, when the humerus is fractured and the bird continues to try to fly, these muscles will be constantly forcing the proximal fragment away from any distal fragments and into the soft tissues causing untold damage.

The only truly successful way of overcoming these forces is with surgery or, in a compound fracture, a shuttle pin. External coaptation is possible by strapping the bird's wing to its body but the outcome is doubtful.

External coaptation

Splinting is out of the question as the humerus is too well covered with muscle mass to be accessible. The wing can be strapped to the body to produce some stability (see Plate 16). However, those pectoral muscles will still continually move the proximal fragment. By keeping the bird quiet, in subdued lighting and without attempts to handle it can mean that it has no necessity to try to fly. This period of inactivity, a maximum of 7 days to deter ankylosis, may give the natural response of the laying down of fibrous tissue time to cement some sort of stability between the fragments. But even then when full healing has taken place there will be some distortion of the flight patterns prohibiting the release of some species.

Shuttle pinning

This is a comparatively new technique being used by some veterinary surgeons to provide stability to fractured bird bones, especially the humerus (Coles, 1997).

As the humerus is a pneumatic bone with a large intramedullary cavity, any intramedullary pin has to itself be large and this can then interfere with the bone healing by obscuring the inside of the cavity from endosteal bone formation. And, of course, an intramedullary pin has to be inserted and removed

through a joint predisposing to fracture disease and ankylosis.

A shuttle pin is inserted through the fractured ends of the fragments and is light enough to be left in place once the bone has healed. The polypropamide rod from the centre of a plastic hypodermic syringe can be cut down to fit inside the humerus and cut short to provide a peg to lock the fragments together. Its cruciform shape allows for some endosteal bone formation and it is sterile.

A suture is passed through one end of the peg and once the peg is pushed into the longer of the fragments the suture can be used to pull it back and into the other fragment. The suture is then removed and a figure-of-eight wire is passed at one end through the bone and the peg and at the other end through the bone only of the other fragment beyond the peg. Carefully tightening this wire will then bring the two fragments together and prevent rotation (Fig. 8.7). The wing is then bandaged to the body for 2–3 days with a typical humerus bandage technique.

Biodegradable bone implants are also available but their cost is prohibitive.

Fractures of the radius and ulna

Probably more often fractured than the humerus, the radius and ulna work symbiotically in the flight patterns of the wing and often both get fractured at the same time.

The cage rest regime of 'no treatment' is not really an option if both the radius and ulna are

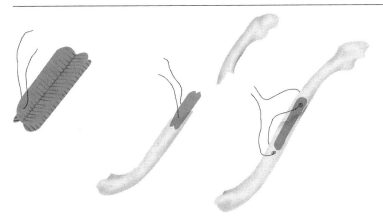

Fig. 8.7 How to install a shuttle pin fixation in a medullary cavity (after Coles, 1997).

broken as these two bones have to move longitudinally to each other. If no control is exercised over their healing, then the callus formation will probably incorporate both bones in a solid mass preventing the bird from ever having control of its flight patterns.

However, if only one of the bones is fractured then the other will act as a very appropriate splint so no further action needs to be taken except for arranging cage rest for 2 weeks to prevent any unnecessary movement (Fig. 8.8).

External coaptation

Using a simple cardboard splint will provide the necessary immobilisation of these two bones. The splint is folded along the length of the folded wing with the fold over the carpal joint. Initially it will be wrapped with a cohesive figure-of-eight bandage including at least one wrap around the humerus to provide support (Fig. 8.9). As all the wing joints are involved in this bandaging there is a great risk of ankylosis so it should be removed after 5 days and the joints physically moved.

The next stage is to make a smaller splint that will support the radius and ulna without involving the elbow or the carpal joint. Using a piece of x-ray film cut to the length of the radius and ulna, it is folded over the radius and down over the ulna reaching about half-way down the secondary feathers. The film on both sides of the feathers is then stapled together including the feathers. The elbow

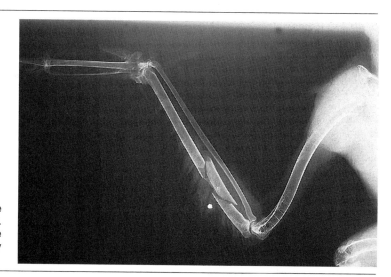

Fig. 8.8 Radiograph of the ulna fracture of a buzzard injured by a shotgun pellet. The radius successfully splinted the fracture and the bird was eventually released.

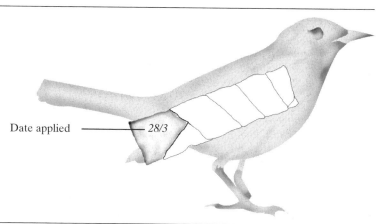

Date applied — *28/3*

Fig. 8.9 External coaptation of a fracture of the radius and ulna.

and carpal joints are then free to move while the fractures, initially stabilised with fibrous tissue formation, should heal reasonably well. Left in place for a further 2 weeks the wing should heal well enough for the bird to fly again.

External splinting

Coles (1997) described an external splint for the radius and ulna using a lightweight plastic material padded with polyurethane foam (Fig. 8.10).

The plastic splinting material, Vet-Lite (Runlite) or casting tape, is cut to the length of the radius and ulna, not including the elbow and carpal joint. A length of polyurethane foam is cut to line the plastic. Four to six separate sutures are then passed through the splinting material down through the skin well behind the ulna and the shafts of the secondary feathers. The sutures should be placed in front of the interremigial ligament which runs along the back of the ulna. The sutures are all tied at the same time so that the splint can be properly positioned. Check the splint with a radiograph after 5 days to confirm the fragments are properly aligned. Two to three weeks should see formation of a stable callus allowing the removal of the splint.

Braille sling

A strip of gauze or soft cloth is folded over the carpal joint. A slit is cut in the fold so that the gauze slips over the carpal joint. The two ends of the strip are then tied medial to the distal humerus then passed over the elbow joint and tied including the metacarpal bones. As with all of these immobilising devices, the author believes it should be replaced after 5 days with the external splint recommended by Coles (1997).

These have been three ways of producing good stability to the radius and ulna where surgery has not been necessary. However, probably the best treatment for fractures of the radius and ulna is with external fixation (Fig. 8.11).

Fractures of the metacarpus

These small metacarpal bones are often dismissed as unimportant. Quite the contrary, the bird uses this part of the wing to control the finer points of its flying ability. They are small and so often get broken and are difficult to align except with an external splint.

Also, the blood supply to this part of the wing is particularly poor and even slight damage can impede this circulation causing necrosis and die-off. To combat this all metacarpal injuries are massaged daily with a human haemorrhoid treatment, Preparation H (Whitehall Laboratories), which does seem to have some beneficial effect.

This susceptibility to circulation damage also often precludes the opportunity for surgical intervention. This leaves external coaptation as the only viable option.

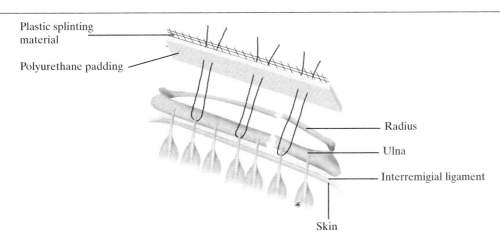

Fig. 8.10 Padded radius and ulna splint (after Coles, 1997).

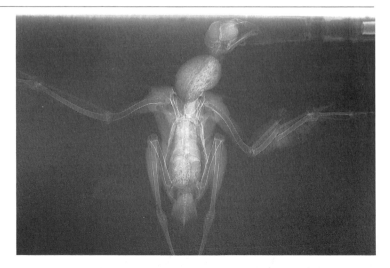

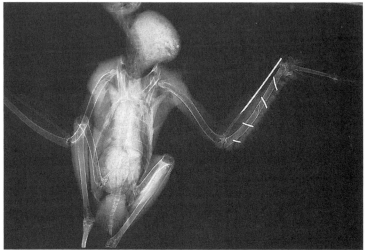

Fig. 8.11 Before (top) and after (bottom). A sparrowhawk showing, on radiograph, fractures of the radius and ulna. An intramedullary pin in the radius (removed after 5 days) provided a rigid guide for extracutaneous fixators to be used to immobilise the ulna.

External coaptation

Very similar to the external splints used for the radius and ulna, this splint is made from a piece of x-ray film cut just wide enough to cover the metacarpal bones but not to interfere with the carpal joint. It is folded down over the metacarpus and secured by sutures through the skin over the shafts of the primary feathers.

Primary feather suturing

In very small birds it is possible to suture together adjacent primary feathers on each side of a fracture. The feather shafts here are attached to the metacarpal bones.

Fractures of the femur

The femur is situated within a muscle mass and is very difficult to immobilise without surgery. Where both legs are essential for the survival of the bird, e.g. birds of prey, swans and waders, then a veterinary surgeon must be involved to carry out the necessary intramedullary pinning.

There are two methods available that are not quite so involved.

External coaptation

The leg is folded in a natural sitting position. The tibiotarsus is strapped to the tarsometatarsus. Do not fold the joints completely as this may impede the circulation. A roll of gauze is taped underneath the body next to the folded leg. The whole leg is then wrapped with cohesive bandage which is passed over the body to support the leg (Fig. 8.12).

The splint should be removed every 5 days and the joints checked for mobility.

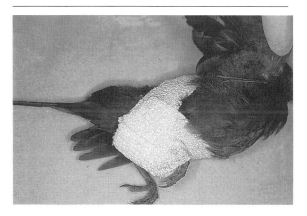

Fig. 8.12 How a body bandage can temporarily immobilise a femur fracture in a blackbird.

Avian bone splints

Cook Veterinary Products now market a range of avian bird splints. Made of PTFE, a biologically inert lightweight material, the splint is inserted across the fracture into both fragments of the bone. A central pin through the splint aids positioning and barbs at each end provide rotational stability. Available in two widths, 1.7 mm and 2.5 mm, they are suitable for femur, tibiotarsus or humerus repair. The one drawback is that they are comparatively expensive.

Fractures of the tibiotarsus

Much easier to stabilise than the femur, the tibiotarsus seems to be the leg bone most likely to be fractured. As with other long bones external fixation would be the treatment of choice but for once external coaptation can be very effective (Fig. 8.13).

Splint

Splints to match the length of the tibiotarsus can be fashioned out of tongue depressers, lolly sticks or, perhaps the best, cut lengths of bamboo or half syringe cases where the leg can fit into the channel. Quite simply the fracture is reduced, a single wrap of conforming bandage (Knit-Fix – Millpledge

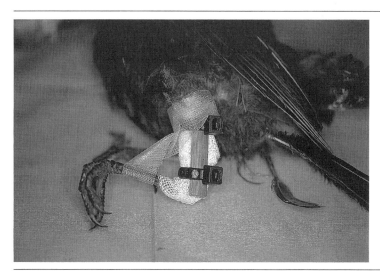

Fig. 8.13 A tibiotarsus splint on a blackbird will provide sufficient immobilisation for healing.

Pharmaceuticals) and then the splint is laid along the bone and the whole thing wrapped in either adhesive or cohesive bandage.

Flex the tarsal joint through 90° at least for the first week of treatment. This seems to provide the right stress on the fracture site and initially stops the bird from using the leg.

Avian bone splints

Just as in the femur, the Cook Avian Bone Splint can be effective for larger birds in immobilising a tibiotarsal fracture without involving the hock or stifle joints.

Plastic splints

Boddy and Ridewood market a pigeon splint, Colomboclip, made specifically for pigeon fanciers to use if one of their birds breaks a leg (Fig. 8.14).

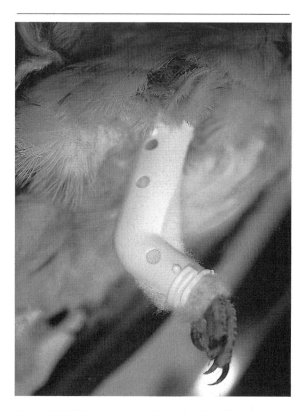

Fig. 8.14 The pigeon Colomboclip (Boddy and Ridewood) is useful for many species.

Used over padding, they immobilise the tibiotarsus, hock joint and tarsometatarsus but do tend to fall short of immobilising the proximal fragment if it is adjacent to the stifle joint.

Not just useful for pigeons, the Colomboclip has been used successfully on kestrels, tawny and barn owls.

It is possible to apply plaster or synthetic casts to tibiotarsal fractures but they are usually too heavy for the bird.

Fractures of the tarsometatarsus

These can be treated in a similar fashion to fractures of the tibiotarsus.

Fractures of the digits

Birds' toes do get fractured but respond well to external coaptation.

External coaptation

Quite simply a piece of cardboard or lightweight plastic is cut to the shape of the foot as if it were placed flat. Each toe is then wrapped to its relevant piece of cardboard and the whole structure wrapped in cohesive bandage.

Casting

Quite often birds do seem to suffer a fracture involving either the distal tibiotarsus or the proximal tarsometatarsus. Simple immobilisation in the flexed position using a malleable lightweight casting like Vet-Lite (Runlite) will render the area stable. Ankylosis may occur in the ankle joint but normally the bird retains full use of its foot.

Fractures of both legs

Many birds seem to somehow fracture both legs. They are usually similar. The fractures can be treated just like any other fracture but the bird needs to be suspended in a sling to prevent the legs being used (Fig. 8.15).

Boddy and Ridewood, once again, produce a sling that will hold a pigeon (the Injury Harness). This can be suspended from a frame until the legs heal. As the legs are not used, much of the strap-

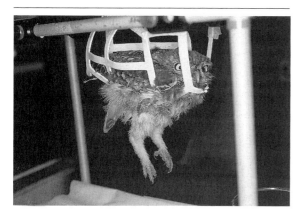

Fig. 8.15 Birds with both legs broken can be suspended like this little owl.

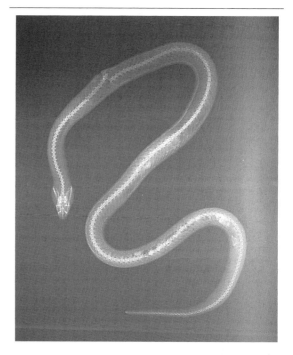

Fig. 8.16 Radiograph of a grass snake whose spine was injured by a dog. The snake coped with the injury.

ping can be removed after 7 days letting gravity provide the traction.

Improvising to suit the sizes of other birds, slings have been made for herons (*Ardea cinerea*), finches and even swans who are notoriously difficult to treat when they have even one leg broken. Keeping the bird in a warm, dark, quiet environment will help it come to terms with its restraint.

Part III: Fractures in Reptiles and Amphibians

REPTILES

In Britain we only have two types of native reptile: snakes and lizards. Until recently not much work had been carried out on rehabilitation of any of the species. However, grass snakes and slow worms are now being presented for care and some of them have obvious fractures.

Unfortunately the main fracture site seems to be in the vertebral column where the fracture is either the result of trauma or from pathological sources, e.g. *Salmonella* infection. Amazingly some snakes can survive with a broken back but it is really up to a veterinary surgeon with experience of reptiles to make a prognosis (Fig. 8.16).

AMPHIBIANS

Frogs and toads appear quite frequently on the agenda of wildlife rescue. Frogs tend to get caught in lawn mowers and strimmers causing fractures to the legs and often the jaw.

Toads, on the other hand, are usually road traffic victims especially during their migration in early spring. They usually have crushing injuries to the legs and pelvis.

An amphibian skeleton is a mixture of true bone and cartilage bones. Fractures will heal but because the animals are ectothermic the healing process can take a considerable time.

Fractures ought to be stabilised with water-resistant materials as the amphibians will take an occasional bath. Synthetic splinting material or Vet-Lite (Runlite) can be used to splint hind leg fractures whereas suturing with non-absorbable sutures will usually be sufficient for the front legs.

The mandibular bones are thin and incomplete but will respond to non-absorbable sutures.

Keeping wild amphibians in captivity for the length of time it takes fractures to heal does not always work. Toads will eat well in captivity but frogs tend to lose weight and condition rapidly. These frogs will do well in an enclosed garden pond area, where they can be monitored and eventually have their sutures and casts removed.

9
Avian Wildlife Disease

British wild bird casualties present a range of problems that can be classified as disease. These include natural phenomena like infections or the regularly seen consequences of trauma. They can affect more than just one species. The aim when dealing with wildlife casualties is not to attempt a diagnosis but the regularity of meeting these conditions makes it practical to have standardised precautionary treatments in place at the time of triage. Of course, the veterinary surgeon may prescribe a differing course of treatment once the casualty is more fully examined.

The drugs and substances mentioned in this chapter may not feature in the standard armoury of a veterinary practice. To offer a comprehensive treatment regime these should be kept in stock for wildlife casualties.

Below are some of the more common problems often seen in wild animals.

ASPERGILLOSIS

Species regularly affected: water birds, pelagic birds, birds of prey and pigeons.

Aspergillosis is the result of a fungal infection by one of the *Aspergillus* species. Relevant to wild birds are: *A. fumigatus*, *A. flavus*, *A. niger*, *A. glaveus* and *A. nidulans*. All have been recorded in birds but *A. fumigatus* is most commonly responsible for the disease.

The problem with the disease is that aspergillosis is hard to detect and by the time that clinical signs are obvious, the disease is so well entrenched that it is nigh on impossible to cure. Often the affected bird will just die without showing any symptoms.

Like any other fungus, *Aspergillus* thrives in damp, decaying vegetable matter especially mouldy or wet hay. Conversely, although the fungus needs damp conditions to flourish, its spores are spread through dry conditions like the bottom of a dusty cage. Both these conditions can be found in some bird-holding facilities so preventive management is required to make sure that damp hay or straw and dry cage debris are not left in the vicinity of birds.

Aspergillus is widespread in the environment and, probably, already present in the respiratory system of many birds. However, it is not always pathogenic and can exist in small amounts without any adverse effects on the bird. Certain circumstances can cause an overgrowth of the fungus, seriously affecting the bird's capacity to breathe. These circumstances can include pre-existing disease, adverse environmental conditions, immuno-suppression or stress.

Once the fungus starts to become invasive it can affect the whole respiratory system including trachea, syrinx, bronchi, lungs and the air sacs which make up 80% of the respiratory system. Once established three forms of aspergillus infection are recognised:

- The *acute form*, which is fatal within 1–7 days. Clinical signs are the moist raëles of a pneumonia and a typically, fluffed up depressed look of a very sick bird.
- The *sub-acute form* may take 1–6 weeks to develop and kill. Clinical signs may show a respiratory wheeze and open-mouth breathing as the disease develops.
- The *chronic form* of aspergillosis takes weeks or months to develop. Clinical signs are similar to

those in the sub-acute phase but with chronic disease the bird will lose weight and become emaciated as well.

However, *Aspergillus* is one of those infections that often shows no clinical signs until post-mortem examination shows the typical lesions in the respiratory tract. Sometimes the open-mouthed breathing gives a chance of prolonged targeted treatments. If there are no outward signs of the disease but the veterinary surgeon has any suspicions then laboratory tests will provide a diagnosis.

For many years it was assumed *Aspergillus* would not respond to treatment and, even now, if aspergillosis is confirmed it can take many months of expensive treatment to possibly bring about a cure. It is now accepted as more convenient and practical to look to prevention rather than cure.

Normally birds that are healthy and kept in a clean environment with good ventilation will not be affected. However, all wild birds taken into care are stressed and often sick, making them ideal candidates for infection. It is not possible to prophylactically treat every bird casualty with antifungal drugs but it is wise and practical to routinely medicate the high-risk species.

Pelagic and seabirds do seem to develop acute aspergillosis soon after they are taken into captivity. In particular, seabirds affected by oil are especially vulnerable and many will succumb to the disease unless treated prophylactically. Diving birds, because of their respiratory technique of the re-circulation of air when diving, seem to be more at risk than others. At The Wildlife Hospital Trust (St Tiggywinkles) all pelagic birds are started immediately on a course of antifungal treatments whether they are affected by oil or not.

Joseph (1996) recommended a prophylactic regime of a 2-week course of itraconazole (Sporanox – Janssen-Cilag) given orally at 10 mg/kg. We in fact provide 20 mg/kg for 2 weeks plus nebulisation of clotrimazole (Canesten Fungicidal Solution – Bayer) in a 3-days-on 2-days-off programme at a duration of 30–45 minutes per session.

Once a bird is open-mouth breathing the disease is well advanced. Treatment can be provided with oxygen therapy, itraconazole and clotrimazole in nebulisation. Bronchodilation can be provided with etamiphylline camsylate (Millophyline-V – Arnolds Veterinary Products) or clenbuterol hydrochloride (Ventipulmin – Boehringer Ingelheim).

Usually aspergillosis is not even suspected until it is too late. Prophylaxis for high-risk birds has proven to be useful and, in pelagic birds, is the only way of preventing the disease gaining a foothold.

AVIAN POX

Species usually affected: pigeons, passerines and birds of prey.

Avian pox is a viral infection that takes two forms:

- A moist form found in the pharynx and upper respiratory tract
- A dry form seen as brown, scabbing lesions on unfeathered parts of the bird

In wild birds it is usually the dry form that is seen on casualties as scales on the beak, cere, feet or sometimes the wing edges.

Avian pox is not a deadly disease in wild birds. In fact it is mild and self-limiting but it is still highly contagious to similar birds. It is spread by contact or by biting insects. This makes it preferable that any bird showing pox lesions is isolated. Generally the birds will recover spontaneously and can be released.

During its stay in captivity the bird may knock the lesions causing a small amount of haemorrhage. The bleeding can usually be stemmed with a caustic pencil or a wound powder.

ECTOPARASITES

- **Fleas.** Wild birds in general do not have trouble with massive flea burdens.
- **Ticks.** Similarly ticks are not often seen on wild bird casualties.
- **Lice.** Lice on wild birds are strictly host specific and live in different layers of the feathers. They exist on feather detritus and are usually not a problem to their hosts.
- **Mites.** Mites usually seen on wild birds, particularly corvids, are visible to the naked eye. Much easier to detect than those on mammals, they have the alarming habit of leaving a bird and

running over a handler's hand and arms. They are not, however, a problem to the handler.

Treatment of affected or suspect birds is with a topical dab of ivermectin (Ivomec Pour-on – Merial Animal Health) on the back of the neck. An estimated dose would be 0.1 ml per crow-sized bird.

- **Biting flies.** These louse flies (hippoboscids) are often first seen when one or two leave their host and land on a handler's face and arms. They have a flattened appearance, sucker-like feet and scuttle sideways at alarming speed. They will not bite humans but their presence and habit of sticking make them very disconcerting.

  Their flattened bodies make them difficult to squash but a mild insecticide powder (WHISKAS exelpet – Pedigree Masterfoods) will extinguish them.

  Unless there are signs that they are causing problems like anaemia or irritation to their host, it is much more comfortable to leave them undisturbed.

FISHING LINE AND HOOK INJURIES

Species most at risk: swans, geese, ducks and other water birds.

Before the introduction of nylon monofilament fishing line, anglers would use catgut which was biodegradable so if it was discarded it would only remain as a hazard until it disintegrated. Monofilament line, on the other hand, does not degrade and, coupled with any hooks or weights still attached, is particularly dangerous to most water birds; and it seems especially to swans.

The line may have been left entangled in a tree or waterside vegetation and may still even have the bait attached to the hook. Birds, especially swans (*Cygnus olor*), will be attracted to the bait and will often swallow it and the hook, and the line, and any weights still attached (Fig. 9.1). Once in the oesophagus the hook easily becomes snagged in the soft oesophageal walls and being barbed is not easily removed.

When the hook is securely embedded in the oesophagus wall, the bird continues to swallow the rest of the line which then forms into a ball of indestructible nylon. As the bird feeds, food gets trapped in the line and ball of line, until finally the oesophagus or proventriculus becomes completely blocked. It does not then take long for the bird to starve to death.

Sometimes, if the bird is lucky, it will be spotted with line still hanging from its beak and can be caught. The hook and line will be so firmly embedded that it will not be possible to easily remove them. The bird should be taken back to a treatment facility where attempts to remove it can be more controlled. Any length of line hanging from the beak will assist in attempts to remove the hook. This should not be cut and preferably should be tied to a stick or clamped so that the bird does not swallow it.

Back at the facility the presence of a blockage in the oesophagus may be suspected if there is a fetid

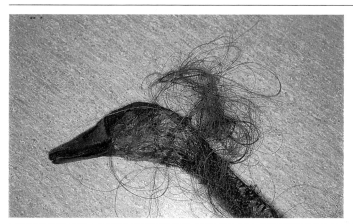

Fig. 9.1 Swans will regularly swallow fishing line, hooks, bait and weights.

smell noticeable in the bird's mouth. A radiograph will establish if there is a hook and where it is situated.

If there is no sign of a hook, check that the line is not trapped around the base of the tongue or glottis. Then gavage into the oesophagus about 20 ml of liquid paraffin. The hookless line and any blockage should then be able to gently, but firmly, be pulled out.

If there is a hook then its distance from the beak should be roughly marked on a plastic stomach tube laid alongside the head and neck. The stomach tube, suitably lubricated, is then slid down the fishing line that comes out at the beak. When it reaches the hook it will stop. Now keeping the line taut a little push on the tube may dislodge the hook which will then be held in the tube. Slowly pulling the tube out while keeping the line taut should bring the hook clear of the bird. Never try to just simply pull the embedded line or else you will only succeed in pushing the hook deeper into the soft tissue.

However, if the hook is not dislodged the veterinary surgeon may decide to operate to remove it. One thing to remember with barbed hooks is that pulling them out against the barb will only cause further injury to the soft tissue. To remove the hook, it has to be pushed further forward until the point and barb are exposed. The barb and point are then cut off with wire cutters leaving the shank free to be pulled backwards and out. Sometimes these hooks have three points and three barbs so each one will need to be cut off and removed separately.

Hooks on other parts of the body also have to be pushed forward, cut and then the shank removed.

Any line wrapped around the wings, neck, body or legs should be unwound and removed (Plate 18). The bird, however, should be monitored for a week in case pressure necrosis prevents its immediate release. All old fishing line should be burned so that it cannot possibly end up back in the environment.

HEAD TRAUMA

Species regularly affected: sparrowhawks, kingfisher, woodpeckers and pheasants.

Head trauma can obviously affect any species of bird especially those in collision with motor cars. However, the species that most regularly suffer are sparrowhawks, kingfishers and woodpeckers that have flown into windows and knocked themselves unconscious.

The key to successful head trauma management is to minimise secondary brain injury by relieving intercranial pressure. For one thing, the old adage of reducing fluid intake to reduce cerebral oedema has now been superceded by a recommendation of maintaining normal fluid levels and even introducing a slight hypervolaemia.

On examination the veterinary surgeon may prescribe very sophisticated treatments and even surgery. However, at triage, a standardised routine will assist recovery by limiting the intercranial pressure. The standard routine we use at The Wildlife Hospital Trust (St Tiggywinkles) is based on procedures to deal with head trauma cases drawn up by Dr JCM Lewis of the International Zoo Veterinary Group (Table 9.1).

METABOLIC BONE DISEASE (MBD)

Species usually affected: collared doves, pigeon, birds of prey and corvids.

Metabolic bone disease (MBD) is a term rehabilitators use to describe birds, or other animals, suffering from an imbalance of calcium and phosphorus, and vitamin D in their diet.

Birds fed on a balanced diet should be receiving the correct intake of vitamins and minerals. However, birds are brought in from the wild showing the classic clinical signs of bent or curved long bones or even spontaneous fractures because of poorly calcified bones.

Birds of prey in the wild receive the ideal ratio of calcium/phosphorus from the bones of the animals they feed on. However, sometimes in captivity a novice may try to hand rear a bird of prey and feed it on meat alone with no bones. These birds never flourish and develop very poorly calcified bones that will bend and spontaneously fracture. Unfortunately chronic cases cannot be rectified and the birds have to be destroyed. Sometimes newer cases can be given a calcium supplement and recover but nothing can replace a

Table 9.1 Wall chart of procedures to deal with head trauma in birds.

St Tiggywinkles
The Wildlife Hospital Trust

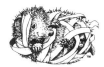

Avian Head Trauma Cases
(i.e. those cases that arrive unconscious)

(1) **ABC:**
Carry out the usual resuscitation Airway, Breathing and Circulation checks and procedures.

(2) **Oxygen:**
If the bird is comatosed, attempt to intubate and instigate slight hyperventilation with oxygen. **This is probably the most important measure to prevent the development of cerebral oedema.** If intubation is not possible, administer oxygen by mask or oxygen chamber.

(3) **Immobilisation:**
Keep the bird immobilised. Do not manipulate the neck, do not take blood samples from the jugular vein.

(4) Check the head carefully for **haemorrhage** or evidence of **CSF leakage**.

(5) Apply anti-shock treatment.

(6) Monitor the **respiratory pattern**.

(7) **Skull x-ray:**
Desirable.

(8) **Release sensitive birds as soon as possible.**

---

balanced diet. It is crucial to remember that birds of prey do not feed just on meat, they feed on whole animals.

Young collared doves (and pigeons) are brought in from the wild suffering from MBD. Symptoms include the classic thin cortex or curved long bones and often an extremely soft beak. Usually these respond to a calcium supplement in tablet form followed by a calcium/phosphorus powder (Stress – Phillips Yeast Products) on their food.

Products available to provide extra calcium include:

- Pet-Cal™ Tablets (Pfizer)
- Stress calcium/phosphorus supplement (Phillips Yeast Products)

Sunshine is also essential for birds to metabolise calcium and phosphorus.

POISONING

Species usually affected: water birds, although birds of prey, corvids and pigeons are sometimes the victims of illegal poisoning that is invariably fatal.

Two types of poisoning are regularly seen in birds, and both seem to occur in water birds:

- *Lead poisoning* – this particularly hits swans who take in and digest lead fishing weights and possibly lead shotgun pellets picked up as grit for the gizzard
- *Botulinum poisoning* – gulls are the main victims of this warm weather phenomenon, but all water birds are at risk

Other poisons may occur and if they have been identified reference can be made to the Veterinary Poisons Information Service (see Appendix 7), who may have records of birds suffering similar trauma.

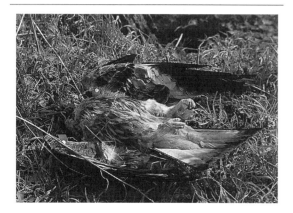

Fig. 9.2 Red Kite found poisoned resulting in a police prosecution.

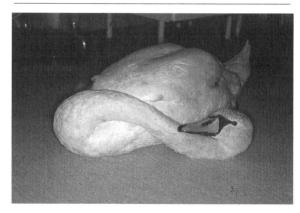

Fig. 9.3 The aetiology of this 'wry-neck' in swans suggests there may be other causes as well as lead poisoning.

There is a charge for the service although the veterinary practice may already subscribe to the organisation.

Intentional poisoning or suspicion of man-made deliberate or accidental poisoning should be reported to the Wildlife Incident Unit of the Ministry of Agriculture, Fisheries and Food on freephone 0800 321 600 (Fig. 9.2).

Lead poisoning (M. Beeson, pers. comm.)

Swans need to ingest grit and small stones which provide their gizzard with grinding stones to break up their food. To do this they sift mud and silt through their beaks, swallowing the grit. A swan's long neck allows it to reach further down under the water and this is why more swans become lead poisoned than ducks or geese. Geese tend to graze more and so are more at risk of picking up gunshot lead rather than fisherman's weights.

If not treated promptly lead poisoning will kill. Legislation was passed banning the smaller sizes of lead fishing weight but there is a huge amount left in river banks and on river floors.

Lead poisoning causes anorexia which leads to emaciation, anaemia, muscle weakness, bright green droppings and general malaise. The gizzard, a muscle, ceases to function and even if the bird can eat, its foodstuffs are not processed and congeal in the proventriculus and oesophagus.

Clinical symptomss

Clinical symptoms of lead poisoning include emaciation, lethargy, bright green droppings and limber neck where the lower part of the neck lies across the bird's back, although other factors may also be involved (Fig. 9.3). Blood analysis can be used but some swans have a naturally high lead reading and are not ill. Radiographs of the gizzard and clinical symptoms are a better guide. Lead shot will appear as radio opaque (Fig. 9.4).

Once x-rayed the swan should be put on to an intravenous drip using a 22 g catheter in the medial tarsal vein secured with lots of adhesive tape. This means that if the bird wishes to stand or change position it can and it also eliminates the need for constant supervision or sedation. 5 ml of Sodium Calciumedetate (Strong) (Animalcare) should be added to a 1 litre bag of Hartmann's solution with 10 ml of Duphalyte (Fort Dodge Animal Health). A 2 ml subcutaneous injections of B_{12} should be given. The thigh is the best injection site as it does not bruise as much as the breast. The intravenous drip should be maintained for 48 hours, with a second bag of fluids and medication running consecutively. A 48-hour break should be taken and then a daily subcutaneous injection of Sodium Calciumedetate (Strong) (Animalcare) and water be given until the appetite has returned. Post lead-poisoned swans very often suffer with absorption and digestive problems and may need to remain in care for a con-

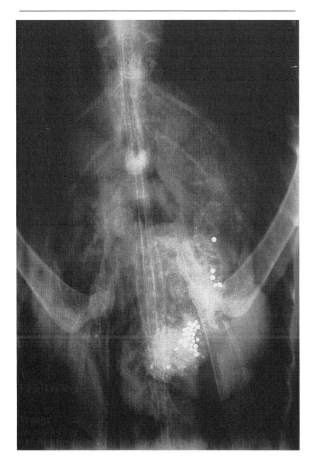

Fig. 9.4 Radiograph of a swan showing lead shot trapped in its gizzard.

siderable time or possibly be rehomed in a safe environment where a good diet can be maintained. It must be remembered that in spells of extreme cold weather swans may appear lead poisoned as the lead laid down in their bones is released, the same may be true of females at breeding time. This is not usually severe enough to require treatment – if it is, a one-off injection is enough.

It used to be common practice to remove the lead from the gizzard surgically. This is now considered too traumatic and surgery on an already debilitated swan is rarely a good idea. The only exception to this is when a large plumb weight or sinker has been ingested, in which case it should be removed through the proventriculus not the gizzard – a procedure that is not to be undertaken lightly.

It is better to encourage both an extra intake of grit through the bird's food and drinking to speedily evacuate any metals.

Lead shot or pellets elsewhere in the bird's body are not considered a lead-poisoning hazard.

Botulinum poisoning

During hot or dry weather when water levels fall, mud becomes an ideal breeding ground for the anaerobic bacteria *Clostridium botulinum*. Water birds, especially gulls, feed from this mud taking in invertebrates and molluscs. The *Clostridium* produces a highly toxic poison that will kill many birds but some will survive long enough to be picked up and taken for treatment.

Clinical signs include flaccid paralysis of the legs, loss of control of the nictitating membrane, a shallow irregular heartbeat and depressed breathing. The temperature may be low, 36.5–37.5°C, and there could be non-smelly projectile diarrhoea. Smelly diarrhoea may point to *Salmonella* poisoning needing antibiotics as a treatment.

Sick birds should be given intravenous or intraosseous fluids at a rate of 50 ml/kg, half being given subcutaneously. Shock should be treated with dexamethasone at 2–8 mg/kg.

Gavaging with a broad-spectrum antitoxin will start the process of washing the poison out of the body. A simple broad-spectrum antitoxin can be made up as follows (Greenwood, 1979):

> 10 g activated charcoal – an absorbent
> 5 g kaolin – an adsorbent
> 5 g tannic acid
> 5 g light magnesium oxide – an antacid
> Water added to bring the total volume to 500 ml

The antitoxin is gavaged at 2–20 ml depending on the size of the bird.

Once the bird's fluid levels are satisfactory, or at least after 24 hours, it can be started on a gavage regime of liquid food. Suitable foods are Poly-Aid (Vetafarm Europe), Ensure (Abbott Laboratories) or Complan (Crookes Healthcare) also at 2–20 ml depending on the size of the bird. This should continue until the bird is feeding itself.

Botulism toxin is very poisonous so do not expect a 100% success rate but 50% success can be achieved.

SYNGAMIASIS (GAPEWORM)

Species affected: all.

Syngamiasis, or gapeworm as it is more commonly known, is one of those naturally occurring conditions that can cause respiratory distress in birds. The culprit *Syngamus trachea* is a nematode worm that infects the trachea of birds often in such numbers as to completely block the trachea. It infects the birds through an intermediate host which may be a slug, snail, beetle or earthworm.

Like many other respiratory problems, it can cause the bird to open-mouth breathe but sometimes the cause can be suspected by the moist raëles coming from the glottis. Also in severe cases the worms may be seen in the opening of the trachea. The worms are red and threadlike (Fig. 9.5).

Control is with fenbendazole (Panacur – Hoechst Roussel Vet) or thiabendazole (Mintezole – Merial Animal Health).

THIAMINE DEFICIENCY

Species affected: fish-eating birds.

The enzyme thiaminase occurs in whitefish, e.g. sprats, whitebait, turbot and white bass. Some birds taken into captivity have to be fed on fish, for

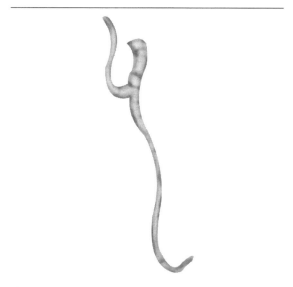

Fig. 9.5 *Syngamus trachea* – the gapeworm, male and female.

instance kingfishers and grebes can be fed on whitebait. The thiaminase in these whitefish breaks down the thiamine (vitamin B_1) in the bird leading to polyneuritis and death.

Clinical signs of thiamine deficiency include a general lethargy and weakness, loss of appetite and a constriction of the pupils followed by convulsions just prior to death. To prevent this happening, all birds fed on whitefish should be given a daily thiamine (vitamin B_1) supplement.

Vitamin B_1 is available in tablet form for humans but a more suitable mix of B vitamins is available as Aquavits (International Zoo Veterinary Group) or Fish Eaters Tablets from Mazuri Zoo Foods. Produced for all fish-eating animals, the dose rates are displayed on the container – a guillemot-sized bird would need one tablet per day.

Birds affected by oil, in particular, are fed on whitefish to help clean their digestive tract of toxins. Each of these birds would need a thiamine supplement daily throughout their stay in care.

TRICHOMONIASIS ('FROUNCE' OR 'CANKER')

Species affected: collared doves (*Streptopelia decaocto*), pigeons and birds of prey.

Trichomoniasis is caused by a flagellate protozoan called *Trichomonas gallinae*. Trichomonads are aerotolerant anaerobes that feed by phagocytosis, absorbing bacteria, leucocytes and cell exudates. No immediate host is required, trichomonads are transmitted by direct contact. Because of this it is usually possible to estimate the source of an infection.

Typically pigeons and collared doves regularly show trichomoniasis lesions presumably because nestlings feed directly from the throat of the parent birds. Trichomonads are very common in the throat area. The author has also seen trichomoniasis in tawny owls, sparrowhawks (*Accipiter nisus*) and a red kite, all of who could possibly have fed on infected collared doves or pigeons. (Plate 19).

The disease manifests itself by causing caseous lesions that may be in the throat, crop, oesophagus and into the roof of the mouth, upper respiratory tract and eye orbits. The lesions are typically deep yellow to brown in colour and may be accompanied by thick saliva and strands of a mucoid material. There is often a fetid smell. Infected birds often starve when the lesions block the throat or suffer respiratory distress if the lesions invade the trachea.

Attempting to remove the lesions before treatment can result in massive life-threatening haemorrhage. However, provided an infected bird receives fluid therapy and is gavaged with liquid nutrition the trichomoniasis can be attacked with medication and will be easily removed in 4–5 days. In fact most of the lesions will be swallowed as they become detached.

The drug to treat trichomoniasis is carnidazole (Spartrix – Harkers) at 10 mg for adult birds and chronic cases and 5 mg for young birds.

Sometimes the infection will have eroded part of the bird's beak or skull. Birds with major defects should possibly be kept in captivity.

So prevalent is the disease in colombids that pigeons and collared doves should be treated prophylactically on admission. Sometimes whole flocks of collared doves are noticeably infected with trichomoniasis. One by one they will fail and be brought into care. It may be possible to treat a regularly visiting flock with dimetridazole (Harkanker Soluble – Harkers) in a drinking bowl. To the author's knowledge this has not been tried but it may be a solution to a mass mortality.

Much of this chapter has mentioned prophylaxis. This is not an alternative to diagnosis but is just a precaution against regularly seen conditions. The ultimate decision on a disease must always remain with the veterinary surgeon.

10
Mammalian Wildlife Disease

Mammals exhibit a whole range of wildlife disease where commonly seen conditions can be expected and possibly treated. The wildlife diseases highlighted in this chapter are more about trauma and metabolic disorders than infection with pathogens in the normally accepted sense of the word.

DENTAL CONDITIONS

Companion animals on a soft food diet are expected to develop dental problems but surely animals in the wild, on a natural diet, should not suffer dental disease. However, some wild animals while being admitted for other problems, are showing enough dental disease that it is a sound protocol to give all mammals a complete dental overhaul before release.

Periodontal disease

Species mainly affected: hedgehogs (*Erinaceus europaeus*), badgers (*Meles meles*), foxes (*Vulpes vulpes*) and otters (*Lutra lutra*).

Periodontal disease should not occur in wild mammals especially the insectivores and carnivores who eat raw meat and invertebrate chitin as part of their natural diet.

However, hedgehogs, in particular, are regularly found with a chronic build-up of calculus on their upper carnassial and first molar teeth (Stocker, 1987). Animals have also been seen with the top jaws firmly cemented to the bottom jaws with this calculus build-up (Plate 20).

Calculus is, in fact, layers of minerals deposited from the saliva in response to plaque on the tooth surfaces. In captivity on a tinned food diet, long-stay hedgehogs can be expected to develop periodontal disease but it has now been shown that some wild hedgehogs also suffer a similar build-up of calculus so each one of them taken in should have its mouth thoroughly checked. Ultrasonic scaling and a few extractions are usually all that is needed to send a hedgehog on its way. In captivity the addition of Hill's Feline Growth or Feline Maintenance pellets will keep the levels of plaque to a minimum and discourage the build-up of calculus.

Similarly, badgers and foxes should have their teeth checked for periodontal disease before release. Untreated periodontal disease can cause infection to spread to other organs. The mouth acts as a reservoir for infection where the bacteria can easily pass through the gingival tissues into the blood. From here the bacteria can be distributed and settle into the heart, lungs, liver and kidneys. Releasing an animal to this future is not acceptable without treatment.

Endodontic disease

Species mainly affected: badgers, foxes, otters and muntjac deer.

Endodontic disease affects the interior of a tooth, the pulp. The pulp is very sensitive and can easily be damaged. Pulp exposure can be seen as a hole in the tooth through which the pulp, either healthy or necrotic, can be detected.

Badgers are more often that not candidates for dental overhauls as their teeth often display great wear (attrition) or else fractures of the canines. These fractures open the tooth to infection and are no doubt extremely painful.

Foxes, otters and badgers all commonly exhibit fractured canines (Plate 21). Wherever possible damaged teeth should be repaired rather than be extracted. Root canal occlusion can provide a good, sound tooth that will stand up to the rigours of a wild existence. There is no place in wildlife treatment for cosmetic surgery such as bridges, crowns or implants. They would not last very long and would leave exposures if they came adrift.

A wild animal released with good sound healthy teeth stands a much better chance of a pain-free survival than does one that is released without dental treatment.

Treatment

Under the auspices of the veterinary surgeon an animal needing dental treatment should be maintained on a course of oral antibiotics both before any treatment and for at least a week after treatment. An antibiotic preparation of spiramycin and metronidazole (Stomorgyl 2 – Merial Animal Health) can be administered at 23.4 mg spiramycin and 12.5 mg metronidazole per kg of bodyweight. Pain relief is provided with carprofen (Rimadyl – Pfizer) at 4 mg/kg for 3 days post-surgery.

Muntjac deer

Deer should not be treated with oral antibiotics and generally their teeth, incisors and molars do not present dental problems. Muntjac bucks, however, have modified upper canine teeth that extend beyond the upper lips as tusks. They feel quite loose in the gum but are in fact anchored with extremely long roots that make it very difficult to use extraction as a method of treatment. The tusks have sharpened edges and are sharply pointed. They are used for fighting with other bucks during rutting. However, muntjac have extremely thick and tough skin so serious wounds are comparatively rare.

Malocclusion

Species generally affected: rabbits (*Oryctolagus cuniculus*), squirrels and other rodents.

Teeth in rodent and lagomorph species continue growing throughout their lives. They are aligned with teeth in the opposing jaw and are constantly being ground down. If, however, for any reason the opposing teeth do not meet, they will continue growing until the upper teeth puncture the roof of the mouth and skull or the animal dies of starvation (Plate 22).

In rodents and lagomorphs it is usually the incisors which cause problems if they become maloccluded. Unchecked the top incisors will curl under, back into the mouth and will eventually pierce the roof of the mouth. The bottom incisors will continue to grow straight out in front of the mouth or up into the roof of the mouth.

In wild animals there is usually one of two reasons for this abnormal growth:

- *Congenital malocclusion* – seen in infants where a congenital deformity of the skull precludes the opposing teeth from meeting properly
- *Traumatic malocclusion* – where the animal has suffered injury which either fractured its incisors or displaced the top or bottom jaw

Once the teeth are maloccluded there are no corrective measures that can be taken to encourage them to grow in alignment. Except, that is, where a single tooth is broken and the opposing tooth has to be kept short until the broken tooth regrows to its normal length.

A rabbit's maloccluded incisors can be extracted but a wild rabbit could never be released with no incisor teeth and could not readily be kept in captivity.

A squirrel's incisors would be too traumatic to remove. The only answer for all these animals is to have their teeth trimmed at regular intervals, for example every month. To a wild animal, this is not humane; the animal should be destroyed.

There will be cases where trimming the teeth might lead to a successful outcome. However, teeth should never be clipped with nail clippers or cutters, they should always be fashioned back to shape with a diamond dental burr. This may even be possible with an unsedated or non-anaesthetised animal.

Clipping with clippers causes major injury (Gorrel, 1996) by:

- the excessive force applied to the crown damaging the tissues and the periodontal ligament
- longitudinal splits often occurring in the teeth
- the procedure being painful
- the pulp being easily exposed
- the teeth being left with sharp edges

and so their use should be prohibited.

Peter Kertesz, the dentist renowned for his pioneering work on animals' teeth pronounces that, 'The mouth is the gateway to existence'. Good healthy teeth are essential for a longer, pain-free life so it is crucial that every wild mammal taken into care has a complete dental overhaul before it is released.

ECTOPARASITES

Usually a wild animal can tolerate a normal burden of ectoparasites: fleas, ticks, lice or mites. However, given the right circumstances, the ectoparasites can multiply out of control and seriously compromise the animals who are infested.

Most wild animals taken into care have a normal burden of ectoparasites but sometimes it is the proliferation of parasites that causes the animal to succumb or vice versa. Typical examples are:

- Foxes with chronic sarcoptic mange
- Young hedgehogs from the nest with massive flea burdens
- Adult hedgehogs with heavy mite infestations
- Emaciated or debilitated badgers with enormous lice burdens

However, sometimes when wild animals are taken into care they are treated for ectoparasites before even the first aid for shock is provided. Often these attacks on the ectoparasites, particularly fleas, are quite inappropriate and actually kill the host as well. Chronic ectoparasite infestation has been affecting the animal for a long time and therefore a more gentle, controlled attack with less toxic weapons will provide a safer outcome.

Fleas

Species usually badly affected: hedgehogs, squirrels, badgers and rabbits.

Fleas are insects and feed on the blood of their host animal. In wildlife most fleas are host specific although the occasional stranger may cross hosts. In particular, the fox does not have a specific flea but may have the occasional badger flea (*Paraceras melis*).

The fleas of wild animals do not normally transfer to dogs, cats or other mammals with the exception of the rat fleas (*Nosopsyllus fasciatus* and *Ctenophthalmus nobilis*) which will interchange between hosts, even humans. Also, the wildlife flea does not complete or start its life cycle in household carpets. This is strictly the domain of the cat flea.

A massive burden of fleas can lead to anaemia. The veterinary surgeon's assessment of that anaemia may suggest treatment with iron dextran. Currently blood transfusions for wild animals are not really an option.

Control of fleas is with insecticides in powder or pump spray form. Aerosol preparations do appear toxic to some animals and are completely unnecessary. The author has used pyrethrum powder for the last 20 years and has found it most successful, and has not been bitten by a wild animal flea.

In recent years fipronil (FRONTLINE – Merial Animal Health) has become available and first reactions seem to be favourable. But as in all uses of chemicals always follow the instructions to the letter.

Myxomatosis

By far the most damaging flea likely to be seen on a rescued wild animal is the rabbit flea, *Spilopsyllus cuniculi*. This is the main vector of the myxoma virus which can kill 40–60% of a rabbit population in an outbreak. In spite of popular opinion, myxomatosis is still rife in the rabbit population with wildlife rescue centres seeing many victims.

Whether a newly arrived rabbit casualty is suspected of suffering from myxomatosis or not, any fleas it is carrying are suspected of being potential vectors of the deadly virus. Consequently, every rabbit that arrives at the Hospital is treated with pyrethrum flea powder while it is receiving triage and first aid. Then it is left isolated in its cardboard box or carrying box for 15 minutes in order for any fleas to die. After that it is put into an isolated cage for at least 24 hours if it has no signs of the disease, or 19 days if it is suspected of being infected. Any boxes or bedding used in its arrival are incinerated.

Suggested products for flea control are:

- WHISKAS exelpet (Pedigree Master foods) – a safe pyrethrum-based flea powder found to be also suitable for birds
- FRONTLINE (Merial Animal Health) – contains fipronil in a pump spray (we have, so far, seen no side effects after its use in small mammals).

Ticks

Species badly infected: hedgehogs.

Ticks are members of the Class Arachnida, Order Acarina, in that the adults have eight legs. They gorge themselves on the host animal's blood and *Ixodes hexagonus* can cause anaemia, particularly in heavily burdened hedgehogs (Fig. 10.1).

Ticks are not normally seen in massive numbers but as they can transmit diseases, including Lyme disease which can affect humans, they should be carefully controlled and definitely destroyed in a deep cup of surgical spirit. Larval ticks are just as infective as adult ticks, but they are much more mobile and can be easily missed as they evacuate from an animal. Luckily, once off the animal they can be seen easily and killed by dropping in surgical spirit; there is a risk of infection when crushing ticks. Somehow most ticks seem to be resistant to chemical control although fipronil is proving useful.

The adult tick will attach itself firmly to its host by penetrating the skin with its barbed proboscis, the hypostome. Clumsy removal of ticks may well leave the hypostome buried in the skin to become a focus of infection. When removing a tick the hypostome must be cleanly plucked from the skin. It can be seen as a proboscis at the front of a removed tick.

There are many methods advocated for the safe removal of ticks. Artery forceps are ideal to get under the tick and remove it complete. However, this takes many years of practice and there are now two simple methods to make their removal that much easier:

- Fipronil, anaesthetic ether, olive oil, surgical spirit can all be dabbed on to the tick with cotton wool and will apparently render it dead or senseless, making its removal possible.
- Alternatively, there are gadgets on the market purely for tick removal. Once of the cheapest and most effective is the O'Tom Hook tick lifter (Fig. 10.2).

Lice (sing. louse)

Species usually badly affected: badgers and muntjac.

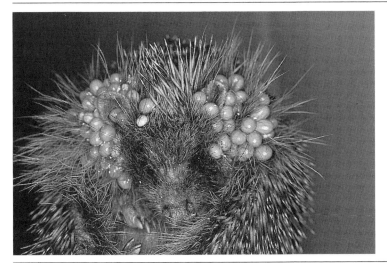

Fig. 10.1 Hedgehogs, more than other mammals, seem to carry heavy tick burdens (*Ixodes hexagonus*).

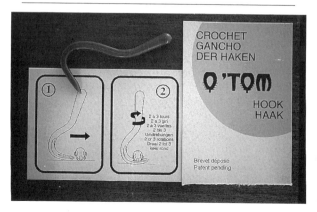

Fig. 10.2 The O'Tom Hook tick lifter.

Lice are insects divided into two groups: biting lice or sucking lice (Fig. 10.3). Lice, even more than fleas, are very host specific and are usually just an irritant causing the animal to sometimes injure itself in trying to scratch the irritation.

Sometimes sucking lice may cause anaemia. Major infestations are seen on old or debilitated badgers or muntjac deer. Lice can be controlled with flea powders.

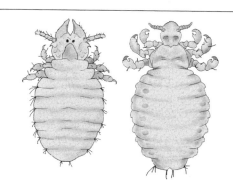

Dorsal view of a biting louse (2 mm long, light to dark brown in colour). If viewed from the side, this louse would appear dorsoventrally flattened.

Dorsal view of a sucking louse (approx. 2 mm long)

Fig. 10.3 Louse species.

Mites

Species usually badly affected: foxes and hedgehogs.

Mites cause mange. They are arachnids, like ticks, and have eight legs. Most of them are microscopic and can infest an animal in their millions. They can even kill large animals such as foxes.

The mite that severely affects foxes is *Sarcoptes scabiei*. It burrows into the skin, first at the base of the tail and the hind feet. They proliferate and gradually spread from the rump forwards until up to 100% of the fox's skin is covered with mites, affected by hair loss and encrusted with scabby lesions. On the face the mites will spread to the eyelids almost completely closing the eyes. An infestation sufficient to kill a fox takes 4 months from start to finish (Corbet & Harris, 1991). Unfortunately by the time the fox is weak enough to be caught the infestation will be so severe that it will have lost 50% of its bodyweight and will be close to death. Initially aggressive fluid therapy may keep the fox alive long enough for it to receive the benefits of treatment both for mange and for the inevitable secondary infections.

Thankfully the mites can be easily eradicated with:

- Subcutaneous injections of ivermectin (Ivomec Injection for Cattle – Merial Animal Health) at 200 micrograms/kg; or
- Intramuscular injections of doramectin (Dectomax Injectable Solution for Cattle and Sheep – Pfizer) at 300 micrograms/kg.

Antibiotics can be broad spectrum but the animal will also benefit from a course of anabolic steroids:

- Nandrolone (Laurabolin – Intervet)
- Ethylestrenol (Nandoral – Intervet)

Sometimes, with an infected fox regularly visiting a garden for food, it has been possible to provide bait suitably laced with doses of ivermectin. This has the advantage that the mange is attacked before the animal is weak enough to be caught. In this situation it is worth mixing the ivermectin in the ratio 1:9 with propylene glycol to provide a more stable additive.

The other wild mammal regularly suffering with mange mite infestation, is the hedgehog. Generally its mange is caused by the mite *Caparinia tripilis*. This is often seen as a powdery mass emanating from the ears and down over the side of the head. It is confirmed by microscopic examination of the powdery substance. Hedgehogs suffer from other mites but their incidence is much more irregular. Once again ivermectin is effective at a dose of 400 micrograms/kg (or 0.4 ml/kg when dissolved 1:9 in propylene glycol).

HEAD TRAUMA

Species affected: all terrestrial mammals.

Mammals presented suffering with head trauma have usually been in collision with a motor car or, as sometimes happens, a train.

Often the animal is comatose or those that are recovering often show nystagmus. Nystagmus is a condition in which the eyeballs involuntarily show constant fine jerky movements. There may also be noticeable swellings or grazes around the eyes. As with head trauma cases in birds, the management is to minimise secondary brain injury by limiting or reducing intercranial pressure. At triage a routine first-aid programme can be instigated (Table 10.1) but the veterinary surgeon should assess the extent of the injury and prescribe any necessary changes to the standard regime.

METABOLIC BONE DISEASE (MBD)

Species usually affected: red squirrels (*Sciurus vulgaris*) and grey squirrels (*Sciurus carolinensis*)

Metabolic bone disease (MBD) is very common in young or juvenile squirrels reared on the wrong diet. It should not happen to wild squirrels although the feeding of peanuts and sunflower seeds can lead to a loss of calcium in a growing animal.

Initially, bottle-feeding squirrels should be fed on the substitute milk formula Esbilac by Pet Ag, an American company who make milk supplements used for other animals. At each feed a little Stress (Phillips Yeast Products) should be added to provide an improved calcium/phosphorus balance. Goats' milk is a readily available substitute milk but will benefit from added Stress (Phillips Yeast Products) and vitamins.

Weaning should be on to good-quality dry puppy food (such as Hill's Canine Growth pellets) or Nutri–Bloc (Rolf C. Hagen). No peanuts or sunflower seeds should ever be given to squirrels – these contain a calcium inhibitor which in a juvenile squirrel can lead to hypocalcaemia which in turn predisposes to fits and an early death. Pecan nuts are more suitable.

To counter a young squirrel that has started to fit, provide diazepam to control prolonged fits and calcium borogluconate (Calciject New Formula 40™ – Norbrook Laboratories) to correct the hypocalcaemia.

POISONING

Poisoning of wild animals usually emanates from one of three sources:

- As a result of the approved use of a product for its intended purpose – e.g. anticoagulant bait put down, legally, for grey squirrels
- As a result of the careless use or storage of a product – e.g. a bank vole (*Clethrionomys glareolus*) taking bait intended for squirrels
- As a deliberate but illegal intention to poison wild animals – e.g. poisoned bait used to attack foxes or badgers

In dealing with wildlife casualties it is very often impossible to confidently identify a poison unless the animal concerned is seen or found by known sources of poison. Generally this occurs when a hedgehog or a mouse has found or fallen into something toxic in a garden or garage. Specific poisons like these may or may not have specific antidotes but if the veterinary surgery has arrangements with the Veterinary Poisons Information Service (see Appendix 7) their general library of incidents may be able to help.

Out in the field all three categories of poison (legal, accidental or illegal) can result in one or many animals being affected. Generally, poisons in

Table 10.1 Wall chart of procedures to deal with head trauma in mammals.

St Tiggywinkles
The Wildlife Hospital Trust

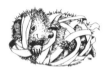

Mammalian Head Trauma Cases
(i.e. those cases that arrive in coma following RTA)

(1) **ABC:**
Carry out the usual resuscitation Airway, Breathing and Circulation checks and procedures.

(2) **Oxygen:**
If the animal is comatosed, attempt to intubate and instigate slight hyperventilation with oxygen. **This is probably the most important measure to prevent the development of cerebral oedema.** If intubation is not possible, administer oxygen by mask or oxygen chamber.

(3) **Immobilisation:**
Keep the animal immobilised. Do not manipulate the neck, do not take blood samples from the jugular vein. When necessary, use a flat board on which to move the animal.

(4) Check the head carefully for **haemorrhage** or evidence of **CSF leakage**.

(5) Assess the state and **responsiveness of the pupils**.

(6) Monitor the **respiratory pattern**.

(7) **Anti-shock therapy:**
As per usual i.e. methylprednisolone (Solu-Medrone V – Pharmacia & Upjohn) can be given at 20–50 mg/kg at 4–6-hour intervals.

(8) **Fluids:**
Give Gelofusine (Millpledge Pharmaceuticals) or equivalent and crystalloid solutions as part of the usual anti-shock treatment.

(9) **Skull x-ray:**
Desirable.

(10) **Dexamethasone:**
For slow recovering patients administer for 2 weeks at 0.25 mg/kg twice daily, followed by a reducing dose to zero over the following 2 weeks. The patient's recovery should be assessed at regular intervals and the dose adjusted accordingly.

(11) **Antibiotics:**
A course of enrofloxacin (Baytril 5% – Bayer) should be instigated.

---

the environment, even legal ones, must be controlled and be of no threat to anything other than the target species. Incidents do occur when wild animals are found dead or dying for no apparent reason. With no evidence it is virtually impossible to categorically decide on poisoning. In fact many wild animals are brought in supposedly poisoned but on close examination are suffering or have been killed or injured by some other cause.

Amongst all the false alarms there will be incidents that do seem like genuine reports. In this case adopt the guidelines of the Wildlife Incident Unit (see Appendix 7), the relevant department of the Ministry of Agriculture, Fisheries and Food (Table 10.2).

The quandary arises if there are live but suffering wild animals in the vicinity. Taking all precautions of protective clothing and driving with the car

Table 10.2 Guidelines by the Wildlife Incident Unit on finding animals suspected of being poisoned.

What to do on Discovering an Incident

- Note the locations, species involved, the purpose of suspected baits or other evidence. A photograph of the location is useful additional evidence.
- **DO NOT TOUCH** any carcasses or bait as the quantities of pesticides in illegal baits are often large.
- If you can without disturbing the evidence, cover it to make it safe.
- Call Freephone 0800 321 600. Your call will be automatically re-routed to the appropriate office.

---

windows open, it may be humane to get the animal to the veterinary surgeon immediately. Humane destruction may well be the only course of action available to the veterinary surgeon. But telephone the poison hotline at the same time, the Wildlife Incident Unit office may well have some advice or instruction.

The two poisons commonly encountered at a wildlife rescue centre are:

- Metaldehyde – which predominately affects hedgehogs
- Warfarin or hydroxycoumarins – which are poisons used against rats, house mice and grey squirrels

Metaldehyde

Metaldehyde is the poison used in slug pellets (molluscides) commonly used in gardens and horticulture. It is usually coloured blue, supposedly to prevent birds and other animals taking it. It is very toxic and in large amounts has been known to kill cattle. Hedgehogs, for one thing are colour blind, but also have the tendency to lick or eat anything nasty. This includes eating the pellets themselves.

Classic signs of metaldehyde poisoning include increased heart rate, anxiety, nystagmus, panting, salivating (probably not a sign in hedgehogs who will salivate freely when they are self-lathering), stiff-legged gait, ataxia and vomiting. The author's experience with hedgehogs poisoned with metaldehyde is that they show severe hypersensitivity. The test is to click your fingers from the other side of the room. A poisoned hedgehog will flinch whereas a healthy one will not. It may also sometimes pass faeces the colour of the slug pellets.

There is no straightforward antidote. However, if the hedgehog dies a post-mortem report with chemical analysis will add fact to the campaign to have these chemicals restricted. Particularly noteworthy is the colour of any gut contents.

There is no definite treatment but as the chemical may contribute to metabolic acidosis the use of Hartmann's solution may help counter this. Further the veterinary surgeon may prescribe bicarbonate of soda.

It may be helpful to flush the stomach with milk or sodium bicarbonate which are said to decrease absorption of the metaldehyde. Also a dose of activated charcoal with a saline purgative may move any unabsorbed metaldehyde out of the intestinal tract. Activated charcoal (Liqui-Char-Vet – Arnolds Veterinary Products) may help remove the poison from the gut. The Wildlife Hospital Trust (St Tiggywinkles) has not found the need to try these purgative treatments so cannot validate their success or failure. They can only help, because if there is metaldehyde poisoning without treatment the hedgehog will die.

Warfarin, hydroxycoumarins

It is not legal to try to treat rats (*Rattus norvegicus*), house mice (*Mus domesticus*) or grey squirrels that have ingested any of these anticoagulant poisons. However, there is always the chance that other wild animals may be incidentally affected. In particular wood mice (*Apodemus sylvaticus*), dormice (*Muscardinus avellanarius*) or voles may take poison bait from a hopper destined for squirrels.

Once again clinical signs are hard to determine but will usually include pale mucous membranes or signs of bleeding in particular from the nose, epistaxis. Vitamin K is antidotal in cases of anticoagulant poisoning. To start with, during the triage and first aid, only administer crystalloid fluids not colloids as these may have further anticoagulant properties. Also avoid cortico-steriods, sulphonamide drugs, aminophylline and frusemide.

An animal under treatment for suspected anticoagulant poisoning should be kept on its own, kept quiet and prevented from injuring itself. Any knock can precipitate internal haemorrhage.

These have been some of the conditions regularly seen in various species of wild mammal. There will be incidents that occur regularly in just one species and also many occasions when the veterinary surgeon will need to make a diagnosis. The re-commendations in this chapter have just been to complement the triage and first aid every casualty should go through. None of the recommendations are harmful if the diagnosis highlights an alternative regime of treatment.

11
Garden Birds

Part I: Common Garden Birds

Species seen regularly:

Wren, goldcrest, tits, sparrows, finches, buntings, wagtails, blackbirds, thrushes, warblers, hirundines, starlings and woodpeckers.

NATURAL HISTORY

All these small birds regularly visit gardens either to feed or to nest. They feed on either live food, such as caterpillars, spiders, worms, snails, aphids and many other invertebrates, or on dry food such as seeds, buds and scraps. All will take live food when they are feeding young in the nest.

Adult birds have specific feeding requirements so it is essential that the species is identified or at least classified by its food preferences. A good, comprehensive book on British birds will assist in their identification. If not available a rough feeding guide can be taken from the shape of their beaks. In time these small birds have evolved beaks shaped specifically for their type of feeding requirements (Fig. 11.1).

Most of these species are resident all the year round except some warblers, hirundines, flycatchers, thrushes and cuckoos (*Cuculus canorus*) who are migratory either for the summer or the winter. All except the summer migratory redwings (*Turdus iliacus*) and fieldfares (*Turdus pilaris*) will nest in Britain during the summer months.

EQUIPMENT AND TRANSPORT

It is very difficult to catch an injured bird even if it cannot fly. Trying to catch it in the hands is even more difficult and if it can fly this becomes quite impossible.

The only sure way to catch a small, injured bird is with a large fine-meshed net, the larger the better. Various sizes of cagebird catching nets are available at pet shops but the most suitable for wild birds is an angler's landing net. These are usually soft and fine-meshed, and have a collapsible handle making them convenient to carry or store.

Transporting small birds should be in a closed, small cardboard box with ventilation holes punched around the bottom edge. A piece of old towel on the bottom will give the bird something to hold on to as it is carried. The darker the box, the quieter the bird will be.

Another useful carrying method is to use the small cloth bag, with a draw string closure, favoured by bird ringers.

RESCUE AND HANDLING

It is comparatively easy to take a small bird away from a cat's mouth but catching a free bird takes a little more planning. The secret is to cut off the bird's escape route which will generally be towards the most open space. Approach the bird from that direction holding the net in front of you. Watch the bird very carefully. When it is about to flee it will flex its body, often defecate and head off away from your approach. Stand still and it may not move but if you are within reaching distance quickly bring the net down over the bird. Put the net to the ground so that the bird cannot escape and hold the bird, through

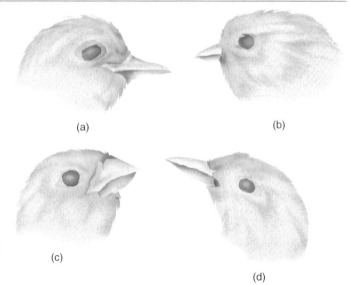

(a)

(b)

(c)

(d)

Fig. 11.1 The various beak shapes of birds found in gardens according to preferred food source. (a) Insects; (b) insects and nuts; (c) seeds; (d) fruit and live food.

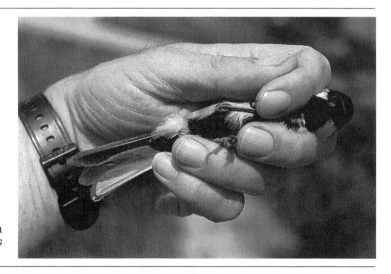

Fig. 11.2 How a licensed ringer holds a small bird. In this case a great tit (*Parus major*).

the net, with one hand. Slide your other hand under the rim of the net and take hold of the bird making sure to grip it around the wings to stop them flapping.

Handling

To examine the bird, use the ringer's holding technique. Lay the bird, on its back, in the palm of the hand. Bend the index finger and middle finger to pass each side of the neck. These two fingers can then hold the bird gently but firmly while it is examined (Fig. 11.2). Try not to keep the bird on its back for any length of time.

While handling the bird watch for any open-mouthed breathing or feel for any change in the heart rate. At either of these signs put the bird *immediately* into the dark box or bag.

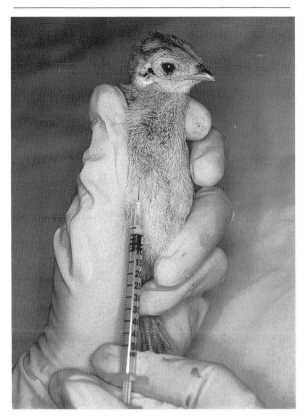

Fig. 11.3 How to give an intramuscular injection to a small bird, here a young pheasant (*Phasianus colchicus*).

ADMINISTRATION OF DRUGS

- *Injections.* Most injectable drugs for birds have to be given intramuscularly. The easiest muscles to access in small birds are the pectoral muscles lining either side of the keel. A bird's pectoral muscles overlay bone so an injection there should not damage any organs unless it is pushed through the bone (Fig. 11.3). Needle sizes should be small: 25 g, 27 g, 29 g being suitable depending on the size of the bird.
- *Tablets or capsules.* These should be pushed down the back of the throat with a cotton bud or a pill giver. Take care to avoid the glottis (which is the opening to the trachea, situated just behind the tongue) (see Fig. 2.1).
- *Liquids.* These should be gavaged (see Chapter 4) well down into the oesophagus, once

again making sure that none flows back into the glottis.
- *Fluids.* Fluids can be intraosseous or gavaged if the bird is really small.

COMMON DISEASES

Garden birds are not very often found alive suffering from infectious disease. This is not to say that it does not happen. There are many references to disease in garden birds but most victims die before they are found (Kirkwood *et al.*, 1995).

There are two diseases regularly recorded in garden birds. One, salmonellosis, is usually fatal, while the other, avian pox, is generally not even debilitating (see Chapter 9).

Salmonellosis

Deaths of garden birds have been reported in the *Veterinary Record* in 1995 (Kirkwood *et al.*, 1995; Routh & Sleeman, 1995). Apparently this type of mortality is still occurring and is being blamed on contamination and infection of bird tables and bird baths. Because these are now used all the year round they should be cleaned at least weekly with an ammonia solution.

Live casualties are not generally found but a sick garden bird with no obvious injury should be suspect. Strict hygiene should be observed and the bird started on a course of a broad-spectrum antibiotic such as enrofloxacin (Baytril 5% – Bayer) at 5–15 mg/kg twice daily, given intramuscularly.

These suspect cases and any other sick but un-injured garden bird should be referred to the veterinary surgeon for diagnosis.

COMMON INCIDENTS

Cat attack

The most common incident that injures a garden bird is being attacked by a domestic cat. For many years it was accepted that a bird caught by a cat was going to die of shock within 48 hours. Since then rehabilitators have discovered that this is not the case and the '48-hour syndrome', as it was called, was in fact a septicaemia that killed the birds. This septicaemia was shown to be caused by a bacteria, *Pasteurella multocida*, a normal bacteria carried on a cat's teeth. Further to this revelation it was also proven that even if the bird was thought to have been caught by a cat it usually succumbed to the septicaemia.

Modern-day practices provide medication for birds both positively caught by a cat and those thought to have been attacked by a cat. A single intramuscular injection of long-acting amoxycillin at 250 mg/kg has markedly reduced the mortality rate.

A single dose of antibiotics is not normally recommended but it was found that to continue a full course was often too stressful for these small birds. Furthermore, rather than trying to weigh these birds and calculate a precise dose of antibiotics, a standard dose for a particular size of bird is:

- Sparrow-sized birds = 15 mg long-acting amoxycillin
- Blackbird-sized birds = 30 mg long-acting amoxycillin

Caught in string or fruit netting

After any ligatures are teased off, the bird should be maintained in captivity for a week in order to monitor for any pressure necrosis (see Chapter 6).

Preparation H (yeast cell extract, shark liver oil) (Whitehall Laboratories) massaged distally to any damaged tissue may help restore circulation.

COMMON INJURIES

Fractures

Garden birds do receive fractures which can be treated just like any other bird fracture (see Chapter 8). In particular, a wildlife rescue centre is likely to see:

- Blackbirds (*Turdus merula*) with broken beaks (Plate 23)
- Robins (*Erithacus rubecula*) with broken legs
- Cat injuries of broken wings

Beak repairs may be attempted under anaesthetic which, as gaseous anaesthetic is not appro-

priate, could be ketamine and xylazine (Rompun – Bayer) (Coles, 1997).

Lacerations

Cat attacks may lead to lacerations especially over the rump. Most of the wounds will heal spontaneously after they are cleaned. Larger and incised wounds may need suturing under anaesthetic.

The anaesthetic of choice is isoflurane (Abbott Laboratories) by face mask. Small face masks can be fashioned out of finger stools or plastic tubing connections glued to an endotracheal tube connector of a suitable size (Fig. 11.4).

ADMISSION AND FIRST AID

Fluid administration of garden birds is quite straightforward either intraosseously, by gavage, or subcutaneously (see Chapter 4).

CAGING

Generally garden birds can be kept in bird cages where three sides are solid. These are called breeding cages. The standard bird cage wire fronts will be suitable for all the birds except wrens which can somehow get through the grilles. A dry fish tank with three sides covered, a 1/4 inch mesh wire top and sand over the bottom will prove suitable for these small birds.

Animal protection legislation states that a bird in a cage must be able to spread its wings in all directions unless confinement is stipulated by the veterinary surgeon. A cage size of 600 mm wide × 380 mm high × 300 mm deep will suit all small garden bird species.

Perches should be provided made out of twigs about 10–15 mm thick. Two perches mounted on blocks about 30 mm above the floor will allow non-flying birds to roost.

Woodpeckers should have vertical logs where they can hang perpendicularly and peck at the wood. To make this, a log about 70–100 mm thick is screwed to a base of exterior-quality timber about 130 mm square.

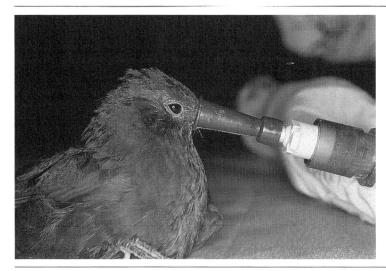

Fig. 11.4 An anaesthetic mask fashioned to suit small birds.

The floors should be covered with bird sand or river-washed sharp sand available from builders' merchants.

FEEDING

Water

Of prime concern in any cage is the availability of drinking water. Wild birds may be able to learn to use a budgerigar water fountain but just to make sure a *shallow* bowl of water should always be available.

Birds do like to bathe to keep their feathers in trim. They will sully their drinking water very quickly doing this. It is important to change the water at every opportunity.

Dry food

For granivorous feeders like finches, buntings and sparrows any good-quality wild bird seed will give the variety they need. A sprinkling of multivitamin powder once a week will stand them in good stead. Foreign or British finch mix is also a good, easily acquired, seed food. However, the birds will benefit from a mixture of wild seed heads picked where there is no danger of insecticide or traffic pollution.

They will also need access to budgerigar grit for digestion of their food in the gizzard.

Live food

Some adult birds live wholly on a live food diet – these include all the thrushes, wagtails, wrens, goldcrests, tits, warblers, hirundines, starlings and woodpeckers. It would be wholly impractical to go into the garden to collect their natural prey so surrogate live food is the answer. The only natural food that is easily collected and could prove to be a lifesaver for wrens and goldcrests is buds covered in aphids that they can peck at.

Earthworms should not be used as they appear toxic to captive birds.

Other live foods that may attract these tiny birds are baby crickets available at pet stores. Medium-sized crickets are also useful for house martins who may not naturally take other live food offered.

Crickets are expensive and so are waxworm larvae, the other food that seems to suit martins and swallows. Both waxworms and crickets should have a vitamin and mineral supplement added, like Cricdet Diet Calci Paste (IZUG).

Generally, feed insectivorous birds on *clean* white maggots available from angling shops. The food in a maggot's intestinal track can be toxic to birds. It shows as a black line along the side of the maggot. Clean maggots have been starved for some days and the black mark should have gone. Do not feed maggots that still have the black line. A vitamin and mineral supplement should also be provided with maggots.

All these live foods should be presented in a shallow straight-sided dish or else they will escape.

RELEASE

Once the bird has recovered, after just a few days in the case of a bird victim of a cat attack, it should be released in a garden area. It is always a good idea to take the bird back to its original garden but if there are resident cats it will probably get caught again. In these cases any safe garden will do.

Some birds, robins and blackbirds, are fiercely territorial so releasing this species should be attempted in vacant territories where there are not likely to be any adversaries.

Migratory birds, hirundines, flycatchers, some warblers, redwings and fieldfares, should only be released in time to join the migration:

- Swallows, martins, warblers at the end of the summer
- Redwings, fieldfares at the end of the spring

LEGAL IMPLICATIONS

It is quite legal to catch an injured or sick wild bird and to tend it until it is fit for release (Wildlife and Countryside Act 1981).

It is not legal to catch a fit and healthy wild bird or keep a fit or healthy wild bird in captivity unless it is close-ringed. Close-ringed means that it was hatched in captivity and ringed before it was 3 days old.

Other rings found on wild birds may give the address of the British Museum. These are not close-rings, they are put on by licensed bird ringers.

Schedule 4

Schedule 4 of the Wildlife and Countryside Act 1981 dictates that any bird on this Schedule found sick or injured should be passed on to a Licensed Person, as defined by para 1 (a-c) of licence WLF

100099 or to a veterinary surgeon. The species on Schedule 4 that have to be reported are shown in Appendix 3.

The Licenced Person or the veterinary surgeon must notify the Department of the Environment, Transport and the Regions (DETR), Bird Registration Section (Fax: 0117 987 8182), within 4 days of taking the bird. The author has produced a standard form that is used at The Wildlife Hospital Trust (St Tiggywinkles) to notify the DETR and includes a veterinary surgeon's statement of the bird's disability (Fig. 11.5).

If the bird has not been released after 15 days it has to be registered with the DETR and a fee paid. Once registered, a DETR inspector will arrive to witness the keeper putting a unique cable tie (supplied by the DETR) on to the bird's leg. When the bird is released the cable tie is cut off and returned to the DETR. The DETR veterinary surgeon's certificate confirming disability of a bird is given in Appendix 4.

Schedule 9

Schedule 9 of the Wildlife and Countryside Act 1981 makes it an offence to release into the wild animals that are listed on this Schedule.

Exotic bird species are now seen regularly in gardens. Should any of these be taken in as casualties they should not be re-released. The most commonly seen are the:

- Budgerigar (*Melopsittacus undulatus*)
- Ring-necked parakeet (*Psittacula krameri*)

In the interests of the environment any exotic species not on Schedule 9 or the British list should also not be released.

Part II: Swifts and Kingfishers

Among the variety of garden birds regularly needing rehabilitation are two species that have quite different requirements to the others mentioned in Part I of this chapter:

- The swift (*Apus apus*)
- The kingfisher (*Alcedo atthis*)

RECORD OF A DISABLED WILD BRED SCHEDULE 4 BIRD
TO BE NOTIFIED TO DETR WITHIN 4 DAYS (FAX 0117 987 8182)

- The Wildife and Countryside Act is the Act that applies to this form

- This form should be kept and every four months copies of all forms are sent to the DETR

- You must return the DETR ring if you are going to release the bird or if it dies

- The bird must be registered before being passed to any other person unless it is for urgent medical treatment

✍ in BLOCK LETTERS   ✓ the appropriate boxes

1) Species:	2) Age:	3) Sex:	4) Number of any ring found on bird:

5) When and where was it found?

6) Name and address of finder:

Postcode:

7) On what date did the bird come into your possession?

8) Describe the nature of the injuries to the bird:

9) What is the date the bird should be registered?
This should be 15 days from the date in question (7)

10) Veterinary confirmation that the bird should be kept more than 15 days:

11) Name of Vet: Signature:

12) If registered: Give date of registration of bird;

                              Ring number of bird;

13) If the bird died or was released, state which and give date:

Fig. 11.5 A suggested version of the record form for notifying Department of the Environment, Transport and the Regions (DETR) of Schedule 4 casualties.

Swifts

NATURAL HISTORY

Swifts feed on the wing by trawling insects with their wide open cavernous mouths. Their beak is too soft to take food by pecking or picking up insects, a major problem when they arrive in a captive situation.

Swifts are migratory; flying here, from South Africa, for a short summer's season of breeding. They nest in high buildings from where the youngsters launch themselves on their maiden flight. They do not then land again for 2–3 years and carry out their feeding, sleeping and most of their mating on the wing. When they do land, after 3 years of aerial existence, they will pick a suitable nesting site high in a building from where the next generation of swifts can launch themselves.

As mentioned they are migratory and visit Britain for the summer but they arrive after all the other migrants and leave before they do. This provides for a short nesting season which does not give swifts the opportunity of annually rearing more than one brood. It also puts pressure on rehabilitation to get any casualties up and out before the migration deadline.

EQUIPMENT AND TRANSPORT

Swifts have very short legs with little clasping feet which have very sharp claws. They can climb walls to gain height and like to hang perpendicularly when they are in captivity. To give the tiny feet something to grip, drape a towel over the inside of a carrying box. This gets the swift off the floor and gives some protection to its extra long, extra thin wings.

RESCUE AND HANDLING

Rescue is just a case of picking the swift off the ground where its short legs and long wings make it difficult for them to move around. With any handling it is important to protect the wing feathers because any damage might delay the release which must be as soon as possible.

DISEASE

There does not seem to be any disease seen in swifts taken for rehabilitation. The only minor problem they have is with their own parasitic louse fly that lives in the nest and crawls onto the birds during their annual nesting. This is *Crataerina pallida*, surely the most repulsive of all bird parasites. Like a giant flattened blue-bottle with padded feet, it cannot fly but crawls in and out of the feathers. Because they are so large they are usually only seen in ones or twos. Any more would be deleterious to the bird and contrary to normal parasite practice. They can be easily picked off and killed but there will be others in the nest site waiting to infest a vacant host.

COMMON INCIDENTS

The usual incident involving swifts is when they accidentally land on the ground. With their long wings they are unable to launch themselves into the air and flutter around almost helpless. They are easily picked up and taken to rescue centres.

Provided there has been no involvement with cats, and there are no obvious injuries, the swift should be released as soon as possible. Taken to a grassy area where there are no hazards, like buildings or pools, the bird is literally tossed underarm as *high* into the sky as possible. Most of the swifts will flap, gather momentum and fly off, gaining height as they circle upwards. Any that cannot fly will come to ground again on the grass. These failures may just be weak and need feeding up for a day or two before trying again.

Swifts are difficult to feed so an added strengthener of anabolic steroid, nandrolone (Laurabolin – Intervet) at 1 mg/kg, will help. The bird should also be completely re-assessed for injuries.

COMMON INJURIES

Grounded swifts do not normally exhibit any injuries. Sometimes, however, there may be damage to the wings which will stop them flying or being released.

Feathers may be broken or dishevelled enough to cause a problem in flying. Normal feather trauma can be smoothed out with the fingers over a stream of steam from a kettle.

Fractures are particularly bad news as it means the swift will have to spend some weeks in captivity which may, in turn, predispose to feather damage and contamination. Also, with serious fractures or those that may not heal correctly, the longer the swift is in captivity the less are its chances of ever being fit for release. Swifts will not survive in captivity so with a candidate for long-term care perhaps euthanasia is the only humane choice.

ADMISSION AND FIRST AID

This should follow the same procedure as for any small bird although there is the distinct possibility that a swift can be immediately released without any need of treatment. Even a swift caught by a cat should have its injection of long-acting amoxycillin and be released within 24 hours.

CAGING

Swifts in captivity thrive much better if they can hang perpendicularly on a towel draped over the inside of their container. Putting them in cages encourages them to climb the wire which can easily damage their precious feathers. Keep any swifts in a plastic stacking box covered with a light wire mesh to stop them getting out over the top.

Swifts, especially youngsters, find that a cat scratching post covered with carpet is ideal for them to climb.

FEEDING

Adult swifts are only able to feed successfully when they are flying. Their soft beak does not have the strength to pick up the types of live food we can offer them. Consequently, in captivity, it is necessary to force feed swifts on waxworm larvae (Fig. 11.6).

Quite simply, the little tufts of feathers under the bottom beak are used to gently pull the mouth wide open. A waxworm can then easily be put into the back of the mouth, the mouth closed and the swift

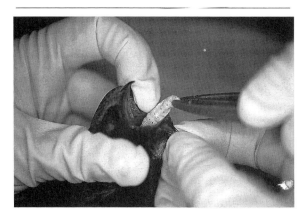

Fig. 11.6 Force-feeding a swift with a waxworm.

seen to swallow. This should be continued until the swift refuses to swallow.

The important thing with captive swifts is to keep their strength up so that they can be released.

RELEASE

Release should be carried out as described above, namely an underarm toss high into the air over a grassy area.

Release should only be during the summer when other swifts are still over Britain. Unlike martins, swallows and other migratory birds, swifts cannot be kept for a year until the next migration. It is imperative that when taken into care they are released within the shortest time possible.

LEGAL IMPLICATIONS

see p. 115.

Kingfishers

NATURAL HISTORY

The kingfisher lives on streams and small pools diving for small fish which it kills by banging them on a branch and swallowing them head first. It usually favours one branch from which to dive into the water. They will sometimes raid garden ponds which is why they can end up as garden bird casualties. They nest by digging a tunnel into a riverbank and laying their eggs in a chamber excavated at the end of it. The young are fed on fish brought by the parents. Eventually the nest becomes a smelly mess of fish parts and fishy faeces. Somehow the young birds emerge as the living jewels that are kingfishers.

EQUIPMENT AND TRANSPORT

Kingfishers are just like any other small bird in its requirements with just one exception, the kingfisher has syndactyl feet in that two toes are joined. This makes it very difficult for the kingfisher to stand on a flat surface. When they are being transported one or two twig perches should be placed in the carrying box off the floor. A cardboard carrying box allows the perches to be pushed through from opposite sides.

RESCUE AND HANDLING

Treat the kingfisher just as any other small bird would be treated.

DISEASE

There are no rehabilitation reports of any infectious disease recorded in kingfishers.

COMMON INCIDENTS

The usual cause of a kingfisher being taken into care is that it will, probably, have flown into a window and knocked itself out. It should be treated as an avian head trauma case (see Chapter 9).

COMMON INJURIES

Concussion is usually the only injury recorded in kingfishers but the author has treated several broken wings, especially where a cat is the first to find the unconscious bird.

ADMISSION AND FIRST AID

As with any other small bird.

CAGING

Caging for kingfishers should be to suit the specialist requirements of their syndactyl feet. Basically a normal three-close-sided rehabilitation cage will suffice with twig perches, about 5–10 mm in width, set at least 40 mm off the floor.

A sturdy stone water bowl will allow the kingfisher to stand comfortably on the rim.

FEEDING

Kingfishers require small fish as their diet and will surprisingly take several at each feed.

Feed kingfishers on whitebait, obtainable individually frozen from fishmongers. Force feed the birds with freshly thawed whitebait as they appear reluctant to feed themselves. They have a very sturdy beak which is held open with one hand while the whitebait, one at a time, are slid headfirst down the bird's throat. It is necessary to make sure that the kingfisher swallows one fish before another is inserted. A thiamine supplement is necessary with whitebait (see Chapter 9).

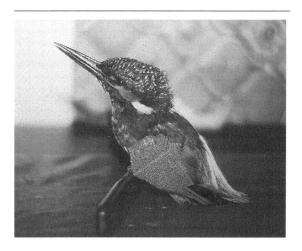

Fig. 11.7 Injured kingfishers can be legally taken into care.

Just like swifts, the secret of success is to get them released as soon as possible.

RELEASE

Kingfishers in care probably have a favourite perch and a territory by a river but invariably they have been found in gardens with no clue as to their origins. To release them on any suitable stream or small river, preferably one that does not freeze in winter, will enable them to forge out new territories.

LEGAL IMPLICATIONS

Just like any other wild bird, both the swift and the kingfisher can be taken into care if they are sick or injured, (Fig. 11.7). They must be released when they are fit enough to do so. It is illegal to keep a wild bird without a close ring in captivity if it is fit for release. Mind you these two birds are so difficult to keep in captivity the question should not arise.

12
The Corn Feeders

Part I: Pigeons and Doves

Species seen regularly:
Feral pigeon, wood pigeon (*Columba palumbus*), collared dove (*Streptopelia decaocto*), stock dove (*Columba oenas*) and, to a lesser degree, the migratory turtle dove (*Streptopelia turtur*).

NATURAL HISTORY

Feral, or 'townie', pigeons are too well known to need an introduction. However, they originated from the rock dove which still breeds on the cliffs on the northwest coast of Scotland. Rock doves were domesticated, first as food and then for pigeon racing, with all the flocks of feral pigeons around towns being descendants or escapees from this ancestry.

The wood pigeon and stock dove have always been native to Britain but the collared dove first started nesting here in the 1950s. Since then they have completely colonised the country and are nearly as numerous as wood pigeons.

The diminutive colourful turtle dove is a summer visitor (Plate 24). Its numbers are now drastically reduced possibly because of persecution as it migrates through Mediterranean countries.

All the pigeons and doves live on seeds and corn as well as any food the human race concedes to them. They build flimsy nests of sticks and normally raise two young at a time. The young are fed on a milky substance (pigeon milk) produced in the adults' crop. All pigeons have the ability to suck up fluids whereas other birds have to take a mouthful and then lift their heads to swallow.

EQUIPMENT AND TRANSPORT

Any cardboard box with ventilation holes will suffice to carry pigeons or doves. In fact small pet carrying boxes are made specifically to suit pigeons and their carriage around the country.

RESCUE AND HANDLING

Pigeons can be caught with a large net and even with the bare hand. Wood pigeons are surprisingly strong and will need extra care to control their flapping wings (Plate 25).

Incidentally pigeon feathers are designed to fall out at the slightest provocation so do not be surprised if in handling one you leave a trail of feathers behind you.

COMMON DISEASES

Pigeons and doves do seem to be ideal candidates for all manner of diseases. In particular avian pox and trichomoniasis are regularly seen (see Chapter 9).

Other diseases, including avian tuberculosis which is zoonotic, may be diagnosed by the veterinary surgeon responsible for their treatment.

Paramyxovirus

The infection of racing pigeons with paramyxovirus PMV-1 has spread into the feral pigeon population. The disease is very contagious although not necessarily fatal if the bird can be supported throughout. Its morbidity is in fact between 30 and 70% of a population with a low 10% mortality rate.

The virus is mainly transmitted by direct contact from the secretions and excretions of a sick bird. It can also be carried on boots, clothing, boxes, baskets and even in the air as a form of virulent dust. It is not surprising that many pigeons suffer from the disease and its transmission is widespread.

When a pigeon first comes into contact with PMV-1 the virus multiplies around the eyes, nose and mouth. From the second or third day the pigeon starts to excrete virus into the environment. After 5–6 days respiratory and ocular symptoms should appear but in the current form of the disease these symptoms are practically non-existent.

It is from the fourth day that the virus multiplies in the gastrointestinal tract and from then can be secreted in the droppings. It is not until watery or bloody diarrhoea is seen that PMV-1 would even be suspected. Only after the gastrointestinal tract has become involved are the neurological or central nervous system signs seen. These are very characteristic:

- Tremor of the head
- Torticollis – head held upside down (Fig. 12.1)
- Loss of balance, tottering and a tendency to fall over
- Loss of coordination – pecking alongside food
- Paralysis of one wing, then both
- And/or paralysis of the feet

These may even occur after no signs of the diarrhoea.

The pigeon will then shed the virus until the disease runs its course, in about 6 weeks. A bird can be kept alive during that period by gavaging liquid food into its crop. Most will make a full recovery.

So PMV-1 is not necessarily a fatal disease but an infected bird is an infectious bird and a threat to any other pigeons in its vicinity. Probably birds showing the nervous signs should not be taken into a care facility with other pigeons but should be passed to the veterinary surgeon for confirmed diagnosis and possible isolation in another building.

Those obviously sick are not the birds that cause great concern. The pigeons that show no symptoms but are shedding virus are likely to pass by all the

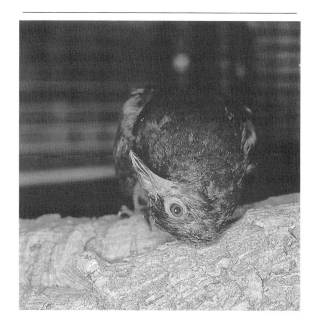

Fig. 12.1 A pigeon with torticollis brought on by paramyxovirus.

safeguards. It is only when they have been in for some days and start showing neurological signs that you realise they have been spreading virus and have probably infected many other pigeons in your facility.

The way to avoid this is to isolate all new pigeon casualties and to vaccinate existing residents. New pigeons can be vaccinated if they show no signs of the disease after 10 days in quarantine. The vaccine (Colombovac PMV – Solway Animal Health) is available in 50 ml or 100 ml multi-dose bottles. Each pigeon receives 0.2 ml of the vaccine by *subcutaneous* injection to the side of the back of the neck. The reason for this is to provide local immunity to the head followed by general immunity throughout the rest of the bird.

Vaccination will also protect pigeons that are exercising in an aviary, prior to release, from wild pigeons who often alight on aviaries.

Ornithosis

Ornithosis is caused by the bacterium *Chlamydia psittaci* responsible for psittacosis in parrots. It is zoonotic so is potentially a dangerous health hazard. The infection is enzootic in feral pigeons and has been reported in collared doves.

Symptoms include ocular and nasal discharge and sometimes dyspnoea. Also the pigeon fanciers' 'one-eyed cold' description of a pigeon ailment could well be chlamydia.

Any bird with symptoms like these must be handled with caution and passed to the veterinary surgeon for definite diagnosis.

COMMON INCIDENTS

By taking in feral pigeons it is sometimes impossible to tell the difference between somebody's racing pigeon and an escaped racing pigeon living in the wild. Both can have rings on them.

Grounded pigeons

Quite often, during the racing pigeon season, a pigeon will be spotted sitting around in a garden apparently sick.

Closer inspection may show a normal plastic ring on one leg and a rubber ring on the other (Fig. 12.2). This is a racing pigeon exhausted during a race. It will just need a few days to rest and feed before it can be let go on its way.

There may be a name and address on the ring or else details may be rubber stamped on the flight feathers (Fig. 12.3). Some fanciers want their birds back, some just want to 'wring their necks'. Con-

tacting the fancier may give you a lead on the pigeon's likely future.

Predated doves

Collared doves are the smaller relatives in the pigeon family wild in this country. They are often caught by cats and are regularly rescued from the clutches of a sparrowhawk. These casualties should be treated as catted birds.

Road traffic accidents

Wood pigeons are regularly hit by motor vehicles. They are large birds and often only lose a lot of feathers. Antibiotics and dexamethasone will help them get over any concussion.

Shot wounds

Pigeons will be presented with shot wounds, either shot gun pellets or air gun pellets. They cause a remarkable amount of damage including comminuted fractures of any bone they are likely to hit. Treatment is the same as for any other bird with a shot wound (see Chapter 6).

Ruptured crop

The injury seen in pigeons but apparently not in other species is a rupture of the crop. Usually the crop is so full that the slightest knock seems to

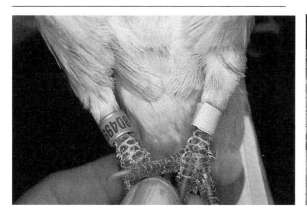

Fig. 12.2 The two rings (one plastic, one rubber) that show a pigeon is in a race.

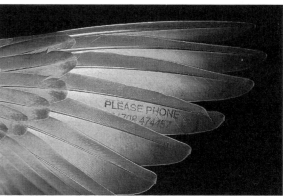

Fig. 12.3 The address or telephone number of a racing pigeon's owner is often stamped on its primary feathers.

explode it. Injury may be obvious with corn seen coming from the defect. Or it may be that the outer skin is not ruptured so the corn coming out of the crop is building up under the skin. Sometimes the injury is quite expansive and often contaminated with food and, sometimes, the lesions of trichomoniasis.

However, if the defects are thoroughly cleaned and sutured most birds make a complete recovery (Fig. 12.4). It should be treated as an emergency as the bird will have been unable to drink since the injury occurred. It could be severely dehydrated warranting extra fluids.

A crop rupture involves two layers, the actual lining of the crop and the fragile skin over the top of it. Both have to be sutured, preferably under anaesthetic. Broad-spectrum antibiotics can be given, usually long-acting amoxycillin at 250 mg/kg daily.

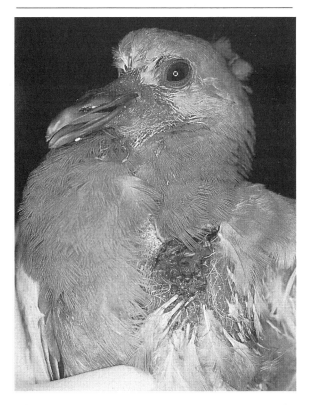

Fig. 12.4 Ruptures of the crop are regularly seen in pigeon casualties.

Fractures

Many pigeons and doves are presented having fractures of any of the long bones of the wings or legs. Most will respond to standard fracture treatment regimes. However, we have found that wood pigeons with fractures that cannot heal properly are not suitable for retention in captivity. Their nervous nature means they will never ever be comfortable, even in an aviary.

Strangely, ringed pigeons often seem to fracture the leg that is carrying a ring. To prevent unnecessary suffering a ring on a fractured or injured leg should be cut off.

ADMISSION AND FIRST AID

After the initial first-aid treatments have been provided, the pigeons and doves are so susceptible to so many diseases it is sound practice to treat them prophylactically against some conditions (Table 12.1).

CAGING

Any large cage will be ample for pigeons. Wood pigeons will need to be kept somewhere quiet or else they will panic. Perches should be provided made of twigs about 10–20 mm in diameter.

A sand base is adequate.

Post treatment in an aviary will provide exercise prior to release. Precautions ought to be taken to stop any feral pigeons breeding. Feral pigeons will pair and make nests, even on the ground in an aviary. They lay two white eggs. Taking away the eggs will only encourage them to lay two more. Replacing the eggs with plastic artificial eggs will put off the ultimate relaying for some weeks. Also by pricking the ends of any eggs with a needle or giving them a shaking may prevent them hatching and deceive the female into brooding rather than re-laying.

FEEDING

Pigeons and doves will eat almost anything. Chicken growers' pellets offer a complete diet.

Table 12.1 Suggested prophylactic treatments for various pigeon species on admission.

Treatment	Feral pigeon	Wood pigeon	Collared dove	Stock dove	Turtle dove
Carnidazole (Spartrix – Harkers) for Trichomoniasis	1 tablet (10 mg)	1 tablet (10 mg)	$\frac{1}{2}$ tablet (5 mg) (10 mg if infected)	1 tablet (10 mg)	$\frac{1}{2}$ tablet (5 mg)
PMV Vaccine (Colombovac PMV – Solvay Animal Health) Should be after 10 days quarantine for new admissions	0.2 ml (subcutaneously)	0.2 ml (subcutaneously)	—	0.2 ml (subcutaneously)	—
Worming capsule (Panacur Pigeon Capsules – Hoechst Roussel Vet)	1 capsule	1 capsule	—	1 capsule	—

Mixed corn is readily available at pet stores but unless vitamins and minerals are added cannot be called a complete diet. There are available specialised pigeon mixtures which offer a varied range of corns and seed.

Pigeon grit should also be provided.

RELEASE

Wood pigeons, stock doves and collared doves can be released in any park, common or country area. Turtle doves will need releasing before their migration at the end of the summer.

If feral pigeons are released locally they will stay around your neighbourhood. Their homing instinct is phenomenal. Feral pigeons are descended from rock doves who live on sea cliffs. Perhaps the best release site for pigeons is near sea cliffs at least 200 km away from where they have been kept. Releasing just before dusk may break the homing cycle and encourage them to stay in their new sea cliff environment.

LEGAL IMPLICATIONS

Under the Veterinary Surgeons Act 1966 and its amendments, only a registered veterinary surgeon and in some cases a veterinary nurse can treat an animal belonging to another person. Racing and fancy pigeons often belong to a fancier so any treatment on these pigeons should be restricted to first aid, life-saving and prevention of pain or suffering unless the person treating is a registered veterinary surgeon or veterinary nurse.

Part II: Game Birds

Species seen regularly:
Pheasant (*Phasianus colchicus*), grey partridge (*Perdix perdix*), red-legged partridge (*Alectonis rufa*) and occasionally quail (*Coturnix coturnix*).

NATURAL HISTORY

'Game birds' means literally that – the birds included in this section, apart from the grey partridge, are bred and released for shooting.

Often native birds, like grouse (*Lagopus lagopus*), are managed for shooting but do not usually arrive for rehabilitation.

More exotic species are occasionally found but are usually escapees from a collection. Although some gamekeepers have been introducing Chukar partridges (*Alectoris chukar*) for shooting, it is illegal to release them.

Exotic pheasant species seen include: golden pheasant (*Chrysolophus pictus*), Lady Amherst's pheasant (*Chrysolophus amherstiae*), Reeve's pheasant (*Syrmaticus reevesii*) and the silver pheasant (*Lophura nycthemera*).

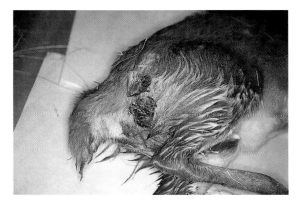

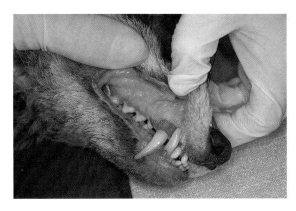

Plate 1 This deer has been attacked by a normally placid family dog. This is one of the dangers imprinted animals have to face.

Plate 2 Foxes may show jaundiced mucous membranes.

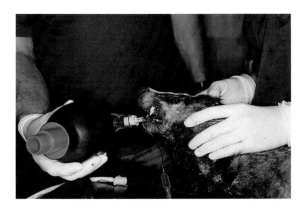

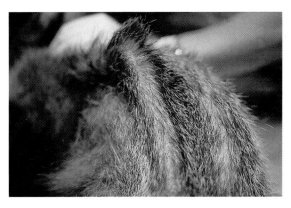

Plate 3 Using an Ambu bag can provide effective artificial respiration to a casualty.

Plate 4 The tenting effect of pinching the skin will show that an animal is dehydrated.

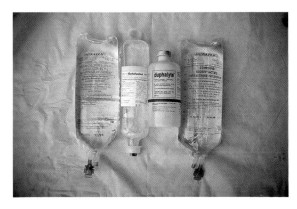

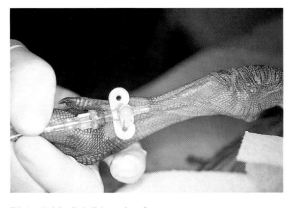

Plate 5 A selection of systemic fluids suitable for wildlife casualties.

Plate 6 Medial tibia vein of a swan.

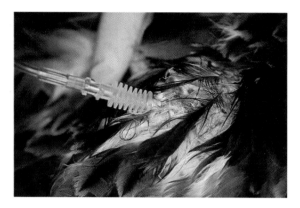

Plate 7 Spinal needle inserted to allow intraosseous fluids through the ulna.

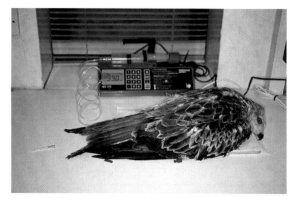

Plate 8 Using a syringe pump can accurately infuse fluids intraosseously to a bird.

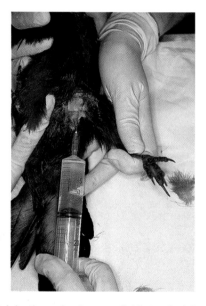

Plate 9 Injecting subcutaneous fluids to a jackdaw in the inguinal area at the top of the leg.

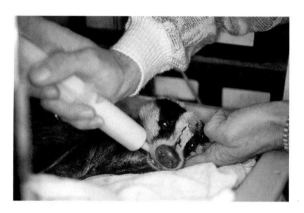

Plate 10 A debilitated badger can be hand fed with liquid food.

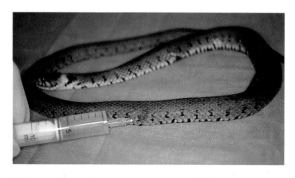

Plate 11 Providing subcutaneous fluids to a grass snake can rehydrate it.

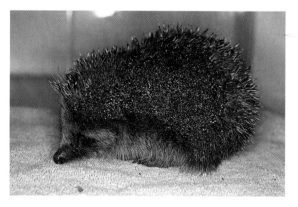

Plate 12 Burnt hair and spines are common hedgehog injuries.

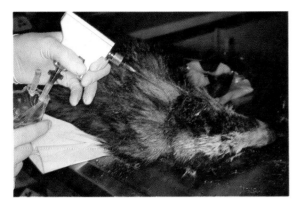

Plate 13 The wound lavage system will safely clean contaminated wounds.

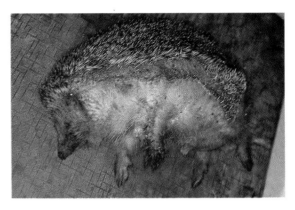

Plate 14 A hedgehog having had major skin lacerations was sutured with surgical staples.

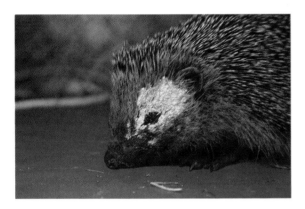

Plate 15 Fly egg infestations are seen in hedgehogs.

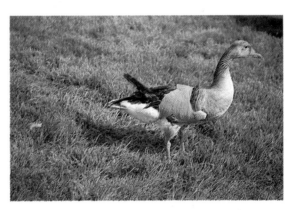

Plate 16 A fractured wing in a bird can be temporarily stabilised with a body bandage.

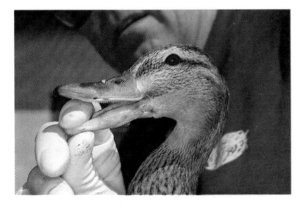

Plate 17 Female mallard 3 months after having a prosthetic bottom beak fitted (see also Plate 27).

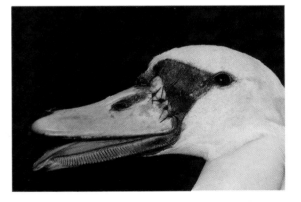

Plate 18 Wound caused by fishing line becoming entangled around a swan's beak. Suturing prevented the wound gaping.

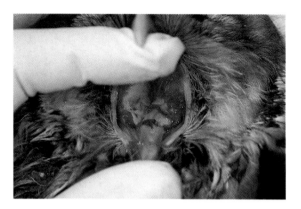

Plate 19 Typical lesions of trichomoniasis – this time in a tawny owl.

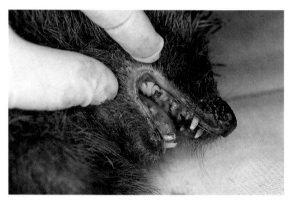

Plate 20 Hedgehogs regularly suffer from a chronic build-up of calculus on their teeth.

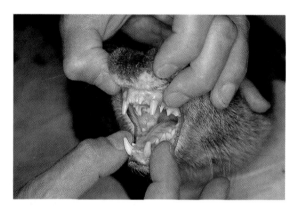

Plate 21 Otters often receive fractures to their canine teeth.

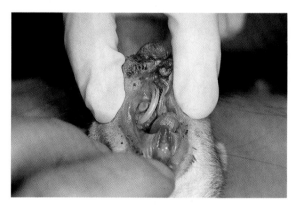

Plate 22 Malocclusion will eventually lead to starvation. This casualty was a grey squirrel.

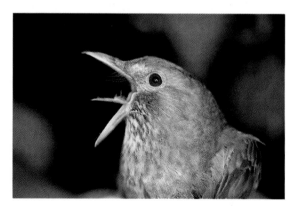

Plate 23 Blackbirds are often found with broken beaks that can sometimes be mended.

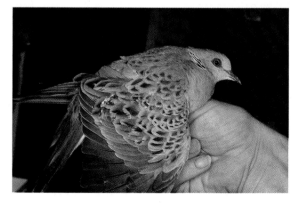

Plate 24 A hanging wing usually means a fractured wing that needs splinting.

Quail are, in fact, a now very rare migrant species that can be confused with the quail sold by pet stores as 'Japanese quail'.

All the species are ground feeders taking a mixture of seeds, corn, shoots and insects. The three regularly seen species tend to skulk in hedgerows and open woodland venturing into fields to feed. All their young are precocial and are fully feathered, able to walk and run and feed themselves immediately after hatching.

EQUIPMENT AND TRANSPORT

Large nets and cat-sized carrying boxes are the order of the day.

RESCUE AND HANDLING

These birds are great runners and do not need to fly to escape capture. A large net with an extra long handle gives the catcher a chance of catching the bird before it has run too far.

Pheasants, especially, are surprisingly strong and should be held firmly around the shoulders. They are also extremely highly strung so should be handled as little as possible. A dark box will quieten them.

In the treatment facility it may be nigh on impossible to evaluate a pheasant as it flaps, kicks and tries to die. Diazepam at 10 mg/kg intramuscularly or intravenously should quieten the bird enough for triage and first aid.

COMMON DISEASES

There are well-recorded diseases of game birds in the shooting world. They are, however, not the subject of a rehabilitation facility that normally only sees trauma victims.

COMMON INCIDENTS

Almost invariably a pheasant or partridge casualty will have been hit by a motor vehicle. The question of ownership docs arise but most of these birds have no identification tags or rings so can be treated as any wild bird casualty.

COMMON INJURIES

There may be occasional fracture of the tibiotarsus but the most usual injury is varying degrees of concussion, especially with pheasants.

Pheasants are regularly presented with no use in either of the legs. Initially they can be treated like any suspect spinal injury case but as bird x-rays are hard to interpret it is often not possible to identify a back injury (Fig. 12.5). If there is doubt the pheas-

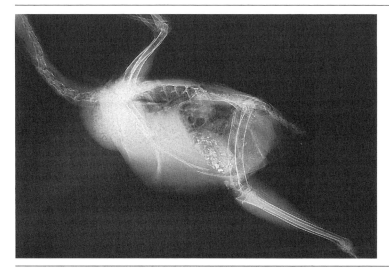

Fig. 12.5 Radiographs of birds, this is a pheasant, are difficult to interpret for spinal injuries.

ant should be treated as a head trauma case (see Chapter 9). However, if no improvement of the flaccid paralysis of the legs is seen in 1 week the bird is probably not going to recover. It should be destroyed.

Some pheasants brought in have part of their top beak missing. This will have been clipped by a game-keeper and should regrow without any problems.

ADMISSION AND FIRST AID

Standard triage and first-aid techniques apply with the addition of diazepam for crazed pheasants.

CAGING

Pheasants, in particular, need a large cage with the front covered to keep them calm.

Once recovered all game birds should be kept in a large aviary for 1 or 2 weeks before release.

FEEDING

Game birds will eat corn, seed and game-bird pellets with the occasional insect supplement, like mealworms, for the grey partridge.

Intestinal worms are often a problem in game birds. Suitable wormers include:

- Fenbendazole (Wormex – Hoechst Roussel Vet) – 12 mg/kg for pheasant and partridges, an oral suspension
- Flubendazole (Flubenvet Intermediate – Janssen Animal Health) – 60 g/tonne of feed for 7 days

RELEASE

Release should be in a suitable habitat of fields bordered by hedges and woods. Be aware of any shooting estates and avoid them or else your patient could end up getting shot.

LEGAL IMPLICATIONS

Under Schedule 9 of the Wildlife and Countryside Act 1981 it is illegal to release the following game birds:

- Chukar partridge (*Alectoris chukar*)
- Rock partridge (*Alectoris graeca*)
- Golden pheasant (*Chrysolophus pictus*)
- Lady Amherst's pheasant (*Chrysolophus amherstiae*)
- Reeve's pheasant (*Syrmaticus reevesii*)
- Silver pheasant (*Lophura nycthemera*)
- Bobwhite quail (*Colinus virginianus*)
- Capercaillie (*Tetrao urogallus*)
- or any other species not indigenous to Britain.

13
Corvids

Species seen regularly:

Carrion or hooded crows (*Corvus corone*), rook (*Corvus frugilegus*), magpie (*Pica pica*), jackdaw (*Corvus monedula*) and jay (*Garrulus glandarius*).

Also the raven (*Corvus corax*) and the extremely rare chough (*Pyrrhocorax pyrrhocorax*) may occasionally arrive at rescue centres.

It is also an opinion that the house crow (*Corvus splendens*) will soon be resident in Britain (Pukas, 1999).

NATURAL HISTORY

The varieties of corvid in Britain have all established their own niches and do not generally compete with each other:

- The carrion crow establishes pairs on farmland in a strict territory
- The hooded crow is the same species seen in Scotland
- The magpie hunts in bands especially amongst hedgerows and light woodland
- The jackdaw often lives around cliffs or human habitation where it nests in chimneys
- The jay, the most colourful crow, is a bird of broad-leaved woodland
- The raven is the giant of the family inhabiting moorland and mountain
- The chough is now very rare, it lives on sea cliffs on the Welsh and northwest coasts

As a family, the crows are very omnivorous and will eat a variety of food from corn, insects, other birds, small mammals and road kills.

Magpies regularly raid birds' nests especially in gardens. They will take any eggs or young birds just the same as great spotted woodpeckers (*Dendrocopos major*). However, they do not generally take adult birds as do cats and sparrowhawks. Therefore their impact on a breeding pair is not as great, the bereaved birds will simply have a second brood whereas the loss of one of the pair would be impossible to replace in that breeding season.

Generally the corvids are very intelligent and quickly adapt to exploit any food source.

EQUIPMENT AND TRANSPORT

A large net, with a long handle, is required to catch any of the corvids because even if they cannot fly they are extremely adept at running and jumping over quite large obstacles.

They will need a sturdy cat-carrying box to hold them and the raven is probably safer in a cat-carrying basket.

RESCUE AND HANDLING

The rescue of these fairly large birds is quite straightforward, although a sturdy pair of gloves will protect against biting or clutching with their very sharp claws. Without gloves an elastic band around the *end* of the beak will prevent a painful bite. This should be monitored closely in case the bird regurgitates or has difficulty breathing. A bird muzzled in this way should never be left unmonitored.

COMMON DISEASES

Corvids no doubt carry a range of diseases, none of which seem to turn up in rescue centres. Routine hygiene should, however, protect other bird patients if it does happen.

Corvids can carry a large burden of parasites both internal and external.

- Internal helminth parasites can be controlled by:
  - ivermectin (Ivomec Injection for Cattle – Merial Animal Health) given orally at 200 micrograms/kg or mixed 1:9 with propylene glycol at 0.2 ml/kg
  - doramectin (Dectomax Injectable Solution for Cattle and Sheep – Pfizer) given orally at 300 micrograms/kg or mixed 1:9 with sesame seed oil at 0.3 ml/kg is the latest drug in this line to become available

    In particular choughs suffer with gapeworm which can be controlled with either fenbendazole or thiabendazole (see Chapter 9).
- Mites are commonly seen on crows and rooks. Their control is with ivermectin (Ivomec Pour-on – Merial Animal Health) at 0.1 ml per bird dabbed on to the skin at the back of the neck.

COMMON INCIDENTS

Apart from jackdaws falling down chimneys, adult corvid casualties are usually victims of careless shooting or of road traffic accidents.

There will also be an annual influx of supposedly orphaned juveniles (Fig. 13.1). Beware for these are probably not orphaned. Young crows and rooks leave the nest long before they can fly. They spend some days hopping around on the ground but still being fed by their parents. Ideally these birds should be left where they are unless there is a real danger from predators or human hazards. Rescued orphans can even be put back as long as somebody watches from a distance to make sure the parent birds are still around.

Other juvenile crows and rooks will be found that have obvious problems:

- Many young birds are found with white or patchy white feathers (Fig. 13.2). These feathers are weaker that the black feathers, easily getting

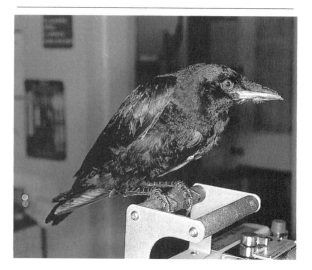

Fig. 13.1 Juvenile corvids are often 'rescued' when there is no need for intervention.

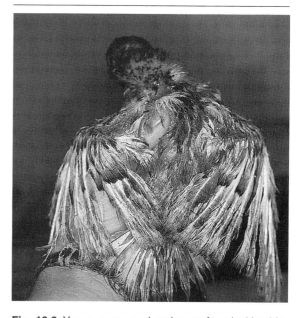

Fig. 13.2 Young crows and rooks are found with white or patchy feathers.

broken and preventing the bird from flying. This may be caused by a nutritional deficiency or agricultural chemicals. To date there seems to have been little or no research carried out on this problem.

When these birds are taken into care there is no short-term solution. The damaged and white feathers have to be moulted out in order to be replaced. This can take up to a year but in that year the keeper can make sure that the birds receive a balanced diet and so are able to produce sound feathers the next time around.

One problem with keeping young corvids for any length of time is that they easily become imprinted on humans. Every effort must be made to keep these birds away from human company or it may be impossible to release them.

- The other young crows or rooks found every summer are those with deformed legs. Both legs seem to folded at the hocks and have fused solid. This probably happens in the nest so when the bird leaves it finds it cannot walk.

   In care there is no remedial treatment or surgery that could be effective so these birds will have to be humanely destroyed.

COMMON INJURIES

With adult corvids the commonly seen injuries are fractures of the long bones of the limbs caused by gun shot wounds or road traffic collisions. Unfortunately, as these birds are fairly capable of living on the ground for a while, without necessarily having to fly, it can be some time before they are spotted, caught and taken into care. By then any fractures will have either fused incorrectly or be totally contaminated, often with lengths of devitalised bone protruding from the skin (Plate 26). There will also be a build-up of fibrous tissue efficiently holding the bones in their new positions. It is often hopeless to try to rectify this but the veterinary surgeon may elect to try an osteotomy in an effort to get the bird fit for release.

One problem being seen at rescue centres is a build-up of disabled corvids who were untreatable because of this type of injury. Some centres destroy their unreleasable birds but those who have a different policy will be eventually totally overcrowded by these disabled corvids.

ADMISSION AND FIRST AID

Standard first-aid procedures are adequate for all the corvids who, generally, are very robust birds. The only modification is that intravenous fluids may be more suitable than intraosseous fluids for the very large raven.

CAGING

Large cages and aviaries with many perches are necessary for any of the corvid family. Even those still unable to fly will want to climb ladders or sloping perches to the highest point, where they will feel comfortable.

They are particularly messy birds and require constant cleaning to keep them hygienically sound.

Crows and ravens tend to be aggressive to each other while being wary of each other. If there are more than two to an aviary their defensive manner never seems to allow them to relax enough to bathe or preen. Consequently an aviary with three or more will become an aviary of birds with substandard feathering which in turn prohibits them from being released until they moult into a new set of feathers the next year.

Rooks seem to be more sociable to each other. Magpies and jackdaws will live together but jays should be kept away from their larger cousins.

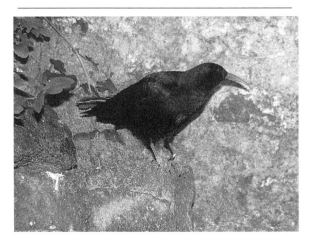

Fig. 13.3 Choughs are very specialised birds.

FEEDING

Most of the corvids will do very well on a balanced diet of dog food, either dry or tinned. They will also take day-old chicks with a vitamin and mineral supplement added.

Jays will benefit from the occasional, once a week, treat of mealworms. They also like small vegetables such as peas.

The chough is very specialised and mainly an insect feeder (Fig. 13.3). If one is taken into care the author would recommend getting in touch with specialists who will be able to advise on the most suitable way of keeping the chough while it is treated.

RELEASE

All the corvids are intelligent enough to cope with being released directly into a suitable habitat.

However, carrion crows are very territorial so should be put back where they were found. If that is not possible a vacant territory should be found or else they might be attacked by a resident pair.

For choughs, once again, please refer to a specialist for the most suitable release procedure. There is a chough re-introduction scheme called 'Operation Chough' which will be able to advise of the best release site (Appendix 7).

LEGAL IMPLICATIONS

Apart from the normal wild bird and animal protection legislation, the only other regulation that applies to corvids is that the chough is on Schedule 4 of the Wildlife and Countryside Act 1981. Any casualties should be preferably passed on to a licensed holder or registered with the DETR, (see page 110 and Appendix 4).

14
Water Birds – Ducks

Species seen regularly:

- **Dabbling ducks** – wigeon (*Anas penelope*), gadwall (*A. strepera*), mallard (*A. platyrhynchos*), teal (*A. crecca*), pintail (*A. acuta*), garganey (*A. querquedula*) and shoveler (*A. clypeata*).

- **Diving ducks** – pochard (*Aythya ferina*) and tufted (*Aythya fuligula*).

- **Seaducks** – eider (*Somataria mollisima*), scoter (*Melanitta nigra*), scaup (*Aythya marila*), shelduck (*Tadorna tadorna*), long-tailed (*Clangula hyemalis*) and goldeneye (*Bucephala clangula*).

- **Fish-eating ducks** (sawbills) – merganser (*Mergus* sp.), smew (*Mergus albellus*) and goosander (*Mergus merganser*).

- **Exotic ducks** – mandarin (*Aix galericulata*), ruddy (*Oxyura jamaicensis*), Carolina (*Aix sponsa*) and others which will need to be identified.

- **Domestic ducks** – muscovy (*Cairina moschata*), Aylesbury, all white ducks and mallard crossbreeds.

NATURAL HISTORY

Obviously ducks are aquatic creatures with a wide variety of adaptation to different environments and feeding methods. Most find their food on the water but the less specialised dabbling and diving ducks will eat from the waterside, especially in parks.

The male duck is called a drake while the female is the duck. She is the only one to 'quack'! Drakes make only little 'quibbling' noises and this difference makes it easy to sex the birds when they are both in their identical drab summer moult. In full-breeding plumage the drakes are very colourful whereas the females have a very drab mottled plumage to make them inconspicuous when they are sitting on the nest.

The duck will lay one egg every 1 or 2 days in a nest lined with her own down feathers. She will not sit and brood the eggs until the full clutch is laid. These unbrooded eggs remain cold and dormant until she starts to brood. By only sitting when all the eggs are laid, the ducklings will all hatch at the same time. Only after the duck has started brooding will an egg be killed if it gets cold.

Ducklings are precocial, so once they are hatched they can feed themselves and follow the duck to her chosen watercourse. When they are on the water the duck makes sure they do not become waterlogged. However, when separated from her or taken into care they seem to become easily waterlogged and hypothermic if they are on water. In captivity ducklings should not be allowed on water until they are 16 weeks old.

In the wild, ducklings fall easy prey to gulls, herons, large fish and even swans.

EQUIPMENT AND TRANSPORT

All ducks are large birds so a large catching net is essential. Ducklings, even the tiniest ones, are also easier to catch with a large net.

Strange as it may seem, a loaf of sliced white bread is often essential equipment for catching ducks, geese or swans. Latex disposable gloves are also essential to protect against polluted water, oil or duck-borne infections such as Campylobacter.

Ducks can be carried comfortably in cardboard cat-carrying boxes or cat-carrying baskets. They are quite messy so a base of newspaper helps keep the box clean.

RESCUE AND HANDLING

Ducks are very difficult birds to catch; unlike geese or swans they have perfected the art of instant vertical take-off. If the net can be dropped over them they will oblige and fly up and into it. On water they have other escape methods like diving out of sight or swimming away at a surprising speed. Even on land a duck that cannot fly can outrun most people.

The technique for capture is to approach as close as possible with the net held in front. Watching the bird will give a clue as to when it is thinking of making its move and fleeing. If you are within reach, and very quick, it is possible to drop the net over it. However, mobile ducks are almost impossible to catch. Sometimes laying a trail of small pieces of white bread may entice the ducks, and all of its contemporaries, to within catching distance.

An added problem is that ducks, geese and swans are very wary of anything resembling a fishing rod or landing net. Many will take one look and swim the other way and there is nothing that can be done about it.

Ducklings may appear easy to catch; they cannot fly and have nowhere near the power of an adult duck. However, ducklings can run at breakneck speed across the top of the water, they can dive in an instant and are superbly camouflaged to hide in the bank where they invariably surface. Try sliding the large net underneath ducklings to cut off diving, their normal escape method.

Ducks on a beach, especially those that are oiled, should only be approached from the seaward side of the beach. This effectively cuts off their escape route because once they are on the sea they are practically impossible to catch.

Handling ducks, always with latex gloves, should involve holding them around the shoulders to control their wings. Some of them may try to bite but their bites are harmless!

COMMON DISEASES

Ducks are susceptible to major epizootic diseases that, given the right circumstances, can wipe out thousands of birds. These diseases include avian botulism, avian cholera, duck plague (or duck viral enteritis) and others. Thankfully massive mortality, seen in some American duck populations, does not often occur in this country. That is not to say that it will not happen. Any mass mortality of ducks should be thoroughly investigated, possibly under the auspices of the State Veterinary Service.

Botulism

Avian botulism does occur in the duck population. *Clostridium botulinum* Type C is usually the bacterial culprit. Temperatures above 20–23°C and anaerobic conditions are required for the bacteria to produce toxin (Wobeser, 1981). The optimum temperature is 28°C (Rosen, 1971) which fortunately is not that common in Britain. Consequently, even during hot weather, we do not see the mass mortality that botulism creates in America.

However, when water levels are low in summer, botulism can still kill many ducks in a population. The toxin is spread by invertebrates, particularly maggots, feeding on the carcasses of birds that have died. It only takes two or three toxic maggots to kill a duck. To prevent the cycle continuing any dead birds in a suspect area should be removed and incinerated. As long as protective gloves are worn when handling live or dead birds, then the botulism is not classed as zoonotic.

Treatment generally given is antitoxin and fluids (see Chapter 9), although the Swan Sanctuary has evolved its own treatment for botulism in swans which may be applicable to other water birds (see Chapter 15).

Other duck diseases are usually seen in wildfowl collections and these should be referred to the veterinary surgeon for diagnosis and treatment.

Parasites

Ducks suffer with the usual quota of helminth parasites including gizzard and proventricular worms. Worming can be with:

- Mebendazole (Mebenvet – Janssen Animal Health) as an oral powder for adding to the food
- Ivermectin (Ivomec Injection for Cattle – Merial Animal Health) at 200 micrograms/kg (or 0.2 ml/kg when mixed 1 : 9 with propylene glycol) given subcutaneously or orally

COMMON INCIDENTS

Before getting involved in any incident involving ducks, it is worth remembering that the domestic species are owned by somebody who is responsible for their welfare. Interfering with owned birds could have legal repercussions. It is safest to refer all domestic duck incidents to the owner.

Fishing hooks and line

Ducks are very often affected by anglers' discarded fishing tackle. The extent of the involvement of any hook can be assessed by radiograph (Fig. 14.1). Attempts can often be made to safely remove a hook or line, or the veterinary surgeon may operate (see Chapter 9).

Mating

Every spring and early summer ducks launch into their breeding season. There always appears to be more drakes then ducks. Consequently ducks will often be assaulted by a number of drakes and may actually be drowned by their mass advances. Many survive the ordeal but are often debilitated and are taken into care.

The tell-tale sign of a mating victim is a bald patch at the back of the head where the feathers have been pulled out by a servicing drake. Usually these ducks just need supportive care and release into an area with fewer drakes.

Road traffic accidents

During the mating season ducks and drakes will venture away from their normal waterside haunts to find suitable nest sites. In doing this they will often cross roads together and both get hit by motor vehicles.

Family groups

The duck often secretes her nest far from any watercourse. Once the ducklings hatch, all on the same day, the duck will attempt to lead them to water. Consequently an adult duck with a line of tiny ducklings following her can be seen in the most inappropriate places.

Rather than trying to catch the group and carry them to a watercourse, it is comparatively easy to shepherd them in the right direction holding back traffic and people until they have passed (Fig. 14.2).

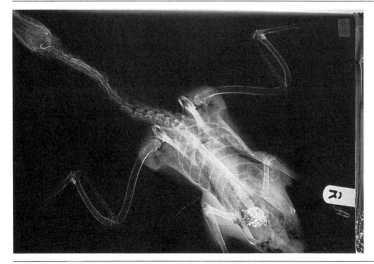

Fig. 14.1 Radiograph showing fishing hook lodged in a duck's throat.

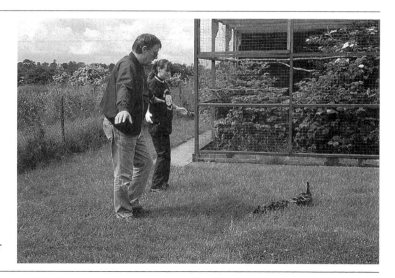

Fig. 14.2 Ducklings will follow their mother and can be gently shepherded.

Orphans

Obviously if the mother is killed or missing, the ducklings will have to be taken into care. But what normally happens is that one of the ducklings either hatches late or is slightly inferior and gets left behind. Its high peeping call and the lack of any other ducklings around means that it does need rescuing.

Other ducks will not accept the ducklings of another brood and will very likely kill them.

Eclipse

All fit birds will moult their feathers once, twice or even three times a year. Normally they will moult two wing feathers at a time, one from each wing. Ducks, however, moult all the wing feathers at the same time and it is during this period, which is called the 'eclipse', when they will not be able to fly. This will happen at various times between mid-July to the end of October.

Oiled ducks

Ducks are almost always involved with any spillage of oil whether it be inland or on the coast. The dabbling ducks inland are quite robust and will normally survive medication, cleaning and rehabilitation. The seaducks, however, are more sensitive and require more sympathetic handling. They will also benefit from prophylactic treatment against aspergillosis (see Chapter 9).

The rescue, treatment and cleaning of oiled birds is covered fully in Chapter 18.

COMMON INJURIES

Fractures of the legs and wings are fairly commonplace, but being large birds they can usually be successfully treated. The pigeon-sized Colomboclip (Boddy and Ridewood) is also suitable for splinting some tibiotarsal fractures suffered by ducks.

Beak fractures

Ducks do occasionally fracture or lose their beaks. Fractures of the bony mandible can often be mended with wire sutures. However, the complete loss of a bottom beak makes it impossible for the duck to continue without it. Without a bottom beak the tongue hangs uselessly and soon becomes necrotic if the bird does not first die of hunger.

Prosthetics for birds, especially for missing beaks, is an area that has hardly been explored. Most efforts are unsuccessful but where a complete beak is missing the bird can only die unless something is tried. A prosthethis for a top beak is not really feasible because it needs a good anchorage and the bones in the region of the front of the skull are not really solid enough. Prostheses have been fitted for the bottom beak and have been successful in ducks, although the birds were never released to the rigours of a wild existence.

Each case deserves an individual approach. Coles (1997) tells of various methods using Steinmann's pins or kirschner wires placed in a cruciate pattern. The wildlife Hospital Trust (St Tiggywinkles) has developed:

The PKP method (Plate 27)

Ducks have fairly substantial lower jaws. If a lower jaw is broken off, just in front of the commisure of the beak (Plate 27a), then a prosthethis could be tried:

(1) A scaffold conforming to the duck's bottom beak is fashioned out of a complete Kirschner wire (Plate 27b).
(2) The two ends of the wire are then pushed through the centres of the remaining fragments of both mandibles.
(3) Where the wires exit the mandibles they are bent and cut to form anchor points to prevent the wire slipping forward.
(4) Then, using a thermoplastic (Hydroplastic – TAK Systems) the scaffold of the bottom beak is fashioned with an impression running in the top to accommodate the tongue.
(5) Prosthetic netting (Ethicon) is then fixed into the thermoplastic before it sets and is sutured to the soft tissue and skin across the two original fracture sites (Plate 27c).

With this prosthesis, ducks and geese can usually start feeding immediately. However, they may gorge themselves so should only be offered dissolvable food like pellets or chick crumbs. Any prosthesis like this should be regularly monitored and serviced.

Prolapsed penis

In captive ducks, bullying will sometimes cause the victim drake to suffer a prolapsed penis (Plate 28). Bullying can happen in the wild but this condition is usually caused by road traffic accidents.

The penis usually sits at the bottom of the cloaca but when extended or prolapsed can cause obstruction to the evacuation of the faeces. The only solution is for amputation.

ADMISSION AND FIRST AID

Fluids

Ducks are normally large enough so that fluids can be infused through the medial tibial vein.

Oral fluids

Oral fluids are called for in ducks with suspect botulism or else victims of oil pollution. Oral fluids help flush toxic material out of the gut.

Amputees

Ducks can manage very well in captivity with the loss of a wing. However, a duck missing a leg will never cope and should be destroyed. Nevertheless, even if the leg bones are badly fractured, compounded and contaminated, it is worth attempting treatment as many birds recover from this apparently irretrievable condition.

Vitamins

Vitamin B$_{12}$

All water birds benefit from an intramuscular injection or oral dose of vitamin B$_{12}$ once weekly at 250–5000 micrograms/kg.

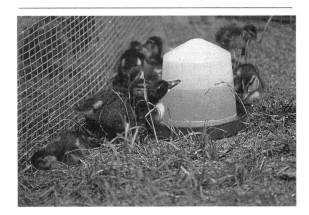

Fig. 14.3 A water fountain – this prevents ducklings getting waterlogged and adult ducks making a mess while in care.

Vitamin B₁

Vitamin B₁

All fish-eating ducks should receive a thiamine supplement (Aquavits – IZUG).

CAGING

Injured ducks have to be kept in large cages, at least until any wounds have healed. Water is provided in a water fountain available from pet stores (Fig. 14.3). If you give them a water bowl, they will sit in it and bathe in it and generally make a complete mess of every clean cage.

It is better to use newspaper on the floor of the cage because it can be regularly changed.

More than one duck in a cage may fight but it is worth trying, just to keep the work-load down.

Once they are healed, ducks must be given facilities to swim and bathe. Sometimes they are not fully waterproof and have to be rescued before they drown. A wet duck is a cold duck so should be dried off in an inside cage. Each time it gets wet it will preen and the more times it preens, the sooner it will be able to swim without sinking.

FEEDING

Dabbling and diving ducks will take white bread off water. However, more goodness can be obtained from duck pellets or mixed corn with added vitamins and minerals. Fish-eating ducks may take seaduck pellets which are scattered on the water. They may even take whitebait from a dish of water.

Seaducks can be offered clean mussels or shrimps. However, although initially frozen, when defrosted shellfish quickly spoil. Seaduck pellets from Mazuri Zoo Foods are ideal if you can persuade the ducks to take them off the surface of the water.

Exotic ducks will have to be identified so that suitable feed can be provided. Most of the ducks are escapees from captivity so will be quite used to artificial diets.

RELEASE

It is best to release ducks back to where they were found if the area is safe.

A female that has been attacked by drakes would benefit from a site with fewer birds on it. A quiet small river or lake is ideal for dabbling or diving ducks.

Fish-eating ducks and seaducks should go back to their original haunts where there is going to be a reliable food source to suit their specialised requirements.

Never release domestic ducks, not even on to a protected stretch of water.

LEGAL IMPLICATIONS

There are no ducks on Schedule 4 of the Wildlife and Countryside Act 1981 but there are some on Schedule 9 which means they should not be released into the wild. The ducks involved are:

- Carolina wood duck (*Aix spousa*)
- Mandarin duck (*Aix galericulata*)
- Ruddy duck (*Oxyura jamaicensis*)

It is also illegal to release or allow to escape any duck that is not ordinarily wild in, or a regular visitor to, Great Britain (Wildlife and Countryside Act 1981, Section 14, part (1)).

15
Water Birds – Swans

Species seen regularly:
Mute swan (*Cygnus olor*), occasionally migrant Bewick's swan (*Cygnus columbianus*), whooper swan (*Cygnus cygnus*) and escaped black swans (*Cygnus atratus*).

NATURAL HISTORY

The mute swan is the familiar swan of watercourses all over Britain. It feeds on grass and water plants but is fairly omnivorous and will take almost anything including insects and small animals. In particular they are regularly fed, by the public, on scraps of bread which many swans grow to rely on.

The male mute swan, with a large black protuberance at the top of the beak, is the cob and the female the pen. Their pair bonding can be for life, a commitment that sometimes causes a singleton, who has lost its mate, to pine and sometimes perish. A pair will be very territorial and will attack any swan that encroaches on their area. In particular, when they have young (cygnets), the cob will attack anything that moves and has been known to kill dogs on the waterside. When their young are grown enough to fly, the adults will aggressively drive them off to clear their territory of swans, ready for the next breeding season.

The mute swan is Britain's largest wild bird with some cobs weighing in at over 12 kg.

Bewick's and whooper swans are winter visitors to Britain. Their nesting grounds are on the Arctic tundra, especially in northern Scandinavia and Russia. They have regular wintering sites in this country and, in particular, the Bewick's swan winter population at The Wildfowl and Wetlands Trust at Slimbridge has been closely studied and monitored for many years.

The black swan is an Australian species introduced to Britain into private waterfowl collections. Many have escaped and joined mute swan populations in the wild and will occasionally turn up at rehabilitation centres.

EQUIPMENT AND TRANSPORT

Nets are generally too small for all but the youngest swans. The only real assistance, designed specifically for catching swans, is the 'swan hook'. This is like a shepherd's crook fitted to a long, extending handle. It is used to catch the swan's neck and pull the bird towards you. A swan's neck is particularly strong so if used briefly and sensibly the swan hook will not cause any injury. But by far the most effective aid for catching swans is a loaf or two of the ubiquitous sliced white bread.

Carrying boxes and cages are too small to accommodate a grown swan. Swans need their own specially designed swan bag. Made of sailcloth, the swan bag is like a conical tube with ties and handles (Fig. 15.1). Once the swan is slid head first into the wider opening, its head and neck are guided out of the smaller opening which will not allow the swan's shoulders through. With just the head and neck protruding from the bag the swan is incapable of movement or flapping its large wings.

A more simple swan bag can be made by cutting a 100 mm hole in the blind end of a sack (Fig. 15.2). Just like the purpose-made swan bag, the bird is slid head first into the sack and its head and neck guided out through the hole. Tying the sack closed

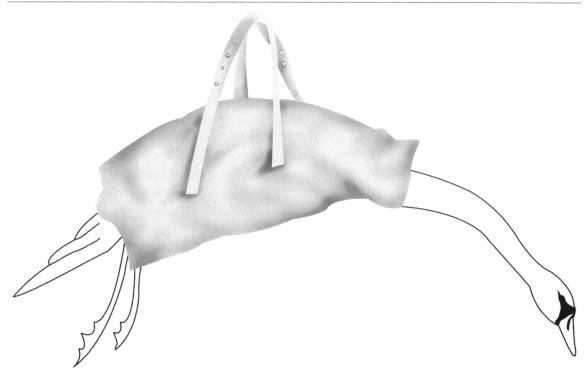

Fig. 15.1 Design for a swan carrying bag.

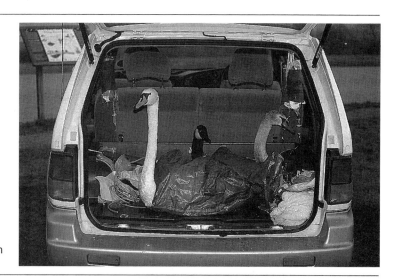

Fig. 15.2 Swans can be confined in converted sacks.

behind the swan also ensures that the swan cannot move.

Another innovation is to use a strong plastic shopping bag such as those available at Ikea stores for about £1.50. Eyelets are placed along the tops of both sides of the bag then, once the swan is sat in the bag, cord is threaded through the eyelets and across the swan. When this is tied only the head and neck will be exposed and the handles will make carrying the swan so much easier.

RESCUE AND HANDLING

Unlike ducks and geese, swans cannot take off vertically. To get airborne they need a considerable run-up whether they are taking off from water or from land. The need for a run-up often gives a rescuer that little bit of extra time needed to apprehend the swan.

By far the easiest way to catch a swan is to use sliced white bread. Scraps are thrown to the swan gradually tempting it nearer to the bank. It will probably come out of the water to pick up scraps thrown on the bank. When it is near, the rescuer simply grabs the bird's head and pulls the bird towards them.

The wings will be flapping and can be painful if they hit you, so the next priority is to grasp the swan's shoulders holding the wings folded to its body.

Once the swan is under control, put it on the ground and kneel astride it, keeping the wings firmly pinned to its body. Then it is comparatively simple to slide the swan bag over the bird and tie it securely.

Cygnets can be caught in a similar manner, although small ones can be caught in a large net. Be aware when catching cygnets that the adult birds will not hesitate to attack, using their wings as weapons.

The swan hook can be used for fully grown or adult swans who will not fall for the bread trick. The one drawback is that swans, like ducks and geese, have been driven away so often with anglers' rods and nets that they are often very wary of anything resembling a rod or a pole.

The swan hook really comes into its own when a swan can only be caught from a boat. Some swans, if compromised, will not venture anywhere near the bank. An inflatable dinghy with an outboard motor is then the only option if the bird must be caught. It takes two people, one to drive and steer while the other kneels in the prow with the swan hook extended and ready to catch the bird. Once the swan is hooked and pulled to the boat its wings must be controlled as it is picked out of the water and put in the bottom of the boat.

Handling swans is just a question of firmness and keeping their wings under control. Even without a swan bag the bird can be tucked under the arm which is held around the bird's shoulders. Generally swans do not bite, although occasionally one might try, but their bite is insignificant.

When a swan is being carried it will usually, if it can, hold its head straight out in front of it.

COMMON DISEASES

Botulism

Swans are susceptible to the usual range of bird diseases but, like other birds, do tend to be relatively free of disease. The only condition regularly seen is botulism in the summer. After a long, warm spell where water levels have dropped, swans will dabble in the exposed warm mud, an ideal breeding ground for the bacterium *Clostridium botulinum* (see Chapter 9).

The Swan Sanctuary at Egham has evolved its own regime for treating swans diagnosed as suffering from botulism (Goulden, 1995):

- 5-day antibiotic cover with a potentiated sulphonamide (Borgal – Hoechst Roussel Vet)
- 3-day administration of vitamin B_{12} as an appetite stimulant
- Intravenous infusion of Hartmann's solution laced with 10% Duphalyte (Fort Dodge Animal Health)
- Caution is needed with bowls of food and water as the weaker birds can easily drown
- A cool, quiet environment is needed
- Recovery can take several weeks

Bumblefoot

Swans are particularly heavy birds and place a great deal of pressure on the plantar region of the feet.

The epithelium can cope with this unless the swan spends time out of the water on hard surfaces like concrete. Then a corn can build up or the skin can be grazed allowing the ingress of pathogenic bacteria like *Escherichia coli*, *Staphyloccocus aureus* or *Proteus* species. Fibrous tissue builds up and as an abscess forms it becomes solidly encapsulated and hard to treat. Liquid and inspissated pus may be obvious under a scab. Before any treatments are started a swab for bacteriological testing should be taken.

Chronic bumblefoot can invade and erode bony tissues and can only really be treated by the veterinary surgeon removing all necrotic and caseous material. A prolonged treatment regime with systematic and local antibiotics can then be instigated to clear the infection. Initially first aid consists of placing a wad of surgical swabs under the foot over a non-stick or paraffin-tulle pad. The whole foot is then wrapped in a cohesive bandage (Co-Flex – Millpledge Pharmaceuticals) and then a waterproof covering to keep the dressing clean in the mess that any swan will make of a dry pen. Unfortunately the swan should not be allowed on to the water until the foot has completely healed.

In a captive situation the use of calf mats and artificial turf will help prevent bumblefoot forming on other swan inmates.

COMMON INCIDENTS

Lead poisoning

Swans have regularly been the victims of lead poisoning from anglers' weights. The incidences of this are now reduced but birds are still being found with the classic 'limberneck' where the swan cannot lift its head. Lead poisoning and its treatment were covered earlier (see Chapter 9).

Anglers' tackle

This is probably the most common cause of swans needing care with practically every swan on well-fished waters being taken into care at one time or the other. Like lead poisoning, the treatment of fishing tackle injuries was covered earlier (see Chapter 9).

Blocked oesophagus

A condition often detected in swans as a result of either lead poisoning, the ingestion of fishing line or plain, simple gorging on feed such as corn, is where the proventriculus and oesophagus is blocked solid. Eventually an affected swan will die, but usually they are seen getting weaker or somebody notices an unusual swelling in the neck. It is then that they are rescued and taken into care.

Sometimes if a blockage is suspected, opening the swan's beak may reveal a fetid smell from the food and vegetation rotting in the oesophagus. Radiographs may reveal the suspected blockage while the use of barium sulphate and an x-ray will show the extent of any mass or, in time, if any food or fluid is being passed through the gizzard.

A lubricated rubber stomach tube can also be used to measure the extent of the blockage.

Once the swan is stabilised with fluids the veterinary surgeon can calculate whether the blockage can be dissolved without any intrusive intervention.

Two options for treatment are available:

- The swan can be anaesthetised using propofol (Rapinovet – Schering-Plough Animal Health) by induction with an intravenous injection and then maintenance on isoflurane through an endotrachaeal tube. The swan is laid on its back on a sloping surgical table. Its head should be at the lowest point. A stomach tube is passed until it stops at the blockage. Warm water is then stomach pumped under pressure to loosen the debris.
- Surgery is the other option and may even be necessary after flushing if a mass of fishing line is still firmly embedded in the oesophagus. An endoscope could confirm its presence and may also be used to try to remove it.

All through the complete treatment of a swan with oesophageal obstruction the use of barium sulphate and radiographs will monitor any progress (Fig. 15.3).

Starvation and emaciation

Once a swan has been unable to feed for any length of time it will gorge itself at the first opportunity. If

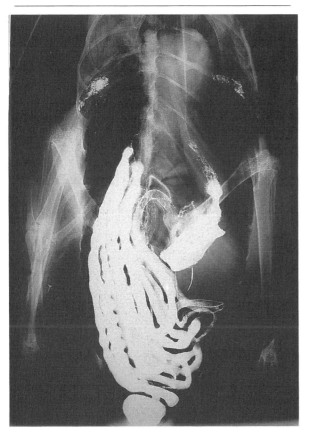

Fig. 15.3 How barium sulphate will highlight the status of a swan's digestive system.

the first meal is corn, or some other insoluble feed, it may well block its own crop and oesophagus with the quantity taken.

The safest way to feed a hungry swan is with dissolvable duck or chicken pellets offered in small amounts at regular intervals. Plenty of drinking water, as well, will make sure the feed is dissolved and digested.

Overhead wires

Other than casualties caused by fishing line, the incidences of swans flying into overhead cables are just as common in some parts of the country. At reservoirs near to Tring swans regularly fly into power lines in their panic to escape the fusillades of shotguns killing ducks and geese.

Injuries can be severe and include fractures of the legs and wings, major lacerations and burns, and damage to the face and neck. The fractures and abrasions usually respond to treatment but often massive lacerations or burns lead to necrosis of parts of the wing which then requires amputation or in severe cases humane destruction (Fig. 15.4).

Crash landing

Swans often mistake wet icy roads for safe landing sites on water. They will fly in and land often

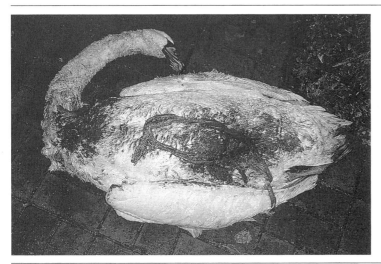

Fig. 15.4 A swan injured and burnt after colliding with electric power lines.

causing themselves injury; a swan's landing is always a heavy, half-controlled affair.

The rescue call is usually from the police because a swan is blocking the road and people or officers do not want to approach it. The swan can usually be caught easily with a swan hook or will run and take off giving the rescuer no chance to see if it was injured. Thankfully, apart from a few bruises, the only thing injured is usually the swan's pride.

Field swans

Calls will be received from the public reporting swans sitting in the middle of a field. 'They can't fly', is always the reason for the call. In fact swans often land in fields to graze. The response to the calls is to tell people who are really worried to approach with caution and ring back if the swan does not move off as they go near.

Rings

Swans often have rings put on their legs by the British Trust for Ornithology (BTO) and other researchers monitoring swan populations. The BTO rings are metal and engraved with the address of the British Museum. The other larger rings are 'Darvik' rings made from a sort of linoleum. They usually have just a consecutive number inlaid into them.

The rings can cause complications if there are any injuries to the swan's legs. In particular a fractured leg may swell and become constricted if the ring is left on. In particular, BTO rings have been known to become snagged and then slide up and into the hock joint (Plate 29). Similarly, Darvik rings can become brittle, break and cut into the swan's leg.

If there is a possible danger from the rings, they should be cut off.

ADMISSION AND FIRST AID

Upon admission, any swan casualty should be put on to an intravenous drip infused through the medial tarsal vein using a $22\,g \times 300\,mm$ over-the-needle type catheter. If there is a problem inserting the catheter then a $21\,g$ or $23\,g$ butterfly infusion set might be more suitable.

Long-acting amoxycillin at $250\,mg/kg$ intramuscularly should be provided and $1\,ml$ of vitamin B_{12} given as a boost to the appetite.

The swan's nostrils, choana and eyes should be checked for leeches. These can be removed with forceps or by flushing with fresh water.

Because fishing tackle is such a hazard to swans, each new admission should be x-rayed to see if there is an underlying problem of a hook, blockage or lead shot. Swans can be easily x-rayed conscious by using tape or small sand bags to hold them in position. Three dorso-ventral x-rays are needed:

(1) Covering the gizzard forward to the top of the sternum
(2) Covering the upper torso and most of the neck
(3) Including the rest of the neck and head

CAGING

Swans are enormous, messy birds that are far too large to be held in normal cages. In many cases they can be given a whole room to themselves. Calf mats should always be provided to protect the swan's feet as these can be easily hosed down and cleaned.

However, rescue centres that take in quite a few swans have to make other arrangements to accommodate them.

The Wildlife Hospital Trust (St Tiggywinkles) has a separate swan intensive care facility that is fully tiled and drained so that it can be easily washed and hosed down (Fig. 15.5). Individual swan pens are used that are easily accessible and also easily washed and hosed down. These give each swan an area of $1.0\,m \times 1.2\,m$ while it is in intensive care. The pens are made from components manufactured for materials handling in warehouses (Fig. 15.6). This also makes them easy to move or store outside if they are empty.

Even if regularly cleaned, swans out of water soon become soiled and lose feather condition. It is imperative to get them on to water as soon as possible. Large pools that are easily cleaned are ideal, especially if they also have access to short grass where they can graze.

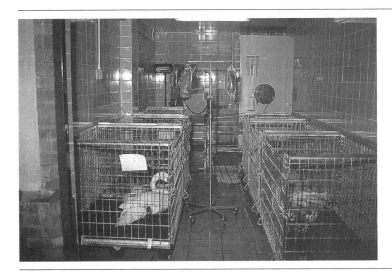

Fig. 15.5 An easily cleaned swan intensive care facility.

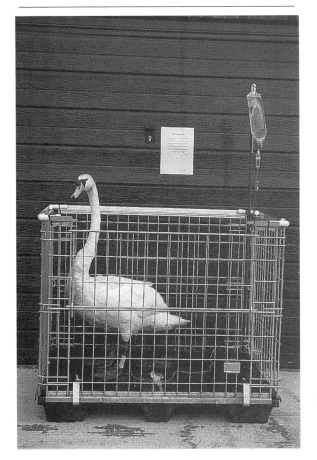

Fig. 15.6 A swan pen made from materials handling equipment.

FEEDING

Many swans, especially cygnets, are used to taking bread from the general public. In care many of them do not seem to recognise other foods and will take only bread. To offer it, break it into small pieces and float it on a bowl of water.

Gradually they can be weaned on to lettuce or cabbage in the water and then on to mixed corn. Once they recognise corn, it and pelleted food can be offered dry next to a clean bowl of water. Swans like to dabble each mouthful of dry food in water before they swallow it.

Large grit should always be available and could be mixed with feed for swans recovering from lead poisoning.

The initial 1 ml of B_{12} they receive at triage should be repeated weekly to improve their appetites and general well-being.

If it is possible, swans should have the facility to graze on short grass before they are released.

RELEASE

Swans must be waterproof before they are released.

One of a pair or a cygnet from a family group should be taken back to its original territory. Other swans with no history of a family should only be released where there are no other swans or, alternatively, where large flocks of mixed adult and young swans are forming.

LEGAL IMPLICATIONS

All swans are protected under the Wildlife and Countryside Act 1981.

However, mute swans in the Thames basin between London Bridge and Henley-on-Thames are seen as Crown property. Hence any offences against these swans may be prosecuted as offending against the Crown.

16
Geese and Other Water Birds

Species seen regularly:
- **Geese** – Canada goose (*Branta canadensis*), greylag goose (*Anser anser*), Brent goose (*Branta bernicla*) and Barnacle goose (*Branta leucopsis*).

- **Other water birds** – Moorhen (*Gallinula chloropus*), coot (*Fulica atra*), grebes (*Podiceps* sp.), herons (*Ardea cinerea*) and bitterns (*Botaurus stellaris*), and water rail (*Rallus aquaticus*).

Part I: Geese

NATURAL HISTORY

Only the greylag goose and the Canada goose are ordinarily resident in Great Britain. However, these have either been introduced or have escaped from collections. Similarly, the Egyptian goose (*Alopochen aegyptiacus*) is another introduced species but is not nearly as widespread. The other goose species are winter visitors who migrate to the high Arctic in summer to nest and rear their young.

Geese feed mainly on grass and aquatic vegetation and can often be seen, in winter, in large flocks feeding on farmland.

In the London parks the Canada goose has now become abundant and, being of an aggressive nature, is said to be displacing other water birds. All manner of control methods are being tried ranging from shooting to pricking the eggs of any nest found. The Canada goose is the most regular visitor to rescue centres but other species may turn up, especially those vagrants from parks or collections.

EQUIPMENT AND TRANSPORT

Would be similar to that recommended for swans.

RESCUE AND HANDLING

Would be similar to that recommended for swans, except that geese can take off instantly. They can often be caught using a large net.

COMMON DISEASES

Like swans, geese seen in care very rarely show symptoms of disease except botulism.

However, there is a range of epizootics that can affect geese: goose virus hepatitis, goose influenza and goose plague. The author has never recorded any of these in our localised intake of casualties.

COMMON INCIDENTS

Fishing line and flying into power lines place geese in the same hazardous existence as swans. Geese, however, have the added hazard in that they are regularly targets of organised shooting with shotguns (Fig. 16.1). Radiographs will, for instance, show practically every Canada goose to have pellets embedded somewhere in its body.

COMMON INJURIES

Most commonly seen are fractures caused by gunshot. The trouble is that often the bird was

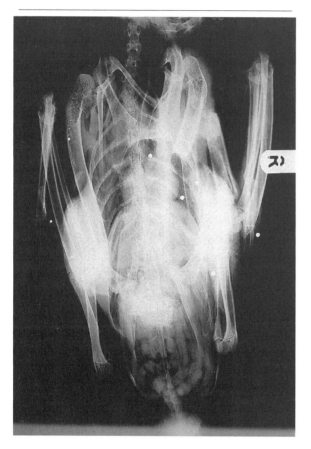

Fig. 16.1 Geese are often the victims of shotguns. This greylag goose has suffered fractures of the humerus.

injured long before it was spotted, caught and taken into care. Many of these fractures will have healed in the wrong place. Unless the veterinary surgeon thinks that osteotomy is possible, the bird will never be fit enough for release.

Broken legs if they heal are fine but if they do not or are already fused incorrectly then the goose will not be able to cope with one functional leg. These birds should be humanely destroyed.

Broken beaks have been repaired with a mixture of healing and inventive metalwork (see Chapter 14, the chapter on ducks).

TRIAGE AND FIRST AID

Standard triage protocol is all that is needed. A radiograph study at this stage should only be

arranged if there is a distinct possibility that a fishing hook or tackle has been ingested.

CAGING

Geese can be kept singly in large cages. The open pens we use for swans are not suitable as geese can usually get out of them.

The same provisions as arranged for swans should also apply to geese. Namely calf mats, artificial turf and access to swimming as soon as possible.

FEEDING

Similar food to that provided for swans is adequate and especially access to short grass for grazing will help bring a goose to a condition suitable for release.

RELEASE

Geese should be released where they were found. However, reference to the legal implications may prohibit the release, in this country, of many species.

Migrant geese should only be released when their species are in this country. This will generally be during the winter months.

LEGAL IMPLICATIONS

Schedule 9 of the Wildlife and Countryside Act 1981 prohibits the release or escape of some non-indigenous species. Geese on the list are: Canada goose, Egyptian goose (*Alopochen aegyptiacus*), and any other species that are not regarded as on the British list.

Part II: Other Water Birds

Coots and moorhens

NATURAL HISTORY

Coots and moorhens are widespread on waterways all over Britain. The coot, with the bold white flash at the base of its bill, is a bird of open water on lakes and reservoirs. The moorhen, with the red and yellow bill, is far more secretive and skulks in the bankside vegetation of small rivers and canals.

Both birds eat a variety of aquatic plants and some animal material. The moorhen will often leave the water to feed in neighbouring fields.

EQUIPMENT AND TRANSPORT

The usual bird-catching nets and standard carrying boxes are all that is needed to catch and transport either of these birds.

RESCUE AND HANDLING

On the water, rescue of coots and moorhens would follow the same procedures as for ducks. The moorhen, however, is quite capable of diving and walking along the bottom until it is out of sight by a bank. It can also sit partially submerged keeping one step ahead of your every move.

Most moorhen rescues are out of the water giving a better chance of catching an injured bird.

Handling each bird is different:

- The *coot* will scratch with its powerful feet which should be kept wrapped in a towel
- The *moorhen* squirts evil-smelling excrement with some force out of its cloaca. To prevent being splattered always hold a moorhen with its rear pointing away from you.

COMMON DISEASES

Apart from individual diagnoses, coots and moorhens seem to be relatively disease free.

COMMON INCIDENTS

Fishing line affects both species (see Chapter 9). Other than that coots are relatively accident free whereas moorhens in their more wandering life-style do get hit on the roads.

COMMON INJURIES

The moorhen regularly suffers from fishing line injuries. Apart from that it is very often found on the road with a fractured tibiotarsus. Most road casualties need treating for this injury. In our experience moorhens cannot cope with just one leg.

ADMISSION AND FIRST AID

A standard admittance protocol is all that is needed for these birds.

CAGING

Standard, fairly large cages with newspaper on the floor are suitable for both species. The moorhen, however, is extremely nervous and should have the front of its cage covered with a towel.

FEEDING

Both birds will take corn and growers' pellets. The moorhen will appreciate regular supplies of live food like clean maggots, mealworms or waxworms.

RELEASE

Both birds should be released back to where they were found.

LEGAL IMPLICATIONS

The usual bird protection legislation and animal cruelty legislation applies to both birds.

Grebes

Species usually seen:
Great crested grebe (*Podiceps cristatus*) and little grebe (dabchick) (*Tachybaptus ruficollis*).

Rarely:
Red-necked grebe (*P. griseigena*), Slavonian grebe (*P. auritus*) and black-necked grebe (*P. nigricollis*) who are winter visitors.

NATURAL HISTORY

The great crested grebe and the little grebe are the two grebes most likely to be encountered. The larger of the two, the great crested grebe, is a bird of open waters, like lakes and reservoirs. It dives for small fish. The little grebe, or dabchick, is more sensitive and keeps to the bankside of open water, It can also be found on small rivers and canals. It dives for small fish but in the summer it will take a lot of insects and crustaceans from the water.

The legs and feet of grebes are designed for fast diving and swimming. Their legs are flattened laterally and their feet have lobes along the toes for propulsion. Because their legs are set so far back on the body, grebes find it hard to walk on land and impossible to take off when they are not on water (Fig. 16.2).

EQUIPMENT AND TRANSPORT

Standard bird catching nets and cat carrying boxes are ideal for grebes. Boxes should have a folded towel at the bottom to protect the bird's keel.

Baskets are not suitable for the larger grebes as they will constantly stab at the wire sides and cause damage to their beaks.

RESCUE AND HANDLING

It is hard to catch a grebe on the water. It will automatically dive and re-surface some distance away.

Driving the bird into shallow, clean water is sometimes successful if it is possible to see which way they are going so that they can be caught underwater with a net.

On land they cannot move very well and are easily picked up.

The larger grebes should be handled with stout gloves as they do not hesitate to stab with their pointed beaks. The great crested grebe is particularly aggressive (Fig. 16.3).

COMMON DISEASES

Grebes are not usually presented for rehabilitation through disease. Like all birds, they are reasonably disease resistant.

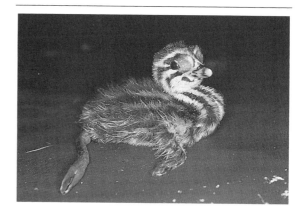

Fig. 16.2 Grebes find it hard to walk on dry land.

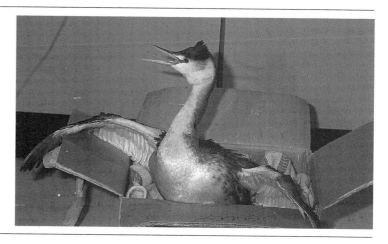

Fig. 16.3 The great crested grebe is particularly aggressive.

COMMON INCIDENTS

Apart from fishing line problems, the usual rescue is of a grebe that has landed in the wrong place. It cannot take off from land. All that is necessary, if there are no signs of injury, is to take the bird to the nearest suitable watercourse and release it.

Preening

Grebes in captivity for any length of time may develop a blockage in the alimentary system. The reason is that when they preen they actually swallow any small feathers that come out. These, in time, will cause a blockage in the gizzard. Liquid paraffin given by gavage should alleviate any problems.

COMMON INJURIES

Grebes, apart from those with fishing line problems, are not usually found injured.

ADMISSION AND FIRST AID

Most grebes can be turned round and released immediately. Any that are injured should receive the standard first-aid measures.

Migratory grebes, red-necked, Slavonian and black-necked, should be started on a prophylactic course of itraconazole (see 'Aspergillosis' in Chapter 9).

CAGING

Grebes should be kept on water for as long as possible. Out of water their keel will become damaged and infected, sometimes leading to euthanasia as the only option.

Thick foam rubber should be used under the birds when they are in cages and this should be cleaned or changed every few hours.

For swimming and feeding of little grebes, fibre-glass garden pools are ideal because they usually have ledges on to which the birds can pull themselves out, especially if they are not fully waterproof.

A bird in for care should not be left swimming when it is not being monitored, especially overnight.

FEEDING

The larger grebe will take whitebait out of a shallow bowl of water.

Presentation of fish feed

Any fish will deteriorate rapidly unless frozen or kept under cold running water. When feeding birds on fish, the birds will reject the fish if it is warm. Our procedures with fish are as follows:

- A few fish are removed from the freezer.
- These are put into a shallow dish or bowl and put into a refrigerator to thaw.
- When the fish are just defrosted they are offered to the bird.
- After 30 minutes any uneaten fish are taken out and disposed of. Any fish that appear to have deteriorated are discarded.

In addition a thiamine supplement is fed to the bird (e.g. a Fish Eaters Tablet – Mazuri Zoo Foods).

Little grebes may take whitebait dropped singly into clean water when swimming. They can be persuaded to dive and take the fish.

RELEASE

Release of grebes should be to suitable water; great crested to open lakes and reservoirs, and little grebes to small rivers or canals with plenty of bankside cover.

Migratory grebes should only be released during the winter when they are normally resident in an area.

LEGAL IMPLICATIONS

Grebes are legally covered by the bird protection legislation of the Wildlife Countryside Act 1981 and the usual animal protection laws.

Herons and bitterns

Species usually seen:
Grey heron and, the very rare, bittern.

Exotic species:
Night heron and little egret.

NATURAL HISTORY

All these heron-like birds feed mainly on fish, although they will take small mammals, birds, reptiles and amphibians.

The grey heron is reasonably common and nests communally in long-established heronries at the top of clumps of tall trees. It feeds on most water-courses and will raid gardens to take fish from garden pools.

The bittern is one of Britain's most endangered birds bordering on extinction in this country. It is a bird of the reed beds where its 'boom' is an easily recognised call.

The little egret is somehow starting to colonise Britain. There are already small groups on some of the estuaries in Devon and Cornwall.

EQUIPMENT AND HANDLING

A non-flying heron is comparatively easy to out run and net. However, a heron that can fly will often evade capture. This can be so frustrating when a heron is seen with a broken leg dangling uselessly and it cannot be caught.

Handling is rather like grappling with a noisy octopus – both legs, both wings, neck and beak all over the place. The most important part of a heron to control is its beak. This can be a lethal dagger which the heron will not hesitate to aim at the face and eyes (Plate 30).

With a heron, always hold the head first and then tuck the harmless wings and legs all under one arm. Then covering the bird's head, while still holding on to it, will tend to quieten it.

COMMON DISEASES

Herons taken into care tend to be trauma cases rather than cases of disease.

COMMON INCIDENTS

Of course, as usual, herons suffer from fishing line accidents and because of their gangling disposition often get tangled into line on bankside trees and bushes.

Similarly, they will often get tangled in the nets people put over their garden ponds to keep herons at bay.

Other incidents include flying into overhead lines and after a prolonged cold spell many are picked up starving and emaciated.

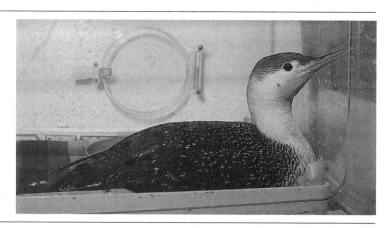

Fig. 16.4 A red-throated diver cannot move on dry land.

COMMON INJURIES

Apart from fishing line injuries, other trauma seems to result in fractures of the long bones of the legs and wings.

ADMISSION AND FIRST AID

Herons can usually be provided with intravenous therapy and, if emaciated, can also benefit from peripheral nutrition or gavaging liquid nutrition (see Chapter 3).

Other first aid includes stabilising fractures that otherwise would be further displaced by the bird flapping and running about.

CAGING

A heron in care should be kept, initially, in a cage where it can stand up. As soon as possible it should be put into an aviary where it can spread and exercise its wings before release.

FEEDING

Initially herons will take fish such as sprats and herrings. They can, however, soon be weaned on to day-old chicks which are more convenient to use.

A reluctant feeder may be encouraged to feed if it can see another heron tucking into its chicks.

Force feeding is possible with whole fish or chicks but herons are one of those species that can easily regurgitate if they become distressed.

Also gavaging with liquidised food or Poly-Aid (Vetafarm Europe) can be useful if the bird keeps it down.

RELEASE

Because herons live and nest in specific areas, it is important to release any back to the nearest watercourse to where they were found.

Herons with one leg or one eye should not be released. A disabled heron will live quite comfortably on an enclosed lake or pool.

LEGAL IMPLICATIONS

Apart from standard animal legislation the only regulation is to prevent the release or escape of night herons under Schedule 9 of the Wildlife and Countryside Act 1981.

Little egrets have no specific legislation so can apparently be considered as any other wild bird.

Other species of water bird

WATER RAIL

Water rails are not uncommon rehabilitation candidates. They can be treated as if they were moorhens.

DIVERS

There are three species of diver on the British list:

- The red-throated diver (*Gavia stellata*)
- The black-throated diver (*Gavia arctica*)
- The great northern diver (*Gavia immer*)

Not unlike large grebes, they are even more specialised for swimming and diving and cannot move at all on land (Fig. 16.4). They sometimes crash land a long way from the sea and cannot take off again.

Divers are a nightmare in captivity and even specialist centres in America can only strive for a 50% success rate.

The major problems are damage to their keels and aspergillosis. Prophylaxis with itraconazole might control aspergillosis. The keel may be protected by foam rubber or air cushions but even that is unlikely to prevent keel damage. If the bird is kept for any length of time it will deteriorate rapidly and euthanasia will have to be applied.

The secret with divers is to get them on to the sea with no delay whatsoever.

In captivity divers will take thawed frozen fish such as sprats, herring or sand eels coupled with a thiamine supplement.

17
Birds of Prey

Part I: Owls

Species seen regularly:
Tawny owl (*Strix aluco*), little owl (*Athene noctua*), barn owl (*Tyto alba*), long-eared owl (*Asio otus*) and short-eared owl (*Asio flammeus*).

Possible escapees:
Eagle owl (*Bubo* spp.) and snowy owl (*Nyctea scandiaca*).

NATURAL HISTORY

Owls are predominantly nocturnal, mainly feeding by catching small mammals in their razor-sharp talons. Although their eyesight is very good in low light levels the unique asymmetry of their ears enables them to locate prey even in full darkness. An owl's ears are set at different levels on each side of its head. They can be found under the feathers as two large scrupulously clean orifices one level with the eyes and the other a little lower. The 'long-ears' and 'short-ears' which describe the two owls of the genus *Asio* are in fact only feather tufts on top of the head.

The short-eared owl and the little owl will also hunt during the day. The little owl diet consists mainly of invertebrates like beetles and earthworms.

Owls, like other birds, cannot move the eyes in their sockets, but they do have the ability to turn their heads through 180°. This probably assists in locating their prey without having to move their bodies.

The tawny owl is the commonest of the owls and the species most likely to be presented for rescue.

EQUIPMENT AND TRANSPORT

Owls can be caught with nets and carried in pet carrying boxes but with a major difference to other birds. To safely handle owls a pair of thick gloves is essential. Welders' gloves or motorcyclist gloves are ideal.

The carrying box should include an old towel which can double as a base for an owl to stand on or as an object it can sink its talons into.

RESCUE AND HANDLING

An owl that needs rescuing is not going to be as evasive as some of the brighter birds like crows and magpies. A large net is the best and safest way to catch an owl. The mesh of a net will not damage the fine soft feathers essential so an owl can fly silently over its prey.

Once it is caught the owl will probably attack with its talons. Often a bird of prey will throw itself on to its back and strike upwards. Without stout gloves the razor-sharp talons can easily penetrate the skin in a vice-like grip. Either the gloves or the towels from the box should be offered to the bird who will hold them securely.

At all times remember that the owl is concentrating on attacking you so do not let it go until it is safely in the carrying box.

Owls do have hooked beaks but like other birds of prey most will not attempt to bite. However, some do bite so be aware that it can happen and keep your hands, arms and face away from the bird. Pick up the owl by holding its two legs in one gloved hand and its shoulders in the other to stop it flapping its wings. In fact tawny owls will often become trancelike if they are laid on their backs; but still keep a hold on the legs.

Back at the care facility the stout gloves should always be used for handling conscious birds of prey. Even the smallest, the little owl or the hobby, can still inflict painful wounds with their talons.

COMMON DISEASES

Trichomoniasis

Tawny owls have been recorded as showing the typical lesions of trichomoniasis (see Plate 19). This was always assumed to be the result of eating infected pigeons or collared doves taken from their nests. Sparrowhawks also contract trichomoniasis and have been reportedly taken off the nest by tawny owls.

Coles (1997) reported that the necrotic foci in the oropharanx may in fact be lesions of owl herpes virus (infectious hepatosplenitis). The veterinary surgeon may be able to confirm one or the other but treatment for trichomoniasis it still called for as this can be a secondary invader. Trichomoniasis is discussed more fully in Chapter 9.

Parasites

Capillaria worms are often visible at the back of the throat. Treatment is with ivermectin (Ivomec Injection for Cattle – Merial Animal Health) at 200 micrograms/kg (or 0.2 ml/kg when mixed 1 : 9 with propylene glycol). This can be given subcutaneously or orally.

Syngamus trachea is the most likely species of gapeworm seen in birds of prey.

These are two specific nematodes. No doubt owls will be carrying a whole range of species but, unless the veterinary surgeon prescribes some other method of control, the ivermectin should be effective against most species.

COMMON INCIDENTS

Road traffic accidents

All the species of British owls are regularly the victims of road traffic accidents. Cooper (1993)

reported that 44.7% of barn owl deaths could be attributed to vehicle collisions.

The vast majority of adult casualty owls seen at The Wildlife Hospital Trust (St Tiggywinkles) are road traffic victims.

Fencing accidents

Tawny owls and little owls are fairly regularly caught on barbed wire fences. Usually there are major lacerations to the underside of one wing. It is often not possible to suture the tears but applications of Intrasite Gel (Smith & Nephew) will encourage granulation.

Orphans

There appear to be more orphaned tawny owls than any other species of bird of prey. Often a young tawny owl is found walking around or lying in a wood. The parent birds are not going to support the youngster in this situation and it will starve if not rescued.

The ideal remedy would be to put the youngster back into its nest, usually a hole in a tree. However, it is not usually possible to trace the nest and even if it were possible there may be legal implications of approaching a wild bird's active nest (Wildlife and Countryside Act 1981). These potential orphans should not be left alone but should be taken into care (see Chapter 19).

Barn owls

Barn owls will arrive at a rescue centre for usually two reasons: either they have been in a collision or else they are starving.

Over the years there have been many misguided attempts to boost the British population of barn owls by breeding them in captivity and then releasing them. It was found that many of these captive-bred barn owls could not cope with a wild existence and many of them starved.

There is now legislation to control the release of barn owls but starving barn owls still do turn up. True it may be a truly wild barn owl but some signs will establish whether it is or not. Any one of these tell-tale signs will point to a captive-bred bird:

- If the bird is comfortable in the presence of humans
- If it has a closed ring (a solid circle rather than a split British Museum ring) on either leg
- If it recognises and readily takes day-old chicks

Emaciation

Barn owls and the juveniles of other birds of prey can be found starving. The breast muscles of any bird can be felt round and plump on either side of the keel (sternum). A hungry bird will lose these muscles so that the keel can be clearly felt as being very prominently sharp without any muscle mass on either side of it.

First aid and treatment of emaciation

The automatic reaction on the presentation of a starving bird is to feed it as much food as possible. However, because the digestive tract has been empty for some time it will have shut down. Any solid food given at this time would remain undigested in the gut leading to an overgrowth of bacteria and a build-up of toxins. This would eventually kill an already weakened bird.

The course of action could be (Neff, 1997):

(1) Assume the bird is 10% dehydrated and provide warmed replacement and maintenance fluids over 2 days (see Chapter 4), i.e. day one: 50% of the deficit plus 50 ml/kg maintenance.
(2) Provide iron dextran at 10 mg/kg intramuscularly weekly for 2 weeks.
(3) Provide B vitamins at 10 mg/kg thiamine content subcutaneously weekly for 2 weeks.
(4) Enrofloxacin (Baytril – Bayer) at 15 mg/kg twice daily for 2 weeks in a 2-days intramuscular/3-days oral programme to protect the muscles from needle trauma.
(5) After 24 hours of fluids then liquid nutrition can be provided either orally with Poly-Aid (Vetafarm Europe) or Ensure (Abbott Laboratories) or intraosseously with Nutriflex Lipid Peri (B Braun Medical).
(6) Once the bird's digestive system stabilises and normal droppings are formed it can be offered chopped mice, about 2–4 pieces for a barn owl. These should be sprinkled with a multivitamin

powder (Vetamin & Zinc – Millpledge Phamaceuticals) and a calcium/phosphorus supplement such as Stress (Philips Yeast Products).
(7) Continue gavaging liquid feed for 2 days in the mornings and afternoon and give chopped mice in the evenings.
(8) For 2 days gavage in the mornings, with chopped mice in the afternoons and evenings.
(9) For two more days feed all three meals of chopped mice.
(10) Resume normal feeding but crush all the bones in the mice.
(11) Leave the mice intact but split open for a week.
(12) Feed as normal healthy bird.

COMMON INJURIES

Apart from the lacerations inflicted by barbed wire fences, most injuries seen with owls are the result of road traffic accidents. Injuries seen include fractures and eye injuries.

Fractures

Fractures of the long bones of the wings and legs are common, as is head trauma normally recognisable by the variation in openness of each eye, by head tilt, unconsciousness or, of course, clinical history. Refer to the head trauma section in Chapter 9 for the emergency protocol.

It is absolutely essential that any bird of prey must be 100% fit to be released. Their legs have to be perfect and coordinated in order to catch prey. Their wings, down to the smallest feathers on the alula, have to be absolutely symmetrical or else the finer movements, needed by a hunting bird, would not be available. Without perfection the bird would quickly starve.

Similarly any ankylosis of any joint would condemn a bird of prey to starvation. Any bird of prey with a deviation in the symmetry of its wings or stiffness of a joint must not be released.

Eye injuries

Boydell (1997) examined 615 rescued owls and found that 189 (30.7%) had some form of ocular lesion. Many owls do appear to have suffered eye trauma of one form or another and many may actually be blind in one eye.

It is commonly assumed that an owl with only one eye can be released and will adequately cope in the wild. There are no records of a totally blind owl surviving but totally blind owls in captivity seem to spend a life of feeling around with the vibrissae and feet, a completely inappropriate lifestyle.

All eye injuries and eye disease, in fact all eye questions, must be the province of the veterinary surgeon. If any eye has to be removed then note should be taken that an owl has bony rings (scleral ossicles) supporting the eye in the orbit and these should be preserved to maintain the contours of the face.

At triage and first aid an injured eye may have a smear of chloramphenicol eye ointment put along the lower lid. Eye ointments with steroids should not be used at this stage.

ADMISSION AND FIRST AID

Owls, at triage, will benefit from the standard intraosseous fluid infusion coupled with antibiotic cover and, if necessary, corticosteroids.

Talons

If the bird is likely to be in care for some weeks, it is a good preventative measure to just clip the tip of both hind talons. This will prevent either of them puncturing the epithelia of the bottoms of the feet and causing bumblefoot infection.

An owl should not be released with clipped talons. It must be maintained in captivity until they grow back to their original lethal sharpness.

Caging

In intensive care owls can be best maintained in a typical veterinary cat kennel with at least one thick perch to keep the birds clear of the floor. The floor can be covered with newspaper.

Perches can be made easily from scraps of wood that can be discarded and replaced when they are no longer able to be cleaned. A straight stout branch about 30–40 mm thick is cut to the width of the cage. It is then drilled and screwed to two cubes of wood 100 mm square by 60 mm high. This can be

scrubbed easily and kept scrupulously clean to avoid any chance of pathogens getting into the feet of the birds (Fig. 17.1).

Once their treatment has run its course owls should be put outside in skylight aviaries to exercise and acclimatise for release. A skylight aviary has no wire mesh where the bird can climb up and damage its feathers. If it cannot fly, the perches, which should be natural branches, can be arranged to provide a ladder to the highest perch.

The aviary by choice should be 8 m × 4 m × 2 m high. At 2 m high planning consent is not necessary. The framework should be fairly substantial, 100 mm × 50 mm tannalised timber covered on all sides by feather-edge timber laid vertically. The top should be covered with 50 mm wire mesh.

A hinged opening at the top of one end will allow for hacking back (see under 'Release' below)

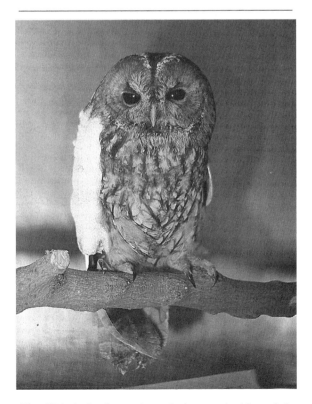

Fig. 17.1 A simple perch made from a stout branch is ideal for many birds.

if the owls are to be released in that area. A peephole at one end or closed circuit television will allow monitoring of the bird's flying expertise without disturbing them.

The addition of baffle barriers down each side of the aviary makes sure that the bird has to fly much further and has to negotiate corners (Fig. 17.2). All this will add to the strength of the flight muscles and the dexterity of those minor wing movements necessary for a change of direction. In fact if the heights of the perches vary, the act of flying upwards to a perch adds even more strength to those vital muscles of flight.

FEEDING

Owls, just like all carnivores, feed not just on meat but on whole animals. In captivity it is crucial that they receive the bone and fur or feather with their meat in order that they can produce pellets which are the indigestible parts of the food animal regurgitated up at regular intervals.

Day-old chicks with a vitamin and mineral supplement added, are easy to obtain frozen. They can be defrosted as needed.

When a wild owl is taken into care it will have no idea what a day-old chick is. It will have been used to eating small mammals and, at first, will only accept similar food. Frozen mice are obtainable but it is no good offering wild birds white mice. They will not recognise these either. When buying frozen mice, always buy dark mice which will be readily accepted by most new patients. After a few days settling in, the owl can be weaned on to day-old chicks, which are a lot cheaper.

Road killed animals that are fresh and unpolluted will also supplement feeding of larger owls like snowy or eagle owls if they are taken in.

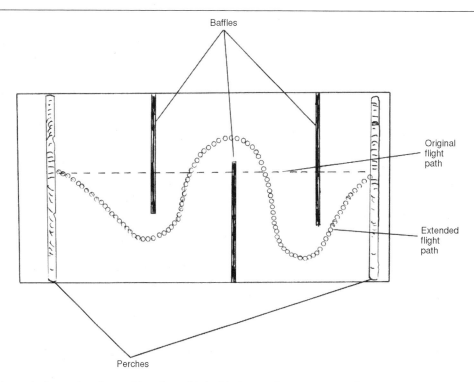

Fig. 17.2 Layout of an aviary to provide a large bird with the maximum amount of exercise.

RELEASE

The life of a hunting bird is never easy. For every prey animal it manages to catch many more will have eluded those lethal talons.

When a bird of prey has been seen to exercise without distress in a skylight aviary it may be considered fit to release. However, there is no guarantee that it is going to survive those first tremulous days of freedom. An attempt to provide for the initial release is to 'hack' the bird back to the wild. What this in fact means is that food is made available for some days after release in the hope that the bird realises it is there.

The bird should be fine. It has been able to exercise from dusk till dawn in its aviary and will have gained enough muscle to face the rigours of flying.

Much is said about using falconry techniques to bring a bird to fitness. The author sees many drawbacks to this theory:

(1) The bird is handled frequently and may become too used to humans.
(2) The amount of exercise it can be given is minimal compared with the exercise it could get in a long aviary.
(3) Many birds escape with jesses still attached to their legs. These are death traps to a free-living bird and can snag on branches or fences.
(4) Most owls do not relish flying during daylight hours.

If the bird is to be released in the vicinity of the aviary it should be fed regularly on a platform level on the inside, with the release flap high at one end. Then as it is fed on the evening it is to be released the release flap should be opened as the food is put on the platform. The flap is then left open and, as before, food continues to be put on to the platform. The bird may or may not avail itself of the food but can return if it fails to kill. The food should continue to be put out until the bird has definitely left the area.

With a territorial species it is preferable that it is returned to where it was found. A similar method of release should be adopted but with a hack box rather than an aviary. All this is really is a scaled down version of the aviary being made portable to the release site.

Barn owls used to be released in wired over barns where a nest box was provided for a pair of owls. They were fed on a hack platform. Barn owls readily breed in captivity and so as soon as they had dependent young the release flap was opened relying on the parental bond to keep the adults returning to feed their off-spring. It is now illegal to release captive bred owls unless a licence is first obtained from the Department of the Environment, Transport and the Regions.

LEGAL IMPLICATIONS

Apart from the usual bird protection laws, there is specific legislation relating to barn owls. They are now included on Schedule 9 of the Wildlife and Countryside Act 1981 and cannot be released without a licence.

But barn owls do still turn up at rescue centres. In order to make sure that genuine wild barn owls were not kept in captivity the, now obsolete, Licensed Rehabilitation Keeper could release any casualties that were truly wild. The Licensed Rehabilitation Keeper is now replaced with a Licensed Person under Licence No. WLF 100099. Presumably the same safeguards for wild barn owls still apply.

As usual it is an offence to release a species not usually resident in Britain. This certainly applies to eagle owls but as there are snowy owls resident on Fetlar in the Shetlands the provision probably does not apply. However, it would be foolish to release any snowy owl other than the very occasional, genuine wild casualty.

Part II: Diurnal Birds of Prey

Species seen regularly:
Kestrel (*Falco tinnunculus*), sparrowhawk (*Accipiter nisus*), buzzard (*Buteo buteo*), hobby (*Falco subbuteo*), merlin (*Falco columbarius*) and peregrine falcon (*Falco peregrinus*).

Other species:
Red kite (*Milvus milvus*), harriers (*Circus* spp.), goshawk (*Accipiter gentilis*), eagle (*Aquila chrysaetos*) and osprey (*Pandion haliaetus*).

NATURAL HISTORY

The diurnal birds of prey hunt or scavenge for their food during the hours of daylight. They, like the corvids, have evolved into their own niches of the environment and tend not to compete with another species in its area of hunting:

- The *kestrel* hovers while hunting for small mammals and the occasional bird in open areas especially along roads and motorways.
- The *sparrowhawk* hunts birds, up to the size of a wood pigeon, by fast acrobatic flying in wood edges and hedgerows. It will also hunt over garden bird tables.
- The *buzzard*, at the moment plentiful in the West Country, Wales, Scotland and the North, is a large bird that will hunt large mammals like rabbits but it will also scavenge road kills and follow the plough for any invertebrates turned up.
- The *hobby* is a true migrant that hunts birds, mainly swallows and martins. It follows these hirundines to Britain in the summer and to South Africa for the winter. It will also hawk insects like dragonflies.
- The *merlin* is now very scarce and confined to the high moorland of Wales, Scotland and Northern England.
- The *peregrine* is said to be the fastest of all birds. It is a bird of the mountains, moors and sea cliffs where it will stoop from a great height at breakneck speed on to larger birds like wood pigeons.
- The *red kite* is still resident in Wales and the subject of a re-introduction programme by English Nature in England. It is slowly getting established in some parts of Britain where it can be seen majestically riding on air currents. It is purely a scavenger feeding especially on road kills and rubbish dumps.
- *Harriers*, *goshawks* and *eagles* are birds of the remotest areas and are not likely to need rescue and care.
- *Ospreys* are very specialised fish eaters and as yet have not been presented for rehabilitation in this country, as far as the author is aware. There is a wealth of experience in America if one should fall sick or injured.

EQUIPMENT AND TRANSPORT

Very similar equipment to that needed for owls is suitable for most diurnal birds of prey. However, if eagles, goshawks and ospreys are involved then much thicker gloves and larger carrying boxes are essential.

RESCUE AND HANDLING

Once again similar to that required for owls but sometimes some of these birds are escapees. These may often respond to a day-old chick being waved in the air.

Extreme care is needed in handling these birds, especially the larger ones. It is said that a strong man cannot dislodge the murderous grip of a goshawk. Hold the legs of all these birds so that they do not get the opportunity to cause any injury.

Sparrowhawks, goshawks and ospreys are particularly nervous and fare better if their heads are covered and they are carried in darkened boxes.

COMMON DISEASES

Naturally these birds are resistant to disease but in a rescue situation the usual conditions seen can include:

- Syngamiasis in all species
- Trichomoniasis in sparrowhawks, red kites
- Helminth parasites in all species
- Avian pox in all species

Other diseases in the wild are comparatively rare.

Metabolic bone disease

Sometimes people misguidedly find and take on the rearing of young or neonate birds of prey. Often they will feed a pure meat diet without the bone, fur and feather necessary for the building of a firm bony skeleton. The result is an imbalance of calcium/phosphorus which leads to poorly calcified bones (seen on x-ray), curved or distorted

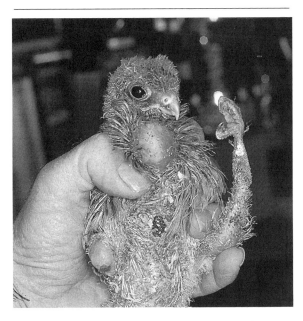

Fig. 17.3 This kestrel has been reared on an inappropriate diet.

long bones and even spontaneous fractures of the long bones.

The condition is probably not reversible although early cases may respond to a balanced diet with an additional calcium/phosphorus supplement. However, usually the bird is incapable of even standing and should be destroyed on humanitarian grounds (Fig. 17.3).

COMMON INCIDENTS

As seen in owl casualties, there is the usual range of collision traumas from kestrels being hit by cars, sparrowhawks flying into windows to red kites and peregrines getting caught in barbed wire fences.

Most other incidents are the result of illegal activity, with casualties being intentionally shot or poisoned. Any incidences of this type of activity should be immediately reported to the authorities: shooting to the local police Wildlife liaison officer and poisoning to the Wildlife Incident Unit of the Ministry of Agriculture, Fisheries and Food on freephone 0800 321 600.

Starvation

In autumn, sub-adult kestrels are often found starving and weak. This is probably because they have not mastered the technical skill of hunting for live prey. On admission they should receive the standard protocol to deal with starvation used for owls in a similar predicament.

It is probably best to keep the recovered birds in a skylight aviary until the spring when the wild food available is on the increase. Hacking back from the skylight aviary will give them a chance to return if they have not been able to kill.

COMMON INJURIES

There will be the usual range of fractures and lacerations as those experienced by the owls. Sparrowhawk casualties, however, are almost invariably head trauma cases from flying into windows. Even if the bird is found unconscious with a flaccid neck, it will still be classed as head trauma since necks are not usually damaged in this type of collision.

Particularly crucial in birds of prey is that they recover 100% of their plumage and 100% of their ability to fly and manoeuvre. In captivity they are very likely to damage their feathers, making their rehabilitation programme a priority to get them released as soon as possible.

Feather damage

Sometimes feathers, which must be perfect in birds of prey before their release, are broken or bent. Missing feathers will grow fairly quickly but a broken or bent feather will be an impediment to the bird's hunting capability until the next moult.

Broken feathers

There is a system of repairing bird of prey feathers called 'imping' which can sometimes help to get a bird released with an adequate feather covering.

A broken feather can be extended by cutting a 'V' shape in the distal end of the stub. A small slither of wood to the diameter of the inside of the

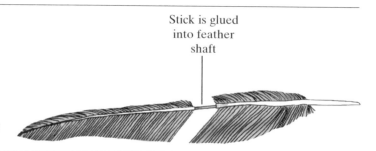

Stick is glued
into feather
shaft

Fig. 17.4 How to repair a feather by 'imping'.

feather shaft is then glued into the shaft with half of it exposed. Another feather, which may be an old moulted feather, a feather from another species or even a chicken feather, is found to match the size and shape of the original feather. The proximal end is cut off in a 'V' shape to match the existing fragment on the bird. The prosthesis is then glued over the exposed wooden peg. This 'make do' feather will then serve the bird until the next moult (Fig. 17.4).

Bent feathers

A bent feather will have a weakness where it is creased. Pulling the feather straight and applying glue from a hot glue gun to the crease will give the feather enough stability, once again, until the next moult (Plate 31).

Eye injuries

Injuries to the eyes must be referred to the veterinary surgeon for immediate diagnosis and treatment.

A diurnal bird of prey, except perhaps pure scavengers like kites, should never be released after the loss of one eye or any impairment of their binocular vision (Fig. 17.5).

Leg injuries

There is a worry that a bird of prey would not be able to cope with the loss of one leg. True it would lose its hunting capability but even in captivity the pressure placed on the surviving leg would predispose to bumblefoot. Coles (1997) assured us that the smaller birds, kestrels and merlins, cope very

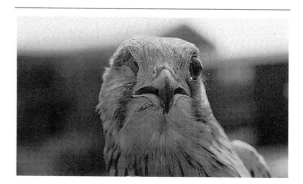

Fig. 17.5 A kestrel with one eye is not suitable for release.

well. With the larger species it can be tried but if it fails the bird cannot be left to suffer the chronic implications of bumblefoot.

ADMISSION AND FIRST AID

Admission of diurnal birds of prey is very much the same as for owls. However, some of the larger birds make the intravenous infusion of fluids much more practical.

On admission sparrowhawks benefit from diazepam at 10 mg/kg intramuscularly.

CAGING

Similar to that required for owls; with, obviously, much larger skylight aviaries required for the largest species.

Sparrowhawks will fare better if the fronts of any cages are 75% covered to give them the privacy this excitable species needs.

FEEDING

These requirements are similar to those of owls in that whole animals are necessary to provide a complete diet. Eventually it is convenient to wean all species on to easily obtained day-old chicks or chickens and rabbits for the larger birds. In order to get the birds eating in the first place, give them food they will recognise. For instance:

- Kestrels – dark mice
- Sparrowhawks, hobbies, merlins – drug-free small garden birds that have died from trauma not disease
- Buzzards – rabbits including road kills
- Peregrine – frozen pigeons or pheasants
- Red kite – rabbits, including road kills

It is illegal in this country to offer live vertebrate prey to birds and mammals in captivity.

RELEASE

The same techniques of hacking, used for owls, are also appropriate for diurnal birds of prey. However, particular attention must be taken of the location of local species and concurrence with the migration timing of hobbies or ospreys. Red kites should be released through English Nature's re-introduction programme (Appendix 7).

LEGAL IMPLICATIONS

All birds of prey are protected by the Wildlife and Countryside Act 1981. Some are on Schedule 4 which means they should be passed to a Licensed Person who then has to notify the Department of the Environment, Transport and the Regions (DETR) within 4 days and register the bird if it is likely to be in captivity for longer than 15 days. Registration also requires a veterinary certificate confirming the need to delay any release (Appendix 4).

Species likely to be involved are: hobby, merlin, red kite, peregrine, goshawk, golden eagle, harriers and osprey. For more remote species please refer to the full list of Schedule 4 species in Appendix 3.

18
Seabirds

Most incidents affecting sea-going birds are generally related to contamination with oil. Other incidents do occur but their impact is occasional and most are beyond our intervention, e.g. massive die-offs with starvation through dwindling fish stocks.

OIL POLLUTION

Major oil spills affecting hundreds, or even thousands, of seabirds are highly documented and reported in the media. The response to this type of disaster is the province of highly organised rehabilitation groups and, although based on the same protocol discussed in this chapter, is beyond the remit of this book.

Many people do not realise that the treatment of oiled birds is not just an occasional media circus. Birds are falling foul of oil every day of every year and each one of these birds needs the specialised treatments developed by rehabilitators since the Torrey Canyon disaster in 1967 when only 2% of the casualties were cleaned, treated or released.

It is not just seabirds that become contaminated with oil and even here, in the centre of England, we have seen robins, kestrels, pigeons, swans, ducks, wagtails, sparrows and even hedgehogs covered in oil. Each was treated using the same protocol used on marine birds such as auks and seaducks.

Britain is still evolving a truly successful oiled bird rehabilitation programme. Chris Mead, the Senior Ringing Officer with the British Trust for Ornithology (BTO), stated (1991), 'All our experience with the rehabilitation of oiled birds points towards a low success rate. . . .'

In the beginning all wildlife rehabilitation was plagued with a low success rate, but by keeping their minds open and challenging preconceived notions about the care of wildlife, the rehabilitators have succeeded in reversing the trend.

More research into the treatment of oiled birds is still needed. Reviews of the American experience, certainly with the Exxon Valdez spill in Alaska (1989) with a great deal of medical investigation into pre-release conditioning of the birds affected with oil, has firmly established the rehabilitation of oiled birds (or mammals) as a medical procedure not just a cleaning process. In this country many groups do still regard oiled birds as simply a cleaning process, but now with the input of experienced rehabilitators, veterinary nurses and surgeons, the medical issues are starting to be given their deserved priority.

Before any oiled bird can receive the treatment it needs, there has to be in place a sequential protocol and a set of suitable equipment and medicaments (Table 18.1).

EMERGENCY PROCEDURES

The protocol for dealing with birds affected by oil or pollutants can be established by means of a flow chart that is easily accessible and can even be incorporated into the bird's record card. The suggested flow chart (Fig. 18.1) can be printed on the back of the individual card so that every bird has with it a record of its progress through the system. The letters denoted in the headings below (in brackets) refer to the various procedures given in Fig. 18.1.

Table 18.1 Suggested equipment and drugs list for treating birds affected by oil.

Equipment

Cloacal thermometer
Haematocrit centrifuge
Haematocrit reader
Scales
Heat lamps

Disposables

I/V infusion sets
I/V catheters and butterfly set 20 g–27 g
Spinal needles 20 g–26 g
Hypodermic needles 21 g–27 g
Syringes 1–20 ml
Feeding syringes 50 ml
Urethral catheters
Paper boottee covers
Plain capillary tubes
Cardboard boxes
Gauze swabs
Assorted sizes plastic numbered rings
Record cards
Tie on labels
Clinical waste bags
Sharps bins
Vinyl gloves and aprons

Drugs

Oral rehydration salts – Lectade (Pfizer)
Hartmann's solution
Amino acids and vitamins – Duphalyte (Fort Dodge
    Animal Health)
Vitamin B_1 (Thiamine) – Fish Eaters Tablets (Mazuri
    Zoo Foods)
Kaolin and neomycin – Kaobiotic Tablets (Pharmacia &
    Upjohn)
Activated charcoal and bismuth – Forgastrin (Arnolds
    Veterinary Products)
Salt tablets – Slow Sodium (Novartis)
Water-based eye drops – Hypromellose (Millpledge
    Pharmaceuticals)
Iron dextran – Veterinary Iron Injection (Arnolds
    Veterinary Products)
Liquid nutrition – Poly-Aid (Vetafarm Europe)
Liquid nutrition – Ensure (Abbott Laboratories)

Rescue (B)

Rescue of oiled birds should be with large nets. It is important to approach the casualty from the sea or water edge to cut off any escape route.

The birds will be contaminated with some sort of petroleum product or crude oil which could have toxic, or at least irritative, properties. It is impor-

tant, therefore, to wear protective gloves and observe health and safety regulations.

All seabirds have sharp beaks and some, like those of gannets and cormorants, can cause serious injury. Whenever handling seabirds do take extreme care to control the heads and so the ability of the bird to bite, stab or slash.

Oil on the feathers of a bird predisposes to:

- Destruction of the waterproofing and insulation properties of the plumage
- The birds will be chilled, unable to stay afloat or fly
- They will have been unable to feed due to their disabilities and the effect of oil on their food

For these reasons the bird must be taken to a first-aid facility without delay. The chemistry of hypothermia is little understood, so if this can be prevented, or at least caught early, the bird may stand a chance of overcoming all the internal problems that oil can cause.

Field first aid (C)

Field first aid is that first response to steady a bird almost while it is still at the waterside. Apart from the external deprivation of oiling, the internal damage is far more life-threatening and needs to be reversed, or limited as soon as possible, to give the bird any chance of recovery.

The bird with oil on its feathers is going to preen in a vain attempt to restructure the feathers and their waterproofing and insulating properties. All it will succeed in doing is ingesting oil and oil fumes. The effect on the bird can be catastrophic and may include:

- Haemorrhage and ulceration of the gastrointestinal tract with a severe loss of digestive and absorptive ability
- Irritation and ulceration to the eyes
- Damage to the trachea and even oil aspiration are not uncommon
- Kidney damage can be severe and fatal
- Affected birds have weakened immunity systems that can allow the progress of fungal and bacterial infections
- The destruction of red blood cells leading to debilitating anaemias

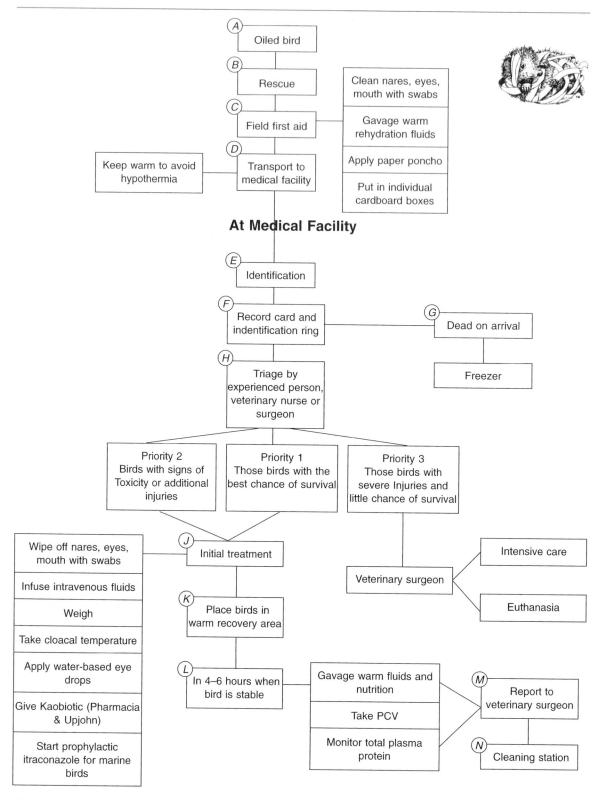

Fig. 18.1 Flow chart for emergency procedures to deal with birds affected by oil or pollutant.

All of these processes will have to be dealt with at a treatment facility, but first aid at the waterside will start the treatment process and will help any bird survive until it can get more intensive assessment and treatment.

Simple procedures should be carried out on every live bird presented for first aid:

(1) The bird's mouth, nares and eyes should be wiped clean with gauze swabs.
(2) A few drops of aqueous eye drops, Hypromellose (Millpledge Pharmaceuticals), will help lubricate the eyes.
(3) Gavage with warmed rehydration fluid (Lectade – Pfizer) at 10% estimated bodyweight.
(4) Gavage bismuth and activated charcoal solution (Forgastrin – Arnolds Veterinary Products) at 5 ml/kg, or a new product consisting of liquid activated charcoal – Liqui-Char-Vet (Arnolds Veterinary Products), could complement a bismuth preparation – Pepto Bismol (Proctor & Gamble).

(3) and (4) can be combined in one syringe.

(5) To prevent the bird ingesting more oil through preening it can be covered with a 'poncho' fashioned from disposable paper surgical theatre bootees. Anything thicker may lead to hyperthermia.
(6) The bird is then put into an individual cardboard box for transport to the main treatment facility. If the weather is cold, hot water bottles covered with towels will prevent hypothermia affecting the coldest birds. Hot water bottles can be improvised out of empty plastic lemonade bottles filled with warm water.

Transport to the main medical facility (D)

After the birds have received their first aid they should be taken to the main medical facility as quickly as possible. This main facility is not necessarily the cleaning station as any washing should be delayed until the birds are pronounced stable and fit for handling.

Many oiled birds succumb to hypothermia during this transfer from the waterside to intensive care. Hopefully the first aid they should have received will provide strength for the journey but even then if the vehicle is cold there will be less birds to receive intensive care unless extra warmth is provided.

If the journey is longer than 1 hour the hot water bottles should be replenished and the birds checked every 60 minutes.

Identification (E)

At the medical facility the birds should be quickly admitted. They must be identified by a person with a knowledge of species even if their distinguishing plumage is heavily disguised with oil.

Species of seabird normally seen include: gulls (*Larus* sp.), seaducks, guillemots (*Uria* sp.), razorbills (*Alca torda*), puffins (*Fratercula arctica*), little auks (*Alle alle*), gannets (*Sula bassana*), shags (*Phalacrocorax aristotelis*), cormorants (*P. carbo*) and petrels (*Hydrobates pelagicus*).

Record card and identity ring (F)

Each bird should be given an admittance code number that coincides with a consecutively numbered plastic leg ring. For each bird a record card (Fig. 18.2) should be made out recording the date and time of arrival, the species, its consecutive number and the leg on which the ring is fitted. The record card will remain with the bird until either its demise or release.

Dead on arrival (G)

Birds which are pronounced dead on arrival should still have record cards made out and a tie-on label giving a consecutive number. They will be stored in a deep freeze for future reference or post-mortem.

Often in oil spills where there are multiple deaths and casualties some immediate post-mortem results may provide guidance on the physiological affects of the pollutant.

Triage (H)

Triage should be by an experienced person who will roughly assess the condition of the bird. A bird, if there are more than one, can then be categorised Priority 1, 2 or 3:

• *Priority 1.* Are birds with the best chance of survival. They can be passed straight on for their initial treatments.

St Tiggywinkles Oiled Bird Record Card

Date:		Time:		Alive/Dead	Consecutive no.	

Species:	Name of rescuer:	Place of rescue:

Triage examined:			Priority 1	Priority 2	Priority 3

Medical record:	Has First Aid Been Provided: Yes/No

Initial examination Time	Examiner

Degree of oiling: None/Light/Moderate/Heavy	Respiration: Shallow/Laboured/Normal

Neurological signs	Mucous Membranes

Other injuries

Treatments			Intravenous fluids: Yes/No	Quantity	

Date	Time	Drugs	Weight	Cloacal temperature	PCV TPP
On admittance					/////////

Veterinary Surgeon Certificate	Bird is to be: Washed/Continue treatment/Euthanised

Signed	Date:	Time:

Fig. 18.2 Record card suitable for an oiled bird.

- *Priority 2.* Are birds with signs of toxicity and additional injuries. They will take a little more time to treat and stabilise but should respond to the standard initial treatment protocol.
- *Priority 3.* Are birds with little chance of survival. They can be moribund and have severe injuries. These are candidates for intensive care under the supervision of a veterinary surgeon or a senior supervisor. A 'trauma team' should be kept on standby just for these, almost hopeless, cases.

Birds in this category may also be beyond help and can be humanely destroyed under the instruction of the veterinary surgeon.

Initial treatment (J)

On being passed through from triage, the Priority 1 and Priority 2 birds will receive standardised treatments:

(1) Initially their nares, mouth and eyes will be checked and cleaned again with gauze swabs. Aqueous eye drops (Hypromellose – Millpledge Pharmaceuticals) will be dropped into both eyes to keep them lubricated after they have been flushed with warm sterile saline.
(2) Any bird is now weighed.
(3) Any bird will be provided with intravenous or intraosseous fluids, Hartmann's solution laced with 10% Duphalyte (Fort Dodge Animal Health) at 3% bodyweight by bolus. Cormorants are particularly susceptible to dehydration and should receive twice as much fluid as other species.
(4) Its cloacal temperature is recorded. Normal temperatures are between 39 and 41°C.
(5) Any bird is given Kaobiotic (Pharmacia & Upjohn) in tablet form. Dose rates are 1 whole tablet per 4 kg. These will be continued daily until there is no trace of blood or oil in the droppings.
(6) All oiled seabirds are going to be more susceptible to the ravages of aspergillosis. Along with other daily treatments should be the prophylactic administration of itraconazole (Sporanox – Janssen-Cilag) (see Chapter 9).

Recovery (K)

The birds are then placed in a recovery area with overhead heating. They must be able to get away from the heat if they wish to (Plate 32).

Second treatment and assessment (L)

After 4–6 hours of recuperation and fluids the birds should:

(1) Be gavaged with warm fluids (Lectade – Pfizer) and liquid nutrition (Poly-Aid – Vetafarm Europe or Ensure – Abbott Laboratories)
(2) Blood samples should be taken to calculate the packed cell volume (PCV) and total plasma protein (TPP)

The PCV is useful in assessing whether the bird is anaemic. Initially when the bird is dehydrated it will show an elevated PCV which may be disguising anaemia. As the bird is rehydrated the PCV will drop sometimes to as low as under 10%.

- Birds with a PCV of 25% or less are not washed until it rises back to normal
- Birds with a PCV of 16% or less would benefit from blood (USA) or plasma transfusions, if these were available
- Any bird showing signs of anaemia should be given an intramuscular injection of iron dextran at 10 mg/kg every 5–7 days.

The TPP for birds is usually 30–50 g/l and similarly no bird should be washed if its plasma solid values are below 20 g/l.

Weight, temperature, PCV and TPP are from then on monitored every day.

Veterinary surgeon (M)

The information gained is then passed to the veterinary surgeon for assessment and direction as to the next course of treatment.

Cleaning (N)

After the assessment the bird will be passed on to the wash station to be cleaned. It should be alert, responsive and stable. Any doubts must be referred back to the veterinary surgeon.

Structure of feathers

The waterproofing and insulating properties of feathers are provided by the structure of the feather. The feather barbs are held together by small hooked structures, barbules. The barbs are situated along the shafts of the feather (Fig. 18.3). When the feathers overlay each other the whole construction provides an impenetrable layer that keeps water out and body heat in. In fact a bird has to lose heat through its open mouth or by fluttering the gular region in its throat.

There is no natural oil involved, so a bird that has lost its waterproofing has not lost the oil of its feathers as is often supposed. The preen oil a bird takes from its uropygial (preen) gland is more of a conditioner than anything else.

The effect of crude oil or petroleum products on the feathers is to break down the structure of the barbs and barbules allowing water and cold to penetrate the coat of the feathers. Hence many birds affected by oil are not waterproof, cannot swim and are often hypothermic.

Washing

Equipment needed:

* Constant running hot water at 42°C
* Fairy Liquid (Procter & Gamble) or Co-op Green washing-up liquid

Fairy Liquid (Procter & Gamble) is the tried and tested product for use in washing oiled birds. Co-op Green washing-up liquid is as useful. Any other product will not work as well. Invariably during any major oil spill people will turn up with their 'wonder product' to try on oiled birds. They never seem to work, so you may lose valuable time in experimenting with them.

The theory behind washing

The purpose of washing an oiled bird is to remove the oil, or other product, from the feathers with a detergent (Fairy Liquid – Procter & Gamble). However, the detergent is as detrimental to the feathers as the oil is. So once the oil has been

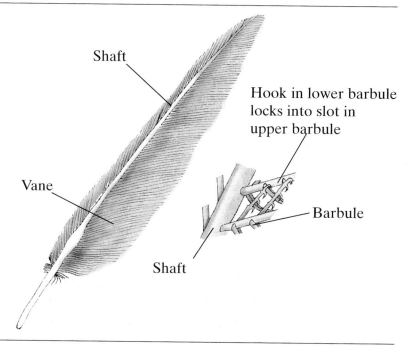

Fig. 18.3 The structure of a feather.

removed any residual detergent has to be rinsed off with clean, hot water. Only then will the feather structure fall into place once more.

The operation of washing

In preparation of washing just one oiled bird, two tubs of hot water (42°C) with a 2% solution of Fairy Liquid (Procter & Gamble) in each are set up. Next to them is another tub of hot water at 42°C but this time it is clean water. After these three tubs should be a rinsing facility with a spray nozzle of constant, clean hot water, again at 42°C.

It will take two people to wash birds the size of guillemots or ducks but a third person should assist with larger birds such as gannets or swans (Fig. 18.4). The procedure to follow is:

(1) Initially place the bird in the first tub of hot water, holding all but its head underwater for 10 seconds. Then while one person holds the bird, the other ladles the hot water over it rubbing it in, only in the direction of the feathers.
(2) The head can be cleaned with a toothbrush dipped in detergent.
(3) When the water is totally fouled the bird is lifted into the second tub and the procedure repeated.

(4) Then it is doused in the third tub for a preliminary rinsing, taken out and held while the hot water spray, at 42°C, is jetted up under all the feathers on each part of the bird.

This is the crucial part of the operation as, slowly, the detergent is rinsed away and the feathers start to regain their properties. After a while the feathers will become drier and the water will bead up and run off (Fig. 18.5). The rinsing has to proceed until the whole of the bird is dry. This can take some time but it is essential because any drop of detergent left on the feathers will be a weak point allowing water in and under the plumage.

If at any time the bird appears stressed it should be quickly dried off with a towel and returned to its pen. Another attempt at cleaning it could be made on the following day.

Drying

The birds can then be put into a room with overhead lamps under which they can preen. Drinking water should be available and they must be able to move away from the heat if they wish.

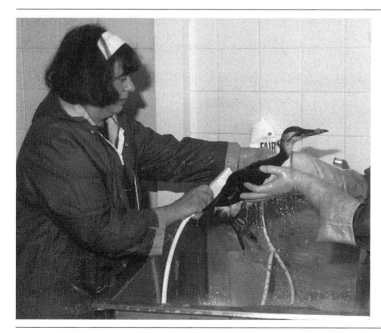

Fig. 18.4 Washing an oiled guillemot.

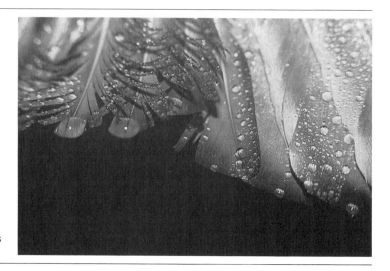

Fig. 18.5 The water will bead on feathers as they are rinsed dry.

All waterbirds are susceptible to bumblefoot and will benefit from soft flooring like foam rubber or calf mats.

Many of the birds will eat at this time and can be offered suitable diets, mostly fish.

Elf Aquitaine bird washing apparatus

In view of the man-hours and stress to birds involved in dealing with cleaning the victims of oil, Elf Aquitaine has designed a machine that can provide washing of oiled birds without unnecessary handling (Fig. 18.6).

The system is designed to clean Alcidae (the auks) perfectly. The bird is placed in a cage in a standing position with opened wings. Its head is kept outside of the cleaning area. The cage is then put into the cleaning and rinsing tank in which the cleaning solution and then rinsing water are programmed to suit particular birds. The cleaning is by nozzles, which are mounted on rotating shafts, spraying liquids under pressure.

The process is very similar to hand-washing an oiled bird but takes only 10 minutes, a fraction of the time normally taken and does not involve handling by two or more people.

Not having seen the machine in use, it would appear to be less stressful to the birds than hand-washing and rehabilitators find that the final rinse leaves a totally, oil- and detergent-free bird (J. De Boer, pers. comm.).

RECUPERATION

Feed

Most of the seabirds encountered are fish eaters and can be maintained in captivity on a fish diet as long as they also receive supplements of Fish Eaters Tablets (Mazuri Zoo Foods).

Initially they will all need force feeding but some will learn to take fish straight from a bowl of cold water or from their swimming area (Fig. 18.7). Whole fish are the most suitable for force feeding. Once again it is a two-person task, one holds the bird while the other pulls open both halves of the beak. The fish, cold, is them pushed head first into the throat and the beak held closed. The bird can be seen swallowing. The Fish Eaters Tablets (Mazuri Zoo Foods) and any other medication can be secreted in the gills of the fish.

Suitable for most seabirds, and easily obtainable from fishmongers, are: sprats, sand eels, herring and sardines. However, any small whole fish are suitable.

Swimming

The next stage is for the birds to swim, which in turn will encourage them to preen, which in its turn re-aligns their vital feather structure.

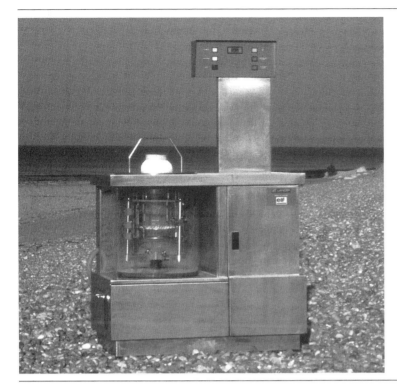

Fig. 18.6 The washing machine for birds designed by Elf Aquitaine (photo: Elf Aquitaine).

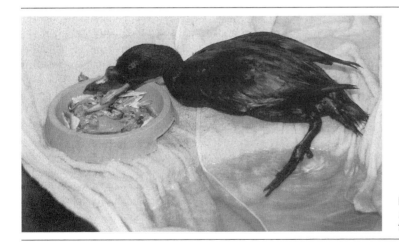

Fig. 18.7 Common scoter (*Melanitta nigra*) will take fish, shrimps and mussels from a bowl.

Indoor swimming

An indoor pool is most suitable for the first swims as at one end, over a climb-out platform, heat lamps can be suspended where any birds feeling cold can stand and preen.

A simple pool of any size can be made from sheets of 30 mm plywood as a frame overlain with a butyl pond liner. Steps can be made at one end to form a climb-out platform as initially the birds will not want to spend that much time in the water (Fig. 18.8).

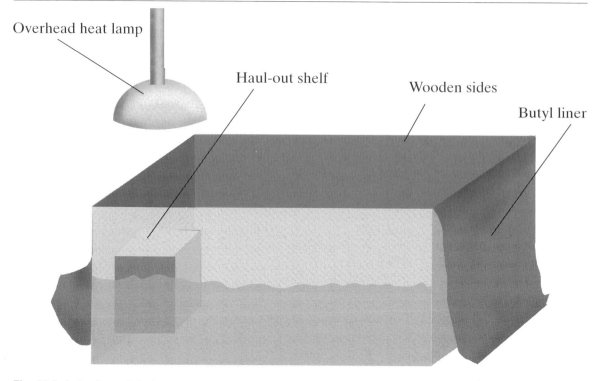

Overhead heat lamp

Haul-out shelf

Wooden sides

Butyl liner

Fig. 18.8 A simple pool design.

Outside swimming

Once the birds look comfortable on the inside pool they can be introduced to an outside pool on similar lines. The overhead lamps should no longer be needed.

The birds will swim but regularly climb out to preen. It is important to keep a close watch on the birds at this stage in case any of them become waterlogged or cold. These should go back to the indoor pool for a few more days.

Eventually the birds should be able to swim for at least 30 minutes without any sign of getting wet.

Salt

Marine birds in captivity are generally kept on freshwater pools. These birds have salt glands which will atrophy if there is no salt for them to excrete. To maintain the integrity of these salt glands these birds should receive doses of salt tablets specially formulated for marine animals. Only birds with salt glands should be given salt supplements as the supplements would be toxic to other birds (Salt tablets – IZUG).

Release

Much has been criticised about the release of cleaned birds. The author's opinion is that they are often released too early. Judging by the severe damage inflicted on a bird's internal organs by oil ingestion, birds should be kept until the veterinary surgeon can confirm by blood tests that as far as is possible the bird is fit for release.

It is very difficult to keep seabirds even as long as 6 weeks and with divers it is impossible. But the longer they are being monitored and remaining comfortable the more chance they have of surviving in the wild.

However, in captivity, the feet of these birds are going to deteriorate. Giving them constant access to clean water and a fresh grass base will give them a better chance of maintaining foot condition. Any creams put on to the feet must be water based and easily soluble or else the feathers will become contaminated all over again.

When the veterinary surgeon finally declares them fit for release they should be taken to a suitable waterfront and be allowed to walk into the water. Do not throw them off cliffs and do not cast them adrift from boats.

OTHER INCIDENTS INVOLVING SEABIRDS

Apart from gulls (*Larus* spp.) being injured and sustaining fractures, the only other regular incidents involving seabirds are crashes.

Crashes occur normally during the autumn or when there are particularly strong gales. They happen all over the country where, miles from the sea, pelagic birds crash land and are unable to take off again to continue their journey. The author believes these 'crashes' are of birds that are totally lost. Normally there is nothing wrong with the bird. They should be put back on the sea as soon as possible. Any delay over 24 hours and the perils of aspergillosis seem to proliferate.

In September it is usually manx shearwaters (*Puffinus puffinus*) that crash inland on their migratory journeys from the Welsh coast to Brazil.

Little auks (*Alle alle*), fulmars (*Fulmarus glacialis*) and gannets (*Sula bassana*) are all regularly found inland.

19
Hand-rearing Orphaned Birds

Before even contemplating hand-rearing an orphaned wild bird it is absolutely crucial to establish that it really is a genuine orphan and it does need help. Many young birds intentionally leave the nest before they can fly. The parent birds encourage their young to disperse into different hideaways where they will carry on feeding them. This is nature's way of spreading the risk of the youngsters getting taken by a predator. Clustered in the nest they would be easy prey for any bird or other animal that has detected it.

This dispersal ploy has worked for millions of years so any youngsters in this situation should be left for their parents to rear. However, the ploy takes no account of man-introduced hazards like cars, cats and humans themselves. Sometimes the fledgling bird is in even more danger out of the nest. This is when it is wise to intervene and take on the task of hand-rearing.

So there are times when to intervene and times when to leave well alone. By watching an apparent orphan from a distance, the parent birds can be observed returning to feed their youngsters. In particular young crows, rooks or gulls spend a lot of time on the ground or beach being fed by their parents. This is perfectly natural behaviour and the fledglings should be left alone, except if:

- There is imminent danger from a predator
- There are nearby environmental hazards like roads or pools
- After observation of about 1 hour the parents do not return
- The fledgling is injured in any way
- The parents have been definitely killed or incapacitated

- The fledglings are of a species known to be ignored once they have left the nest prematurely, e.g. tawny owl, heron or swift

Only if one of these conditions occurs is it opportune to intervene and pick up the fledgling for hand-rearing.

NATURAL HISTORY

There are two types of baby bird, altricial or precocial. More commonly it is the altricial birds, those that are hatched with few or no feathers, with their eyes closed and entirely dependent on their parents for food and warmth, that require rescuing.

The other type of baby bird, the precocial chick, hatches with a good coat of down feathers and an ability to immediately leave the nest and follow its parents. Some, like ducklings and pheasants, are able to feed themselves while others, like moorhens and partridges, will need some encouragement to feed or have food supplements from their parents. Once again a precocial chick on its own is not necessarily an orphan. By watching from a distance the parents can be seen returning to brood their youngsters. But, as always, there are exceptions to the bland 'leave them alone' rule. Occasions when we can intervene with precocial chicks include if:

- There is imminent danger from a predator or the environment
- There is an obvious injury to the chick
- There is a straggler.

With large hatchings of precocial chicks, seen in birds such as ducks and pheasants, the mother bird will lead the chicks away from the nest to other areas. Often there appears to be a 'runt' chick that cannot keep up with the rest and is left behind. This straggler chick is the orphan that is often taken to rescue centres. However, it appears that being left behind was no accident by the mother as these stragglers often have no idea how to feed or look after themselves. Perhaps there is a genetic problem we know nothing about. But the author knows that it is very difficult to keep these stragglers alive.

Whatever happens it must be remembered that it is a long-term commitment to hard, and often heartbreaking, work to take on the hand-rearing of an orphaned wild bird. The parent birds make a much better job of it so leave them to it and only adopt an orphan if there is no other way.

EQUIPMENT

Before even thinking about taking on an orphaned wild bird it is essential to have a stock of supplies and utensils to complement any of the species that may turn up (Table 19.1; Appendix 6). Once people know that you have adopted one baby bird then many, many more will land, literally, in your lap.

CAGING

Various species require different forms of caging. However, every cage should have an overhead heat lamp of the ceramic type that does not emit any light. The cages should be open topped so that the birds can be fed from above and the heat can be directed to one end of the cage allowing mobile youngsters to move out of the way if they so wish.

Cages available at pet stores for other animals as part of the Hagen range (Rolf C Hagen) are eminently suitable and easy to keep clean; known respectively as a 'Zoo Zone 1 and 2' which has enclosed clear plastic sides and a 'Ferret Cage' which has wire sides, they both have plastic bottoms (Fig. 19.1).

Table 19.1 Suggested utensils and supplies required for hand-rearing orphaned birds.

Utensils

Electronic or diabetic scales (increments of 1 g)
Shallow plastic food bowls with lids (Ashwood Timber & Plastics)
Teat cannulas (Jorgensen Laboratories)
Non-sterile syringes 1–20 ml
Coffee stirrers (plastic)
Used clean giving sets to make gavage tubes
Various mixing jugs
Food processor
Fridge/freezer
Plastic forceps
Feather dusters
Ceramic heat lamps
Plastic pudding bowls (for nest pans)
Clockwork alarm clock
Plastic numbered leg rings (must be removed before birds are released)

Supplies

Tropican Rearing Mix (Rolf C. Hagen) available in pet stores
Pedigree Chum Puppy dog food (Pedigree Masterfoods)
Prosecto dried insects (Haith)
Avipro Paediatric (Vetark Animal Health)
Waxworm larvae (Mealworm Company)
Pancrex Vet (Pharmacia & Upjohn)
Chick crumbs
Paper kitchen towels

On the bottom of all the cages use river-washed sharp sand which is easily obtainable from builders' merchants. It can be changed regularly.

Nesting altricial birds

Old nests should never be used as they are a base for many parasites. In their place small plastic feed bowls or pudding bowls, lined with paper towel, make ideal nests. Placed in an open-top cage they can be positioned so that the birds with the least feathers get the most benefit from the heat lamp (Fig. 19.2).

As they start to develop the altricial birds will often get out of their nests. The sand base is going to cause them no harm but a few twig perches, just above the sand, will give them something to stand on or roost on.

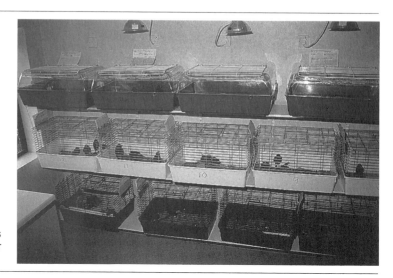

Fig. 19.1 Zoo Zone and Ferret Cages by Rolf C Hagen provide facilities for many species of orphaned birds.

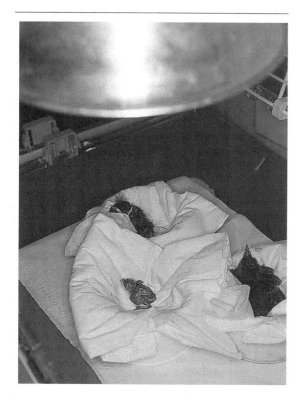

Fig. 19.2 Nest bowls for altricial species need to be under a heat lamp.

Once they have most of their feathers they can be moved out to a wire-topped cage without the need for extra heat. A selection of perches will provide exercise for both their feet and their wings.

Precocial birds

Precocial birds will not need nest pans. They will be able to walk around and find their own food. Initially scattering some of their feed on the sand may encourage them to peck at it. However, a shallow bowl for their feed will allow an estimate of how much they are taking.

Initially, when they are very small, a heat lamp at one end of the cage will give them somewhere to huddle together.

There are two tips that often encourage precocial chicks to settle:

(1) A feather duster stood on the feather end will act as a surrogate mother, especially to ducklings (Fig. 19.3)
(2) Game bird chicks and other terrestrial birds may well home in on a clockwork alarm clock ticking under a feather duster

As they move more away from the heat lamp, they can be moved into wire-top cages without any heat. Their feather dusters and alarm clocks should go with them.

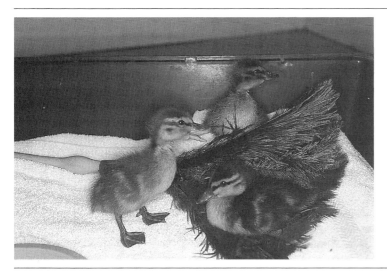

Fig. 19.3 A feather duster will serve as a surrogate mother to ducklings.

Water

Even young water birds should not be allowed to bathe until they have a substantial plumage of adult feathers. Giving them water to drink in a bowl may lead to drowning or hypothermia. Far more suitable are budgerigar drinking fountains and for duck, geese and swans the larger waterbird fountains (Fig. 19.4).

Grit

When the birds start feeding themselves they should have access to various suitable sizes of grit for ingestion to their gizzards. At pet stores sizes are available to suit small birds (budgerigar grit), large birds (pigeon grit) and really large birds (chicken grit). This can be presented in an open bowl and topped up as necessary.

Quarantine arrangements

Cross infection, if there is an infection, in baby birds is easily transmitted in the warm, humid atmosphere of a rearing cage. Also the use of the same feeding utensils for different birds will readily transmit infection from one bird to another.

In an ideal world each bird would have its own cage, its own food and its own feeding utensil. However, with the number of baby birds that can arrive to be reared, it is impossible to provide these

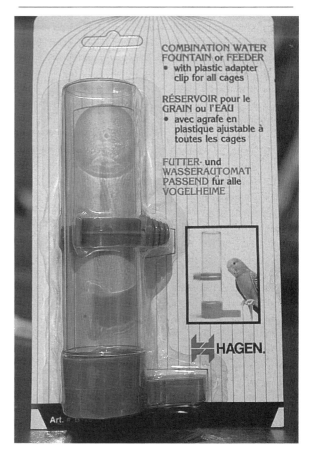

Fig. 19.4 Drinking fountains (Rolf C Hagen) prevent small birds from drowing.

optimum conditions. Yet some quarantine can be provided as a damage limitation exercise so that if disaster does strike its impact will only affect a few birds. And even then the problem will be highlighted so that emergency diagnosis and treatment can be arranged.

As birds are admitted they are naturally split up into similar species, i.e. small garden birds together, ducks together, birds of prey together and so on. By also splitting these groups, for instance, the garden birds into those received on a certain day into one cage and those received on another day into another cage, if any infection is unknowingly introduced only one day's orphans will be affected. The time period is flexible and can be birds brought in over a week.

The birds are then kept in the same groups all the way through the system until they are weaned and ready to go into outside aviaries for acclimatisation before release. During their stay they will be kept to their own food supplies with their own utensils. Once again this stops the opportunity for cross infection from another group.

ADMISSION AND FIRST AID

At the admission stage baby birds should receive the same first-aid treatments as adult birds. However, the use of intravenous or intraosseous fluids is usually out of the question. Instead gavage or subcutaneous fluids will provide some stability before introduction to the nursery.

At this stage the bird should be identified and aged:

(1) A hatchling with little or no feathering (we call these plastics)
(2) A nestling, a little older with its eyes open and some feathering
(3) A fledgling with almost a full quota of feathers
(4) A precocial species

A plastic numbered leg ring should also be fitted and referred to on the admittance card. Any bird with suspected disease or injury should be isolated and highlighted for treatment.

FEED

Altricial birds

Young altricial birds pass through two stages of hand-rearing. Initially they are fed a prepared mixture to suit a variety of species. Once they are more mature and starting to peck at the feeding utensils they can be offered a more appropriate adult diet.

Small garden birds

Species seen regularly:
Tits (*Parus* spp.), sparrows (*Passer* spp.), finches, wagtails (*Motacilia* spp.), flycatchers (*Muscicapa* spp.), buntings, goldcrest (*Regulus regulus*) and wren (*Troglodytes troglodytes*), warblers, swallows (*Hirundo rustica*) and house martins (*Delichon urbica*).

Food mixture
These small birds are fed on the proprietary Tropican Rearing Mix (Rolf C Hagen) available at pet stores. Each group will have its own mix freshly made each day. Keep refrigerated between feeds.

Larger garden birds

Species seen regularly:
Thrushes, corvids, woodpeckers, cuckoos, nuthatches (*Sitta europaea*) and starlings (*Sturnus vulgaris*).

Food mixture
'St Tiggywinkles Bird Glop' provides a balance of meat, roughage, pro-biotic and digestive enzyme. Mixed in bulk it is made up of:

> One dog food tin of Pedigree Chum Puppy Food (Pedigree Masterfoods)
> One dog food tin of water
> One dog food tin of dried insects (Prosecto – Haith)
> One pinch of Pancrex Vet (Pharmica & Upjohn) enzyme
> One pinch of Avipro Paediatric (Vetark Animal Health) pro-biotic

This is liquidised to the consistency of soft ice cream and frozen in *shallow* dishes with lids (Jonipax – Ashwood Timber & Plastics). The mixture is not used until it has been frozen and then allowed to defrost at 4°C as it is needed (see Fig. 28.3). It should not be defrosted with heat or a microwave.

Once again each group of birds will have its own dish of glop which will be discarded after 24 hours and a fresh one defrosted. In between feeds all the glop dishes should be kept in the refrigerator. It has been proven that feeding chilled mix to baby birds has no adverse effect whereas warming or allowing it to warm only encourages the proliferation of harmful bacteria.

The use of shallow glop dishes is to discourage the growth of deadly anaerobic bacteria that can thrive in the bottom of a deep dish. Similarly any food processors must be thoroughly washed and then the bowls soaked in a bactericidal cleaner such as Trigene (Medichem International).

Precocial birds

These birds should be offered an adult diet of a manageable size, e.g. mini-mealworms or foreign finch mix.

FEEDING

Imprinting

The logistics of feeding baby birds varies with the different species involved. However, all species are susceptible to imprinting. It is always necessary to form a loose bond with any orphaned bird that is being hand-reared. Imprinting occurs when that birds identifies itself as your offspring. It, in fact, becomes tame and will never more interact with its own species.

It is therefore essential that contact with these orphans should be kept to a minimum and on no account should they be picked up to be fed after they are in care. This is particularly important with birds of prey or waterfowl who are easily tamed. An imprinted or tamed wild bird should never be released.

Altricial birds

These birds are usually fed in a nest and will readily raise their heads, open their mouths wide (gape) and call to elicit feeding.

Those on Tropican Rearing Mix (Rolf C Hagen) will have it gavaged, via a syringe and teat cannula, directly into their crop (Fig. 19.5). They should be observed swallowing it.

The glop-fed birds are given, into their crops or their throats, a 'spatula-full' of the glop mix. Plastic coffee stirrers are ideal for feeding the thrush-sized birds while tongue depressors serve the larger helpings demanded by the corvids.

At the first cropful of a session the baby bird will turn round, point its rear roughly over the edge of the nest bowl and pass a faecal sac. This should be a sealed little packet that can be taken with forceps. It gives a good indication of the suitability of the diet. If the diet is not suitable the faeces will not be contained in a sac.

After the first cropful the baby bird will probably turn and gape again. More food can be given until it stops gaping. Repeat cropfuls will not produce more faecal sacs at that session.

The smaller birds should be fed as often as possible but at least every 10 minutes from dawn till dusk. The corvids will cope with 30-minute feedings.

As the birds open their eyes they will gradually start pecking at their food supplier. They can then be offered a more appropriate adult feed

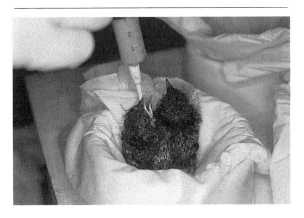

Fig. 19.5 Altricial birds are fed by gavage.

and be supplemented by the hand-feeding. Generally allow 2 weeks for garden birds to become weaned.

The faces and beaks of the birds should be kept clean with baby or pet wipes. A dirty face will lead to bacterial infection.

Pigeons and doves

These birds will not gape but may well respond to a short gavage tube being offered up to their beaks. If they take the tube in, it should be slid into the crop and a measured amount of Tropican Rearing Mix (Rolf C Hagen) syringed in. Birds that are reluctant to take the tube have to be assisted by opening the beak and then sliding the tube into the crop. Feeding every 30 minutes should be ample.

Birds of prey

These birds can be taught to peck and take quite large portions of chick or mouse from a pair of forceps. It will be swallowed whole so should not have any sharp bones protuding from it. A reluctant feeder can be encouraged to take the morsel by touching it to its beak or wiping it across its feet.

As they mature they will pick up whole food from the floor and tear it themselves.

Precocial birds

These species should be feeding themselves from the time of hatching.

WEANING

Garden birds

As they wean garden birds are split into two categories of adult diet:

- *Seed eaters.* Sparrows, finches and buntings are offered either British finch mix, foreign finch mix or, as a last resort, budgerigar or canary mix. They will also appreciate mixed wild seeds collected from the garden or organic fields.
- *Insect eaters.* Tits, wagtails, flycatchers and warblers can be fed on clean white maggots or pinkies, mini-mealworms or waxworms.

Swallows and martins will take any of these but can be offered middle-sized crickets if they prove to be reluctant feeders.

Thrushes, woodpeckers, cuckoos, starlings and nuthatches will take similar food especially the cheaper clean white maggots.

Corvids (crows, rooks, jackdaws, etc.) will thrive on tinned dog food but can also be offered occasional day-old chicks or mice.

Swifts

Swifts offer a difficult challenge in hand-rearing (Fig. 19.6). They are strictly insect eaters but can be hand-reared on either the Tropican Rearing Mix (Rolf C Hagen), the glop or on whole waxworms with a vitamin and mineral supplement added.

As swifts get older they will always be unable to pick up their own food; they naturally feed on the wing. Their forced diet of waxworms or glop can continue all the way to release.

Pigeons and doves

In the wild these Columbids feed their young on a milk substance produced in the throat of the adults. We cannot reproduce this but the Tropican Rearing Mix (Rolf C Hagen) gavaged into the crop of young

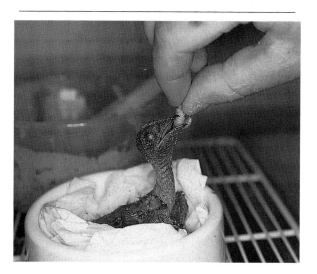

Fig. 19.6 Swifts are particularly difficult to rear.

pigeons and doves serves to bring them up to weaning.

At weaning collared and turtle doves will take small seed or chick crumbs and pigeons and larger doves require either a proprietary pigeon mix or mixed corn or pellets.

Birds of prey

All bird of prey chicks require a whole animal diet which includes meat, bone, fur or feather. Orphans can be reared successfully on chopped day-old chicks or mice with added vitamins and minerals. Larger birds can be offered chopped rabbit or chicken.

As they get older all birds of prey will take day-old chicks or mice. Once again the larger birds can be offered rabbits or chickens.

Birds of prey must not be offered live food (Protection of Animals Act 1911).

Precocial birds

Ducklings, goslings and **cygnets** will feed on a mix of corn and chick crumbs offered in a bowl near to a water fountain so that they can dabble in between beakfuls of dry food. It is best to vary the feed between corn and pelleted food, to slow the rapid growth that may lead to slipped carpal joints. Grit should be provided as it should with all birds. As they mature these birds will feed on mixed corn or a proprietary waterfowl mix. They will always need a bowl of water near to the feed.

Other precocial birds will peck at seeds and chick crumbs scattered on their sand substrate. However,

some, such as partridges, may only start pecking at live food. Waxworms and mini-mealworms can also be scattered on the sand. However, at weaning they can all be fed on corn or a proprietary game bird mix.

Moorhens and **coots** will often feed themselves on waxworms, clean white maggots or mini-mealworms. Some may take a little time to get the hang of it and should be offered live food in forceps. Painting the tips of the forceps red and yellow will often encourage moorhen chicks to peck at them. When they mature moorhens and coots will take a variety of foods including mixed corn, clean white maggots and water plants.

Waterbirds, namely **grebes** and **sawbill ducks** can be offered cold whitebait from forceps until they will take them from a bowl of cold fresh water. Remember to add the thiamine supplement.

Seabirds should be offered larger fish like sprats, sand eels and herrings. Thiamine supplementation is required with sprats and sand eels. Both of these latter categories of birds will remain on a fish diet, with thiamine supplement, until they are released.

Gulls can be offered the cheaper options of dog food or day-old chicks.

RELEASE

All these species of young bird should, on weaning, be encouraged to fly in an aviary, or swim in a pool, for 1 or 2 weeks. They can be released into a suitable habitat with methods similar to those used for their adult contemporaries.

20
Small Mammals

Part I: Mice, Voles and Shrews

Species seen regularly:
- **Mice** – Wood mouse (*Apodemus sylvaticus*), yellow-necked mouse (*A. flavicollis*), harvest mouse (*Micromys minutus*) and house mouse (*Mus domesticus*).

- **Voles** – Bank vole (*Clethrionomys glareolus*), field vole (*Microtus agrestis*) and water vole (*Arvicola terrestris*).

- **Shrews** – Common shrew (*Sorex araneus*), pygmy shrew (*S. minutus*) and water shrew (*Neomys fodiens*).

NATURAL HISTORY

These are the small mammals that live in the woods, hedges and fields under the leaf litter or under anything that gives them cover from predators. In particular, voles are probably the major prey item of foxes, owls and kestrels.

Features that help to identify different species are:

- Mice have long naked tails, large eyes and a semi-pointed snout.
- Voles have short tails, small eyes and a very blunt snout. The water vole is as large as a rat, but has the typical vole blunt nose and short tail. In contrast the brown rat has a pointed snout and long tail.
- Shrews are dark grey in colour and have a very pronounced long snout.

The water vole is the mammal most rapidly disappearing from our countryside. Therefore its care and re-establishment are absolutely crucial (Fig. 20.1).

Wood mice are different from house mice in:

- Having much larger eyes
- A mid-brown coat rather than a brownie-grey coat
- It has a white chest and abdomen
- Its hind legs are very long allowing it to hop a bit like a miniature kangaroo

Wood mice can be found in houses so identification is essential.

Shrews are incessantly eating so in care or captivity must always have a constant supply of food and water. Their metabolism is so highly charged that they could die quickly if they cannot feed.

EQUIPMENT AND TRANSPORT

If these small, very fast mammals have to be caught, then a small bird catching net will suffice. However, with practice of the speed-of-hand they can sometimes be caught manually.

They will escape from cardboard boxes and anything that is not secure. Ideal carrying containers, and later on in their rehabilitation suitable cages, are the Hagen range of plastic aquaria available in pet stores. They have a small trapdoor in the lid which allows food and water to be put in without the animal shooting out (Fig. 20.2).

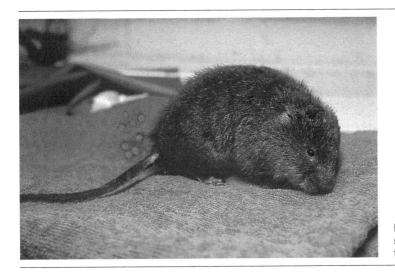

Fig. 20.1 The water vole is now very scarce and should not be confused with the brown rat.

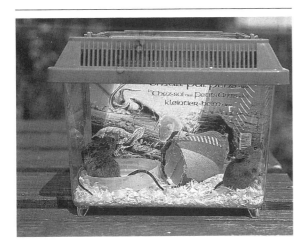

Fig. 20.2 Various sizes of small plastic aquaria (Rolf C Hagen) are ideal for small mammals.

RESCUE AND HANDLING

With these small mammals, rescue is just a question of being able to get hold of it. Some of them will bite so lightweight gloves give the catcher more confidence to hold the animal in a clenched hand. This is the best way of holding these little, speedy escape artists. The secret is to get the animal into a container as soon as possible after capture.

COMMON DISEASES

We do not normally see disease in these small mammals. Probably their metabolism is so finely balanced that any pathogenic disease will kill them before they are found.

COMMON INCIDENTS

By far the most common reason for getting these small mammals is capture by a cat. Most of them are killed but cat owners will often rescue a live one and bring it in for care.

A new worrying phenomenon in this country is the use of glue traps for house mice. In America, where glue traps are widely available, the rehabilitators are seeing all manner of small birds or mammals stuck to these devices. The author has seen glue traps covered in struggling, still very much alive, house mice. These traps are not selective in which animal they catch (Fig. 20.3). The glue is hard to remove so the live animal has to be gently prized off the trap and kept long enough to grow new fur or feathers.

COMMON INJURIES

Usually resulting from an encounter with a cat, the injuries seen include fractures of the legs which can

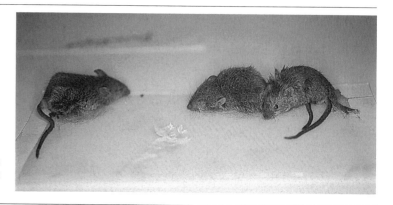

Fig. 20.3 Glue traps – but house mice are not the only animals to become stuck to them.

be splinted, and prolapsed intestines which can sometimes be successfully treated.

ADMISSION AND FIRST AID

All these species should be given subcutaneous fluids as other routes of vascular access are probably impossible to use.

The cat-injured mammal should receive an initial injection of amoxycillin at 100 mg/kg. Given subcutaneously the amoxycillin should be repeated daily for a further 2 days when it should be superceded by long-acting amoxycillin trihydrate for the rest of the week.

CAGING

These mammals are so small that they will easily escape from most cages. The Hagen animal aquarium is ideal because it has a latticed top with a hinged trapdoor in the centre.

Sand or clean wood shavings can be used as a substrate. All of the small mammals like to hide and can be given rocks to get under. A very useful small mammal house can be the cardboard tube centre of a roll of kitchen towel. This will also make moving the animal much easier as with a hand over each end it is effectively trapped. The tube and the animal can then be moved easily.

FEEDING

Mice and voles will eat dry food such as seeds, dry porridge oats, crumbled digestive biscuits or a pro-prietary mouse food. Voles take some green food and can be offered leafy twigs with buds and hay. Shrews have to have a constant supply of insect food. Clean white maggots, mini-mealworms or waxworms are suitable.

RELEASE

All of these small mammals can be released into clean hedges or even gardens. Harvest mice appreciate being near a field edge with tall grasses to enable them to build their spherical nest suspended off the ground.

Water voles should be released in good water vole habitat at the side of small rivers or canals. Contact the Mammal Society (see Appendix 7) for any water vole projects in your area.

LEGAL IMPLICATIONS

Shrews are protected under Schedule 6 of the Wildlife and Countryside Act 1981.

In 1996 the Wild Mammals (Protection) Act came into force. This was the first British legislation to protect all wild mammals from acts of cruelty.

Part II: Squirrels and Dormice

Species seen regularly:

Red squirrel (*Sciurus vulgaris*), grey squirrel (*S. carolinensis*), hazel dormouse (*Muscardinus avellanarius*) and edible dormouse (*Glis glis*).

NATURAL HISTORY

Of these four species only two, the red squirrel and the hazel dormouse, are true natives of Britain. Both are now in serious decline, not necessarily from the competition of the two introduced species, but from other factors that are not yet fully understood.

The red squirrel was in decline even before the grey squirrel was introduced to Britain. It is an animal of the ancient Caledonian pine forests which have now virtually disappeared. It is very slow at adapting to the deciduous woodlands especially as it is not able to easily digest the acorns and other nuts on which the grey squirrel thrives. There has also been quite a lengthy history of disease not normally seen in the more robust grey squirrel. The red squirrel is now confined, in England and Wales, to small pockets of population. Its main stronghold is in Scotland.

The hazel dormouse is a small arboreal animal that rarely descends to the ground. It prefers to live at about 5m above the ground in coppiced hazel woodland. With the demise of ancient forestry practices, such as coppicing, the habitat of dormice is disappearing or, at best, becoming islands with no overhead connecting pathways. Like all dormice the hazel dormouse hibernates in winter when it is said that four out of five get eaten by opportunist predators.

Both animals are the subject of concerted conservation and re-introduction programmes which should be considered before either is released.

The grey squirrel is a much more robust squirrel, 500–600 g compared with 270–320 g of the red squirrel, and is now widespread throughout Britain. Introduced from America in the nineteenth century this squirrel has a bad reputation with forestry workers and is actively trapped, shot, poisoned and killed. Black (melanic) or white (albino) grey squirrels are not uncommon.

The edible dormouse, also known by its scientific name *Glis glis*, is rather like a small version of a grey squirrel (Fig. 20.4). Released around Tring in Hertfordshire at the turn of the century it has not spread more than about 10 miles. It is accused of causing damage to trees but is most often encountered when it moves into houses in order to hibernate in the winter. In particular, hibernating *Glis glis* have often been found in switchgear installations and on one occasion in a Royal Mail post box.

Dormice have nocturnal habits while squirrels are active during the hours of daylight.

EQUIPMENT AND CAGING

The most important equipment when dealing with squirrels or *Glis glis* is a pair of extra thick gloves. These animals do have a dangerous bite

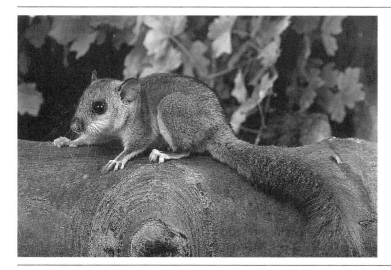

Fig. 20.4 Edible dormice (*Glis glis*) are not unlike small grey squirrels.

that once inflicted does not stop until it reaches the bone.

Nets and cat carrying baskets are also needed. These animals will quickly gnaw their way out of cardboard or wooden containers.

RESCUE AND HANDLING

Rescue is not usually needed with squirrels or *Glis glis*. But if one has to be rescued then the net followed by controlling the animal with thick gloves is the recommended procedure. Quite often though grey squirrels or *Glis glis* are inside the roof space of houses and have to be caught in humane cage traps.

Handling is with great care and a grey squirrel is a surprisingly strong animal. It is extremely fast and will not hesitate to bite or rake an arm with the long sharp claws of its back feet.

The hazel dormouse, on the other hand, is hardly ever aggressive and is easily picked up and put into a carrying box. Give it warm towels in the box and it will probably go to sleep.

COMMON DISEASES

Following on the work of Sainsbury and Gurnell (1995) and Duff *et al.* (1996) disease in the red squirrel is now being documented. However, disease records of the other three species are sparse and in need of more investigation; although, occasionally, infected animals are found and require treatment (Plate 33).

The three main diseases discussed in red squirrels are a parapox virus, metabolic bone disease and infection with coccidia species.

In grey squirrels in Britain only one parapox infection case has been confirmed. The other diseases seen are ringworm and malocclusion (Plate 22).

There is little or no reference to disease seen in either dormouse species.

Parapox virus

Parapox virus is seen as pathogenic in red squirrels. Characterised by pox-like lesions around the eyes, face and other parts of the body, the author can find no reference to treatment for the condi-

tion. However, if the veterinary surgeon suspects the parapox virus then reference could be made to other veterinarians with experience of the disease in live animals. In particular Tony Sainsbury at the Institute of Zoology, Regent's Park, London has been carrying out research for some years.

Metabolic bone disease (MBD)

Metabolic bone disease (MBD) is also regularly recorded in wild red squirrels and is caused by an imbalanced diet where the calcium/phosphorus ratio has too high a phosphorus content. Affected red squirrels may show lethargy, weakness, loss of weight and curvature of the spine (Sainsbury, 1997).

Prevention in captivity should be with a more balanced diet such as a rodent pellet (Mazuri Zoo Foods) and a small amount of fruit and nuts. In America, where many squirrels are raised, it has been found that peanuts and sunflower seeds predispose to MBD. On no account should peanuts or sunflower seeds be fed to any wild bird or other animals, especially squirrels who, as a species, seem to be particularly susceptible to MBD.

Grey squirrel juveniles that have had access to peanuts and sunflower seeds may develop fits and seizures and die. Immediate calcium supplementation by injection seems to be the only way to prevent fatality.

A suitable diet for squirrels and *Glis glis* is a good-quality dry puppy food (Hill's Canine Growth) supplemented with spinach, curly kale and pecan nuts.

Coccidiosis

Most red squirrels seem to be hosts to the coccidia *Eimeria* spp. It may or may not be debilitating but can be identified by faecal parasitology and treated with sulphonamides.

COMMON INCIDENTS

Grey squirrels and *Glis glis* are regularly taken from houses. Amazingly they are also often caught by cats although an adult grey squirrel could inflict serious injury even on a master predator like the cat. Sadly hazel dormice are also caught by cats but reports of red squirrels suffering a similar fate have not been found.

Grey squirrels are often seen with limb or spinal fractures caused by falls or road traffic accidents. Younger squirrels regularly fall from trees and are often seen with epistaxis. This can be as a result of a fall or spontaneous haemorrhage caused by ingesting warfarin-type baits.

Glis glis adults are sometimes accidentally disturbed while in deep hibernation. These can be carried easily and allowed to wake up in captivity.

ADMISSION AND FIRST AID

On admission all these species will benefit from subcutaneous fluid infusion. Only if the animal is comatose will an intravenous or intraosseous infusion be tolerated.

Squirrels may have heavy flea burdens that can be controlled with pyrethrum-based powder (WHISKAS exelpet – Pedigree Masterfoods).

If any of these animals is prescribed antibiotics for any reason then a pro-biotic (Avipro – Vetark Animal Health) will regulate the sensitive gut flora.

CAGING

All of these animals are rodents with tremendous gnawing ability. Metal cages are essential with a mixture of logs and branches to climb and gnaw. Hazel dormice will appreciate clumps of leafy hazel or sycamore branches.

FEEDING

As mentioned in the section on diseases, a balanced diet is absolutely crucial. Good-quality dry puppy food (Hill's Canine Growth), pecan nuts, curly kale, spinach and hazel nuts for dormice and red squirrels will be ideal.

Never feed peanuts or sunflower seeds.

RELEASE

The only two of these species allowed to be released in this country are the red squirrel and the hazel dormouse. Because of the endangered nature of these animals any release, if at all possible, should be included in one of the re-introduction programmes where ideal habitat will give them a much better chance of survival.

The Mammal Society will be able to provide details of the nearest re-introduction programme (see Appendix 7).

LEGAL IMPLICATIONS

The red squirrel and hazel dormice are fully protected under the Wildlife and Countryside Act 1981 and the Wild Mammals (Protection) Act 1996.

The *Glis glis* and the grey squirrel are also protected from illegal cruelty. However, the *Glis glis*, by a slip of bureaucracy, is protected under Schedule 6 of the Wildlife and Countryside Act 1981 from being killed or taken by certain methods. It is also on Schedule 9 which states that it is an offence to release one or allow one to escape.

The grey squirrel has all manner of legislation heaped against it:

- Destructive Imported Animals Act 1932 – Grey Squirrels (Prohibition and Keeping) Order 1937 makes it an offence to keep a grey squirrel and to release one or to allow one to escape without a licence
- Schedule 9 of the Wildlife and Countryside Act 1981 makes it an offence to release one or to allow one to escape into the wild
- Grey Squirrels (Warfarin) Order 1973 allows for warfarin poisoning in areas where red squirrels are not at risk

And still the grey squirrel keeps surviving. In fact it has been stated that no matter how many squirrels are killed in a year the same number will be there the following year (S. Carter, pers. comm.).

21
Hedgehogs

NATURAL HISTORY

The hedgehog (*Erinaceus europaeus*) is the most regularly seen of all British mammals. It regularly visits gardens where it feeds on beetles, worms and other invertebrates, including many that gardeners see as pests. It is also the mammal most often seen in need of rescue and rehabilitation (Stocker, 1999).

The hedgehog follows a nocturnal lifestyle and has the ability to hibernate during cold winter spells. In this country it has only one major predator, the badger, although dogs do account for many of the injuries seen.

As far as anybody knows, the hedgehog only has one litter each year, which may produce four or five urchins, between May and September. These stay with the mother and are independent at 8 weeks. After the mating, the male hedgehog has nothing to do with the females or the urchins.

EQUIPMENT AND TRANSPORT

The equipment needed to rescue hedgehogs will include: a pair of stout gloves, a pair of scissors, fencing pliers and two pairs of ordinary bull-nosed pliers.

Carrying hedgehogs is fairly simple and only requires a cardboard box or pet carrier and an old towel.

RESCUE AND HANDLING

Hedgehogs are generally easy to rescue. The criteria to consider when deciding if a hedgehog needs rescuing are:

- Is it obviously injured?
- Is it out during the day?
- Is it underweight in winter?
- Is it trapped?

On most occasions the hedgehog can simply be picked up and put into a carrying box. They do, however, regularly get trapped needing various scissors and pliers that are part of the hedgehog rescue kit:

(1) Hedgehogs will get trapped in bean netting, tennis court nets, cricket nets, in fact any kind of soft net they can find (Fig. 21.1). It is usually impossible to unravel the hedgehog without anaesthetic so they have to be cut free with scissors. After cutting them free they should not be immediately released but should be monitored, for at least 7 days, in case there is evidence of pressure necrosis from constriction injuries.

(2) Similar, but more difficult to deal with, is the hedgehog that gets trapped in wire netting or fencing. This time the fencing pliers will cut most metal strands. The precaution of monitoring in case of pressure necrosis also applies.

(3) The third type of rescue is the hedgehog who has fallen down an uncovered drain. Curled into a ball the hedgehog exactly fits most garden drains. It is often impossible to get underneath the hedgehog in order to lift it out.

This is where the pliers are useful. By clamping the pliers on to some of the hedgehog's spines it is possible to use these to lift the hedgehog free. There seem to be no ill effects after this rescue technique.

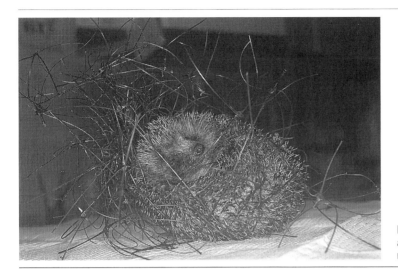

Fig. 21.1 Hedgehogs may require anaesthesia to be unravelled from netting.

Handling should be with some form of glove which will protect against the sharp spines.

Hedgehogs in the garden or on the roadside at night, unless they are obviously injured or tiny, are behaving perfectly naturally and should not be rescued. However, a hedgehog apparently asleep and not in a nest is ailing and needs rescue. Similarly, hedgehogs only ever hibernate in nests. They do not hibernate on a lawn, in a hedge or anywhere out in the open. Hedgehogs in these situations need rescuing.

Hedgehogs seen crossing a road can be helped to the other side but they should not be picked up and taken elsewhere. A hedgehog may have a dependent family nearby which will be left to starve if she does not return.

COMMON DISEASES

There are some conditions so regularly seen in hedgehogs that their treatment, once instigated by the veterinary surgeon, can become part of a standardised protocol. Some demand treatments that are well recognised in saving lives.

Lungworm infestation

Probably the most insidious of hedgehog complaints is lungworm infestation with *Crenosoma*

striatum and *Capillaria aerophila*. Starting before birth by crossing the placental barrier, *Crenosoma* sp. seem to affect most hedgehogs and particularly juveniles during the autumn. Symptoms are not always obvious but a moist chesty cough in some cases does point to lungworm problems. Sometimes there is respiratory distress, usually when a pneumonia has set in.

The lungworm can be verified by parasitological examination of the faeces or by post-mortem. Practically every hedgehog that dies of natural causes in the autumn is a victim of the infestation. The Wildlife Hospital Trust (St Tiggywinkles) and Mean (1998) have over the years carried out studies of the efficacy of various anthelmintics and have now recommended a course of pro-active treatments which includes corticosteroids and antibiotics (Table 21.1). Corticosteroids are used because when the lungworms are killed an inflammatory reaction can result and become an even greater problem. The corticosteroids are to reduce the inflammation.

Pneumonia

Hedgehogs are often found suffering from severe respiratory distress. Apart from the lungworm there are also going to be pneumonias caused as a direct result of heavy parasite burdens and other factors. Various drugs are at the veterinary surgeon's disposal and here are some of those we have used

Table 21.1 Hedgehog worming regime.

St Tiggywinkles
The Wildlife Hospital Trust

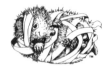

Drug	Dose	Frequency	Effect
Levamisole (Levadin – Univet)	20 mg/kg	Three injections (1 week between each)	Wormer
Etamiphylline camsylate (Millophyline-V – Arnolds Veterinary Products)	28 mg/kg	One dose given on admittance then given with each levamisole dose, and on the day following each dose	Bronchodilator
Methylprednisolone (Depo-Medrone V – Pharmacia & Upjohn)	Up to 4 mg/kg	One off injection given with first levamisole	Corticosteroid
Amoxycillin (long acting)	40 mg/kg	Given with methylprednisolone and every third day after, for a total of three doses	Antibiotic

without seeing any adverse side effects (Stocker, 1998):

- Enrofloxacin – Baytril 5% (Bayer)
- Bromhexidine – Bisolvon (Boehringer Ingelheim)
- Etamiphylline camsylate – Millophyline-V (Arnolds Veterinary Products)
- Clenbuterol – Ventipulmin (Boehringer Ingelheim)

Hedgehogs with respiratory distress are kept in plant propagators fed with oxygen. Respiratory drugs can also be nebulised if the patient is seriously distressed.

Balloon syndrome

Another, possibly respiratory, condition seen in hedgehogs is described as 'balloon syndrome' (Plate 34) (Stocker, 1987). With this condition the hedgehog's normally flexible skin covering is inflated like a balloon. The skin is stretched taut and the hedgehog cannot reach the ground with its legs. It is helpless.

No reasons have been found for this condition but possibly damage to the respiratory system has allowed inspired air to escape and fill the subcutaneous cavity. Relief is provided by a veterinary surgeon either making a scalpel incision over the back of the animal, or aspirating with a large gauge needle and syringe and a three-way tap, between its spines. Release of the air may need to be repeated several times but eventually the condition will resolve itself.

Antibiotic cover by long-acting amoxycillin is usually adequate.

Intestinal flukes

Hedgehogs, especially juveniles, will occasionally show a green, mucus-like faeces. In most cases this seems to be caused by the fluke *Brachyleamus erinacei* in the intestines (Mean, 1998). Treatment can be provided by a one-off injection of praziquantel – Droncit Injectable (Bayer) at 5.68 mg/kg (0.1 ml/kg).

Tumours

Hedgehogs are seen with quite extensive tumours especially around the throat and within the mammary glands. The veterinary surgeon will decide whether to operate or use euthanasia.

There is scant information on the nature of these tumours so any histopathology results would be welcome to add to our existing records.

Spondylosis deformans

Some older hedgehogs will show a paralysis or reluctance to use the back legs. In the absence of a history of trauma there may be bony overgrowths (osteophytes) around the intervertebral joints. Treatment can be attempted with corticosteroids and analgesics but the condition is irreversible.

Dental conditions

Hedgehogs do suffer from dental disease seen both in wild and captive animals. All hedgehogs should receive a dental examination on admittance and, if necessary, be treated before they are released.

A pre-treatment and post-treatment course of antibiotics is always to be recommended. Oral medicines are difficult to administer to some hedgehogs but we have found it useful for dental cases. The antibiotic of choice is metronidazole and spiramycin – Stomorgyl 2 (Merial Animal Health), at $\frac{1}{2}$ tablet/kg given orally.

Paraphimosis and penis trauma

The hedgehog has an extraordinarily large penis. Occasionally it becomes extruded and because of its size is often seriously damaged. Urethrostomy may be necessary so all cases should be immediately referred to the veterinary surgeon.

Skin conditions

All these conditions will require definite diagnosis but three of them are regularly seen in hedgehogs and can possibly be the subject of standardised treatments.

Zinc deficiency

This may occur leaving the hedgehog with no spines and no hair. A completely bald hedgehog can be given a vitamin and zinc supplement (Vetamin & Zinc – Millpledge Pharmaceuticals) which might just encourage a regrowth of the pelage.

Ringworm

A fungal condition ringworm in hedgehogs, usually *Trichophyton erinacei*, does not fluoresce like common pet disorders. Lengthy dermatophyte tests may or may not confirm the Trichotophyte. In the meantime any hedgehogs with flaky skin and debris at the base of the spines can be started on antifungal treatment using enilconazole (Imaverol – Janssen Animal Health) in the form of a spray mixed 1:50 with sterile water and administered on a daily basis.

Mange

Mange caused by mites, in particular *Caparinia tripilis* (Fig. 21.2), can be identified under the microscope. Visually, in hedgehogs, it occurs as a powdery deposit around the ears and cheeks (Fig. 21.3). Treatment is with ivermectin (Ivomec Injection for Cattle – Merial Animal Health) at 400 micrograms/kg or mixed 1:9 with propylene glycol at 0.4 ml/kg.

Ear mites

Ear mites are very common and seem to be resistant to ivermectin. Relief for the hedgehog can be provided with one or two drops in each ear of neomycin and permethrin (GAC Ear Drops – Arnolds Veterinary Products) or ivermectin mixed 1:9 with propylene glycol.

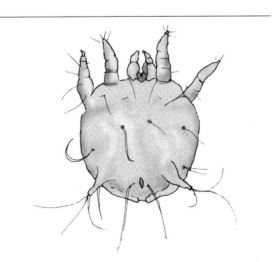

Fig. 21.2 *Caparinia tripilis* – a mite found on hedgehogs.

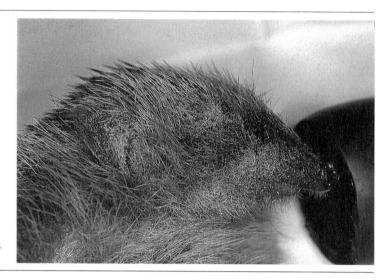

Fig. 21.3 Hedgehog mites may show as powdery deposits.

Other diseases

Some conditions have been reported in hedgehogs with very little opportunity for decisive treatments. These include:

- Protein-losing nephropathy causing extreme oedema on the ventral surfaces
- Avian tuberculosis in the mesenteric lymph nodes
- Salmonellosis

There are, undoubtedly, many more diseases to be found in hedgehogs. The database of information on this most regularly rehabilitated mammal is constantly growing. Any more data, new information or news of treatments are always going to be welcomed.

COMMON INCIDENTS

Already mentioned earlier in this chapter are the incidences of trapped hedgehogs. There are, however, many more situations that the unfortunate hedgehog will find itself in.

Road traffic accidents

Hedgehogs are renowned for getting into trouble on the roads. Most of them are killed outright but some do survive and are brought in as casualties. Their injuries are usually peripheral, to legs and head, so many of them do survive after treatment.

Dog attacks

Hedgehogs are often attacked by dogs, both large and small. The hedgehog under attack will curl up and manage to deter most dogs. Some dogs however, do press home their attack and cause the hedgehog serious injury usually resulting in major skin wounds or snout damage. The dog owners, full of remorse, tend to bring the hedgehog in for treatment.

Poisoning

Hedgehogs eat slug pellets which contain metaldehyde for which there is no antidote. The symptoms observed are mainly hypersensitivity where the hedgehog flinches at the slightest sound. It may also pass blue/green faeces from the dye in the slug pellets.

The hedgehog is probably going to die. Treatments can be tried including:

- The usual fluid therapy using Hartmann's solution (metaldehyde does lead to metabolic acidosis warranting the administration of bicarbonate of soda)

- Milk or sodium bicarbonate tubed straight into the stomach may decrease absorption of the metaldehyde
- Activated charcoal (Liqui-Char-Vet – Arnolds Veterinary Products) may absorb some of the metaldehyde

Other than these measures, supportive treatment and warmth may help overcome the toxicity but do not be too hopeful.

Hedgehogs will often enter garages or garden sheds and help themselves to any concoction lying around. They have been known to drink weedkiller, lick acid from a car battery or fall into tubs of oil or tar. The oil or tar can be treated as you would an affected bird but other poisoning will require the veterinary surgeon's input and possibly the Veterinary Poisons Information Service (see Appendix 7). Tar can be removed with warm water after it has been softened up with the hand cleanser 'Swarfega' (Deb).

Out during the day (ODD)

By far the most common incident that warrants a hedgehog being rescued is that it is out during the day (ODD), i.e. it has been seen out and about during the daylight hours.

Hedgehogs are very strictly nocturnal. They will only venture out during the day if:

- They are juveniles and have not been able to find enough food. This happens especially near the onset of winter
- They are sick or injured and have been unable to feed and build a nest
- They are young and have lost contact with their mother
- They are blind and have lost the concept of night or day

All the hedgehogs in these situations will fail if they are not taken into care.

Too small to hibernate (TSTH)

Nobody knows why a hedgehog picks a time to hibernate. It may be daylength, it may be temperature, it may be food shortage or some other reason. What we do know is that hedgehogs under the weight of 450 g have less chance of surviving hibernation than one of 600 g. For this reason many juvenile hedgehogs weighing less than 450 g at the end of November are taken into care and fed through the winter.

If they reach 600 g they are given the opportunity to hibernate in an outside pen. They are closely monitored with food available if they come out of hibernation. Eventually they are released in April or May.

Experience has shown that hedgehogs generally hibernate between January and March, but in some years, in warmer parts of Britain, they do not hibernate at all.

COMMON INJURIES

Fractures

Analgesia for all fractures can be provided with:

- Carprofen (Rimadyl – Pfizer)
- Flunixin (Finadyne Injection for Dogs – Schering-Plough Animal Health)
- Buprenorphine (Temgesic – Reckitt & Colman)

Leg fractures

Hedgehogs are often presented showing fractures of one or more legs. Usually the fracture is compound and grossly infected.

A simple fracture of the tibia, radius and ulna, metatarsal and metacarpal bones can be stabilised using old-fashioned plaster of Paris casts. Plaster of Paris seems to be more manageable in hedgehogs than the more modern materials.

Of course, even the simplest cast will not be able to be put on without the hedgehog being anaesthetised. A small face mask fashioned out of a sphygmomanometer bulb is ideal for administering isoflurane and oxygen or halothane and oxygen (Fig. 21.4).

Fractures of the femur or humerus may be internally fixated using suitably sized hypodermic needles as pins. Compound fractures, usually of the tibia or radius and ulna can be stabilised with extra-cutaneous fixation even while the wounds are being treated. This method is also useful as a last resort when an infected compound fracture will not

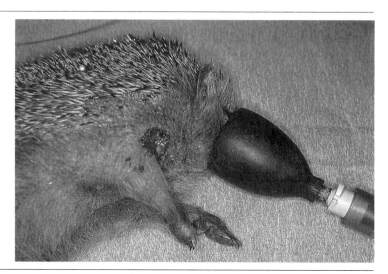

Fig. 21.4 A face mask for hedgehog anaesthesia can be fashioned from a sphygmomanometer bulb.

respond to treatments. With an extracutaneous fixator in place the wound can be left open and treated topically with hydrogels like Intrasite Gel (Smith & Nephew).

Most antibiotics show no adverse effects on hedgehogs although cephalexin has not been proven with regular use. Soluble antibiotics for addition to the drinking water have been found to be a complete waste of time.

Jaw fractures

Often caused by dogs, fracture of both the top and bottom jaw are fairly common. The top jaw can be wired and usually the palate is torn and needs suturing. The bottom jaw and symphysis can be wired.

Spinal fractures

A hedgehog with a fractured spine will not be able to use its back legs and is usually presented showing its hindquarters protruding from beyond its spiny coat. These are the exact same symptoms seen in a hedgehog with another condition I have called 'pop-off syndrome' which *can* be cured (see page 192).

An x-ray is needed to confirm a fractured spine or not, as the case may be. At the veterinary surgeon's decision, the hedgehog may have to be humanely destroyed by euthanasia.

Euthanasia is from the Greek meaning 'painless death'. It is impossible to provide a painless death to a hedgehog unless first it is anaesthetised and then given intracardiac barbiturates. Without anaesthesia, and certainly without unrolling the hedgehog under anaesthetic, there is no way the lethal injection can be given painlessly.

However, if a vein could be accessed then an intravenous injection of barbiturates would not cause the hedgehog unnecessary suffering as would an injection into a sentient hedgehog.

Crushed foot disease (CFD)

Hedgehogs often appear with injuries that defy reason. Quite a lot of hedgehogs have just one foot with all the bones crushed, full of infection and leaking pus (Plate 35). It is still a mystery how these injuries happen and why no other part of the hedgehog is injured.

Treatment is very difficult as the infection will have spread right through the foot to be almost a cellulitis. Bacterial sampling of any exudate may indicate a suitable antibiotic but, even when the infection is cleared, the best the hedgehog can hope for is a solid foot. The leg may have to be amputated and the hedgehog kept in captivity.

Skin wounds

Major wounds

Usually as victims of road traffic accidents or dog attacks, hedgehogs are often admitted with extensive skin wounds sometimes covering 60–80% of the back spiny coat. It is probably because the hedgehog has a very loose skin covering that the skin is ripped away with very little damage to underlying tissue. The wound may look horrendous but if the hedgehog is kept on continuous fluids the loose skin can be pulled over and sutured. There is very seldom any skin lost. Usually these wounds are freshly inflicted and are clean but contaminated making treatment that much more feasible.

To prepare the wound for suturing it should be filled with hydrogel (Intrasite Gel – Smith & Nephew) or K-Y Lubricating Jelly (Johnson & Johnson) while the spines surrounding the edges are cut back and the wound flushed with sterile saline. The edges can then be sutured or stapled together (Plate 14).

Face wounds

Just as alarming as the massive skin wounds are the face wounds that hedgehogs seem to suffer presumably from lawn mower/strimmer injury or dog attack.

Usually the skin is intact but pulled out of place exposing the nasal bones and soft tissues. After preparation the skin can usually be carefully sutured back into place using fine Vicryl (Ethicon) with swaged-on needles.

It is important that as a starting point the skin surrounding the eyes, simply a hole in the skin, is put back in place and held while the rest of the face is reconstructed. Daily dressing with Intrasite Gel (Smith & Nephew) will speed the healing process.

Fly strike (myiasis)

During the summer months every hedgehog casualty is likely to have been the victim of attack by blow flies. The evidence may be in the form of eggs or larvae from fresh hatches up to full-grown maggots. These will kill the hedgehog unless they are controlled.

Fly eggs

These may look like minute grains of rice and can be anywhere there is a likelihood of moisture. The eyes, ears, nose, mouth, face and underarms are all favourite laying sites. They can be picked off with forceps or brushed off with a stiff washing-up brush. Those in the eye sockets can be expelled by sliding the fingers from behind the socket pushing the eggs out of the eye socket. Filling the eye sockets with bland chloramphenicol eye ointment will smother any eggs that may have been missed.

Sometimes the eggs will have recently hatched into the same situations. Brushing them off will remove the larvae and the chloramphenicol in the eye sockets will suffocate them. The mouth can be flushed with a proprietary mouth wash. One or two drops of GAC Ear Drops (Arnolds Veterinary Products) in each ear will cover any maggots missed.

Coumaphos, propoxur and sulphanilamide (Negasunt – Bayer) seems to be the best preparation for killing fly larvae. Unfortunately it does appear too toxic for hedgehogs. An effective larvacide that can be used topically in small amounts on hedgehogs is ivermectin (Ivomec Injection for Cattle – Merial Animal Health) mixed 1:9 with water. It is not very stable once mixed and should be used immediately. Restrict the topical use of this mix to a maximum of 1.0 ml/kg.

Hedgehogs with fly strike should also be given a subcutaneous injection of ivermectin at 400 micrograms/kg to cover any straggler maggots not discovered.

Maggots

The fly eggs hatch into maggots often within hours of being laid. Contrary to popular opinion maggots will attack sound flesh as well as necrotic material. As they grow the maggots will burrow into the animal and are seen as groups buried deep in the tissues with their hindquarters only showing.

Each maggot should be picked off with forceps and destroyed. Large infestations covering massive areas of the body can be flushed out using warm saline in a Water Pik (Teledyne).

A covering injection of ivermectin will deal with the occasional straggler maggot. Broad-spectrum antibiotics, such as long-acting amoxycillin, should be provided.

Maggots do create toxins that can be taken up by the affected animal. If there is a massive maggot build-up then a drug with antitoxin, anti-inflammatory and analgesic properties will help the hedgehog recover. The drug we have found to be suitable is flunixin (Finadyne Injection for Dogs – Schering-Plough Animal Health) at 2 mg/kg intramuscularly for a maximum of 5 days.

Other injuries

Prolapsed eyes

Presumably caused by collision, prolapse of the eyes is far more common in the hedgehog than in other animals. The hedgehog's eye seems to be a very simple structure and when prolapsed withers almost immediately. Hedgehogs in semi-captivity can manage adequately without eyes. In cases of prolapse, the eye stalk can be simply ligated with absorbable suture material and the ball cut off. Broad-spectrum antibiotic eye ointment will control any infection.

Pop-off syndrome

This is one of those hedgehog-only conditions encountered in the mid-1980s (Stocker, 1987). With this condition the main orbicularis muscle, which is responsible for curling the hedgehog, seems to slip over the top of the pelvis (Fig. 21.5). This is usually self-induced by the hedgehog particularly in its struggles to escape after getting stuck in fences. It renders the hedgehog helpless and produces the same symptoms as the paraplegia of a fractured spine. X-rays will confirm the diagnosis one way or the other. If the orbicularis has popped-off it will not be possible to pull it back over the pelvis without the assistance of anaesthesia. Once it is replaced 'pop-off' should not recur.

Ligatures

Ligatures from garden string, netting or anything hazardous are found on lame hedgehogs. Usually it requires anaesthesia to release them. Pressure necrosis is always possible so any afflicted hedgehog should be retained and monitored for at least 7 days.

Sometimes a ligature will have actually removed a leg completely. Hedgehogs can manage very well on three legs but it is best to keep them in semi-captivity where they cannot find another hazard to cause them even more injury and where they can be regularly checked for soreness.

ADMISSION AND FIRST AID

On admission all hedgehogs should receive fluid therapy either intraosseously, subcutaneously or in

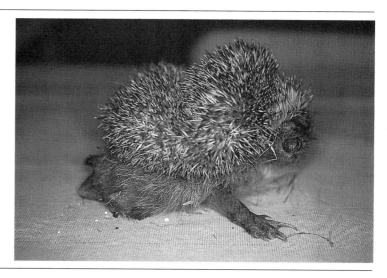

Fig. 21.5 Pop-off syndrome should not be confused with spinal injury.

large cooperative hedgehogs intravenously. Venous access in hedgehogs can be via the superficial veins of the hind legs.

It is sometimes impossible to assess a hedgehog's injuries because it curls up into a tight ball. Holding and rocking the hedgehog may encourage it to open up sufficiently for its underneath to be checked. However, if there is any suspicion of a life-threatening problem the hedgehog should receive its fluids, be left to stabilise for 30 minutes and then quickly anaesthetised with isoflurane and oxygen so that the full extent of any problems can be realised.

All hedgehogs once stable and not on any further medication should receive the full regime for lung-worm treatment.

Hedgehogs with more than one leg missing should be humanely destroyed.

CAGING

Hedgehogs are solitary animals that will often fight or attack others. During a stay for treatment they should be kept on their own. Provide newspaper on the floor and a clean towel each day for them to get underneath. Hay, straw or shredded paper do not suit hedgehogs who will often circle and end up with ligatures around their legs. Any that are classed as seriously ill should be provided with a metal heat mat at one end of their cage.

Once they have recovered they should be kept in much larger outside pens for at least 2 weeks before being released. If the pens are large enough more than one hedgehog can be kept together. A large sleeping box, this time with hay as bedding, will be used by all the hedgehogs.

For overwintering youngsters that have been cleared of illness and disease, we provide indoor cages (Ferret cages – Rolf C Hagen) with three to four hedgehogs in each cage. These are kept in a room with an ambient temperature of 18°C. Once these hedgehogs reach a weight of 500 g, and because of the numbers involved, they are put into large outside pens with other hedgehogs of similar weight. They are provided with communal sleeping boxes with hay bedding. They are all physically examined each day. Food and water are provided at all times. The hedgehogs are maintained in these pens until their release in April or May.

FEEDING

In the wild, hedgehogs feed on all manner of invertebrate prey. In captivity it is neither feasible nor affordable to provide this type of diet. Hedgehogs will receive a suitably balanced diet by being offered tinned dog or cat food. Fishy cat food is not suitable.

Each hedgehog will consume at least a third of a tin of dog food each night. In captivity they can overeat and become obese. Their weight in captivity should be restricted to about 1200 g. The problem with a long stay on a soft diet is the inevitable build-up of calculus on their teeth.

To combat this add to their soft food a dog or cat pellet that is palatable to hedgehogs. In particular hedgehogs relish Hill's Canine Growth or Feline Growth or Maintenance Food while often rejecting other dry foods. The Feline Growth pellets seem to be particularly favoured by juvenile hedgehogs and those reluctant to take the normal dog or cat food.

Adult hedgehogs should only ever be offered water to drink. Milk is likely to cause intestinal problems and, in fact, should never be considered for any adult animal.

Hedgehogs with mouth problems or other disabilities can be offered complete liquid nutrition. Vanilla-flavoured Ensure (Abbott Laboratories) is eminently suitable especially for animals recovering from food deprivation.

Biscuits, nuts, cheese or vegetable matter should not be offered to hedgehogs. They are insectivores without the intestinal refinements to cope with these inappropriate foods.

RELEASE

Hedgehogs are not territorial and need not be released specifically where they were found. That is unless the particular hedgehog is obviously a nursing mother and can be returned within 24 hours. Apart from this proviso hedgehogs can be released in gardens subject to the following conditions:

- That there are hedgehogs in that area – showing good habitat
- That they have unfettered access to at least 10 other gardens

- That there are no badger colonies in the immediate vicinity
- That there is a reasonable chance of the hedgehogs avoiding roads – complete avoidance of roads is not possible in this country but major A and B roads are the greatest hazards
- That generally the neighbouring gardens are reasonably free of molluscicides and dangerous dogs
- That any ponds should have escape ladders for hedgehogs

The hedgehogs should be released via a suitable nest box where they can return if they so wish. Marking the hedgehogs with correction fluid will identify any that do return.

Studies have shown that reared or rehabilitated hedgehogs do comfortably make the transition from captivity to freedom (Morris, 1999). However, recent blood assays taken from hedgehogs due for release from The Wildlife Hospital Trust (St Tiggywinkles) are showing that a seemingly perfectly fit hedgehog may be disguising internal problems (JCM Lewis, pers. comm.).

We are now considering that each hedgehog should be given a clean bill of health by the veterinary surgeon before it is released. In particular:

- Teeth should be cleaned and overhauled
- Blood samples should be taken and assessed

On release hedgehogs should weigh at least 450 g during the summer, 500 g up to the end of November and at least 600 g up until the middle of December. Hedgehogs would benefit from not being released from the middle of December to the middle of April.

LEGAL IMPLICATIONS

In the wild the hedgehog, like all wild mammals, is protected from some kinds of cruelty by the Wild Mammals (Protection) Act 1996. In captivity it is completely protected from cruelty by the Protection of Animals Act 1911.

Under the Wildlife and Countryside Act 1981 it is on Schedule 6 which prohibits its taking by certain methods.

22
Rabbits and Hares

Species seen regularly:

Rabbit (*Oryctolagus cuniculus*), brown hare (*Lepus europaeus*) and mountain or Irish hare (*L. timidus*).

NATURAL HISTORY

These three species are very similar to rodents in that they have open-rooted teeth that grow continually throughout life. They are, however, not classed as rodents but as a totally separate order, the lagomorphs.

Rabbits are well known and live underground in groups of burrows called 'warrens'. They will eat a wide range of herbage and, in particular, have been responsible for keeping the grass of open areas cropped short therefore moulding much of the landscape.

However, within 2 years of the introduction of the viral disease myxomatosis, in 1953, 99% of the population had died causing much of the grass landscape to grow longer and eventually revert to scrub. The change had drastic consequences for many species of wildlife the most severe of which was the extinction of the large blue butterfly (*Maculinea ariou*) as a British breeding species. Hares were one species that may have benefited from the longer grass as it offered more cover for their open nests, their 'forms' which are no more than shallow depressions, in the ground.

More recently the rabbit population has shown an increase, probably due to an increasing immunity to the various strains of myxomatosis.

Brown hares, on the other hand, are showing a rapid decline in numbers possibly due to mod-ern arable farming methods (Corbet & Harris, 1991).

The mountain hare is smaller than the brown hare and favours higher ground in Scotland and Ireland, where it has replaced its larger cousin. There is also a scant island population of mountain hares on the fells in Derbyshire. The mountain hare adopts a pure white coat in harsh, winter conditions and can regularly be seen glaringly dead by the sides of winter roads.

Rabbits and hares are noticeably different in that adult hares are much larger than rabbits and generally have a more athletic gangling make-up. Hares also give birth to young that are fully furred and have their eyes open. In contrast baby rabbits are born underground in 'stops'. They are naked, helpless and have their eyes and ears closed.

EQUIPMENT AND TRANSPORT

The only equipment that is functional for catching these animals is a large net with a long handle.

Carrying boxes should be enclosed, with ventilation holes low down, and made of cardboard or wood. Both rabbits and hares will remain quieter if they cannot see out of the box.

RESCUE AND HANDLING

It is generally rabbits that have to be rescued. These fall into three categories:

- Those injured in road traffic accidents
- Young rabbits caught by cats
- Rabbits infected with myxomatosis

All these incapacitated animals are still going to be elusive and need the long-reach net to be sure of catching them.

The difficulty often occurs when a rabbit with myxomatosis is spotted on the road and there is no net available. Its eyes may be closed but it can still have some hearing and sense of smell and will run blindly if anyone approaches it. The thing to do is to creep up on it from the road, so that if it does run it will not run into other traffic. Then when near enough to reach it, it should be grabbed securely around the body.

It will not bite but will struggle and possibly scratch with its hind legs. It is crucial that both rabbits and hares are controlled, as they are very susceptible to damage of the spine. Holding them should be with one hand clutching the scruff or around the shoulders. The other hand must be used to support the rump and stop the animal struggling (Fig. 22.1). The animal can then be gently put into a box and covered with a towel or blanket.

Rabbits and hares must never be picked up by their ears.

Both hares and rabbits have been known to die of cardiac arrest brought on by stress or fear of being caught. Diazepam at 1 mg/kg given intramuscularly will calm the animal during transport to the medical facility.

Hares are generally road traffic victims although some do survive being shot. More usual though is the arrival of supposedly orphaned young hares, leverets, which have been found sitting in the middle of a field (Fig. 22.2). This is quite normal behaviour, the leverets would remain unattended in their form until the female hare returns once during

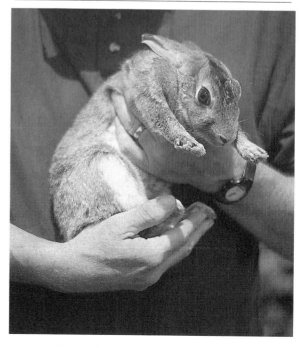

Fig. 22.1 Rabbits and hares must have their backs supported as they are handled.

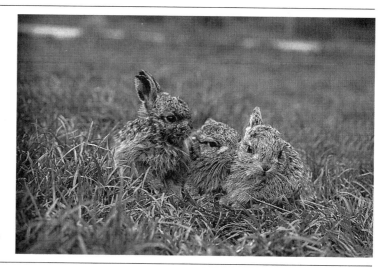

Fig. 22.2 Leverets should not generally be 'rescued'.

the night to suckle the youngsters and to stimulate and clean any faeces or urine.

Unfortunately it is not always possible to relocate the form and replace the leverets. They then have to be hand-reared, a particularly daunting task with such a sensitive animal. This is where the cry of 'Leave them alone' really does hold true.

COMMON DISEASES – RABBITS

Although infectious diseases in wild mammals should be natural phenomena, the two diseases that regularly kill wild rabbits are present in Britain solely through the action of man.

Myxomatosis

The myxoma virus is found naturally in the South American forest rabbit *Sylvilagus brasiliensis*. In this species it only causes mild, non-lethal disease. However, when the virus was introduced to Britain, in 1953, its effect was devastating. Within 2 years 99% of the rabbit population had perished.

Since that initial onslaught there have been frequent outbreaks of the disease, but with more animals being able to survive. These survivors are passing on their immunity and gradually the mortality rate has been reduced to between 40 and 60%. If this trend continues eventually the rabbit will enjoy the resistance to the virus seen with the forest rabbit. The myxomatosis virus does not affect any other species.

The virus is spread from rabbit to rabbit by fleas or biting flies. The incubation period is from 2 to 8 days after which the eyelids become swollen and closed. A purulent conjunctivitis further inflames the eyes and peri-orbital tissue followed by subcutaneous swellings and abscesses around the ears, neck, head, nose and anogenital region (Fig. 22.3). Although the affected rabbits will continue feeding and mating as normal, death usually intervenes within 11–18 days. However, some rabbits do survive to pass on any acquired immunity to future generations.

Myxomatosis is the most common reason why rabbits are caught and taken into care. Euthanasia has always been the recommended treatment for affected rabbits and, certainly, if we receive an animal exhibiting extreme suffering or having fits we will euthanase it. Some rabbits, though, are now recovering from the disease and can be given supportive treatments to bolster their active immune systems. Many of the animals in care show no distress and continue feeding and drinking normally until they either recover, die or are humanely destroyed.

After the stabilising treatments offered on admission, where all rabbits receive fluids and flea control, any apparently infected rabbits are started on an intensive course of treatment (Table 22.1). If they survive for 19 days they are presumed to have

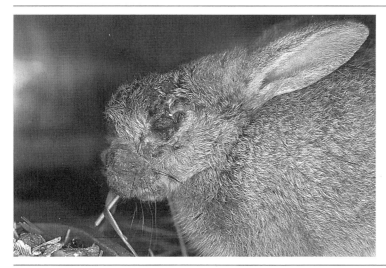

Fig. 22.3 Rabbits with myxomatosis will continue eating and drinking and may recover.

Table 22.1 Routine treatments for rabbits affected by myxomatosis.

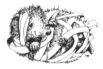

Drug	Dose	Frequency	Effect
Hartmann's solution	50 ml	Twice daily	Fluids
Enrofloxacin (Baytril 5% Injection – Bayer)	0.2 ml	Daily	Antibiotic
Etamiphylline camsylate (Millophyline-V – Arnolds Veterinary Products)	0.2 ml	Daily	Bronchodilator
Bromhexine hydrochloride (Bisolvon Injection – Boehringer Ingelheim)	0.3 ml	Daily	Mucolytic
Flunixin (Finadyne Injection for Dogs – Schering-Plough Animal Health)	0.15 ml	Daily for 5 days, than a 2-day break	Anti-toxin
Avipro (Vetark Animal Health)	Pinch	Daily on food	Pro-biotic

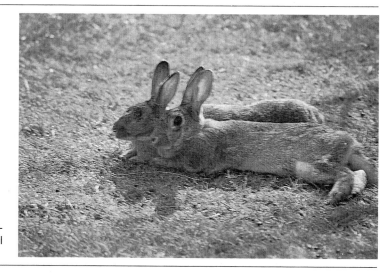

Fig. 22.4 Rabbits surviving myxomatosis may be blind but can settle to a full existence in captivity.

survived the infection and are prepared for release or retention in semi-captivity.

Those retained will be the animals with irretrievable damage to their eyes which usually require enucleation. It has been found that blind wild rabbits, having survived 19 days of intensive care, in fact become very steady and thrive with similar rabbits in open pens proofed against foxes (Fig. 22.4). They exhibit no signs of stress but should be neutered so as not to needlessly increase the population of rabbits.

Viral haemorrhagic disease (VHD)

This is a comparatively modern horror inflicted on rabbits. The viral disease emanated, in around 1984, from domestic rabbits in China. It took 10 years to finally be confirmed in Britain's wild rabbit population as recently as 1994 (Anon, 1994).

Transmission of the virus is by direct contact with infected rabbits or by rodents, insects or birds. Once in captivity it can be transmitted mechanically on equipment, feed or clothing. It is not transferable to humans or other species.

The symptoms of the disease include:

- Loss of appetite
- Depression
- Symptoms of respiratory distress
- Incoordination
- A blood-stained mucus discharge
- Death within 1–2 days

The disease has a high morbidity and a mortality rate in domestic rabbits close to 90% (Capucci *et al.*, 1997).

The incubation period is 24–72 hours followed soon after by death. Its affect is obviously devastating and probably too severe to be treated.

As it is there have been no confirmed cases being offered for rehabilitation but strict precautions should be taken if any sick rabbit is taken into care. A quarantine system similar to that used for animals affected by myxomatosis would be suitable with extra precautions to prevent mechanical transfer of the virus. Vaccination is available with Cylap (Fort Dodge Animal Health).

Coccidia

Both rabbits and hares may be infected with coccidia, especially *Eimeria* sp., which may cause diarrhoea especially in young animals. Confirmation of their presence can be from identifying oocysts in faeces samples.

Treatment can be provided in drinking water by mixing in sulphadimidine to give a 0.2% solution. Of course this may only be effective if the animal deems to drink.

Sulphamethoxypyridazine (Bimalong – Bimeda) may be a useful injectable to treat coccidiosis.

Now some proprietary rabbit foods contain a coccidiostat which may prevent the disease but these are unlikely to cure it.

Generally enteric problems, particularly in rabbits, are more complicated than simple coccidiosis. Any other symptoms will require an urgent and definitive diagnosis and prescription by the veterinary surgeon.

Endoparasites

Both rabbits and hares will carry a burden of endoparasites and may benefit from being treated with ivermectin (Ivomec Injection for Cattle – Merial Animal Health) at 200 micrograms/kg.

Hares in particular may well have a problem with the nematode *Graphidiem strigosum*.

Fly strike

Rabbits produce two types of faeces in pellet form. The caecal pellets are moist and expelled at night to be re-consumed by the rabbit. If they are not cleared they may leave a damp area which in daylight will be attractive to flies.

Similarly a rabbit with loose or diarrhoeic faeces may also attract flies to its anal region where most fly strikes in rabbits occur. The anal region on both newly admitted and captive rabbits should be checked for evidence of fly strike. If there is a history of diarrhoea or an obviously damp area then the whole hindquarters can be protected with an insect powder (WHISKAS exelpet – Pedigree Masterfoods).

Mycobacterium avium subspecies paratuberculosis

Greig *et al.* (1997) found evidence of this disease in 67% of a batch of wild rabbits killed on Tayside in Scotland. There is no evidence that this high incidence is repeated throughout Britain but, as there is a possibility, handlers should be even more aware of the essential hygienic conditions necessary when handling any wild animal.

COMMON DISEASES – HARES

European brown hare syndrome

A disease reported in hares is the viral disease European brown hare syndrome. It is apparently extremely virulent rather in the mould of VHD in rabbits. The author has no records of wild hares ever being presented for treatment at rescue centres suffering from EBHS. Just like VHD in rabbits, death is fairly rapid after contracting the disease. This is probably why no living, affected animals have been found and rescued.

Treponemal infection

Scabby lesions around the mouth and noses of brown and mountain hares, in central and southern Scotland, have been recognised for some years. During 1995 sections from 9 out of the 11 carcasses collected in the period 1992–93 were re-examined (Munro *et al.*, 1995). Spirochaetes were found in the epidermis of one brown hare and two mountain hares. This was probably the first record of treponema-like organisms in wild hares. More examples of hares showing scabby lesions are needed to establish the extent of the condition.

COMMON INCIDENTS

Apart from the three examples, road traffic victims, cat victims and disease victims, there are not many other regular occasions when lagomorphs may be presented for care. The only other situation likely to occur is the rescue of a survivor after being shot either with a shotgun from long range or an air rifle when one pellet may cause injury.

Malocclusion is unlikely to be seen in wild rabbits or hares. If it does occur it can be treated as it would in a domestic animal. However, the affected animal should never be released and may need regular treatment making a life in captivity untenable.

Spinal fractures requiring euthanasia are the most regularly seen fracture injuries in both rabbits and hares. However, young animals in particular may receive treatable fractures of the long bones in the legs.

Other injuries are likely to be particular to a situation and should be evaluated when they arise.

Antibiotics for rabbits should be supplemented with a pro-biotic to reinstate the gut flora.

Enrofloxacin (Baytril – Bayer) and amoxycillin with clavulanic acid (Synulox – Pfizer) have both been used systematically without any adverse side effects. Lincomycin, however, has been shown to be toxic in rabbits (Flecknell, 1991).

ADMISSION AND FIRST AID

Initially rabbits and hares should receive fluids intravenously. Access to a rabbit's cardiovascular system can be through the marginal ear vein with a butterfly infusion set that can be glued with tissue glue (Vetbond – 3M) into place. The vein can be dilated by applying digital pressure to the base of the ear. Hares are large enough to allow access to the cephalic veins.

Diazepam at 1 mg/kg is helpful in calming down a hare and a vitamin E/selenium (Dystosel – Intervet) intramuscular injection will help combat post-capture myopathy, a condition common in sensitive wild animals like hares and deer (see Chapter 25).

Broad-spectrum antibiotics, long-acting amoxycillin, can be provided as a cover for the effects of shock.

All rabbit admissions are potentially carriers of myxomatosis or infective fleas whether they are obviously diseased or not and could pass infection on to other rabbits. An admission protocol will keep disease transmission under control:

- After fluid administration a rabbit must be dusted with flea powder (WHISKAS exelpet – Pedigree Masterfoods). In 1997 Cooper & Penaliggon reported that the manufacturer (Rhone Merieux) of fipronil (FRONTLINE Spray) recommended that the spray was unsuitable for use in this species.
- The rabbit should then be put into a cardboard box for 15 minutes so that the fleas can die off.
- The rabbit is then put into a quarantine cage where it is held for 10 days.
- Myxomatosis victims, after their initial medication, are put into bird-holding facilities where no fit rabbits are kept.
- Any carrying boxes, hay or bedding used in admitting the animals are incinerated.

CAGING

Rabbits can be kept in any large cage. The use of wooden rabbit hutches should be avoided as it is almost impossible to keep them sterile.

Once they have recovered, rabbits should be put out on grass inside a wire pen with housing at one end. A chicken ark without any floor is ideal.

However, it should be moved every day or else the rabbits will burrow out.

Hares should be kept in isolated sheds well away from the hubbub of general practice.

FEEDING

All these species will appreciate fresh grass, chickweed and, favourite of all, dandelion leaves. For a more balanced diet there are proprietary foods available at most pet stores and agricultural merchants.

Rolf C. Hagen produces two rabbit products:

* Rabbit pellets in a 5 lb polybag
* Gourmet rabbit mix in 1 kg packets

However, as soon as possible, rabbits should be put out on to grass or weedy areas.

RELEASE

There is obviously going to be controversy from farmers about releasing rabbits on to farmland. We overcome these objections by finding release sites with no farming interest. In particular upland areas with open grassland and other rabbits tend to be amenity areas that welcome natural lawn mowers.

Hares are more suited to farmland but can be persecuted if they are not welcome. They do not damage crops on the scale of rabbits so many farmers will be only too pleased to allow the release of hares on their land.

Rabbits blinded by myxomatosis should always be kept in semi-captivity. They settle really well (Fig. 22.4).

LEGAL IMPLICATIONS

With no formal protection specifically for these three species they are, however, protected from cruelty by the Protection of Animals Act 1911 and the Wild Mammals (Protection) Act 1996.

23
Red Fox

NATURAL HISTORY

The red fox is the only canid native and resident in Britain. It was never a plentiful predator until its numbers were artificially swollen by Scandinavian and other European foxes introduced for hunting in the nineteenth century.

In Britain, since the demise of the wolf, the fox is seen as the foremost predator and top of the food chain. After the scourge of myxomatosis in the 1950s, the field vole has replaced the rabbit as its chief prey item but the fox is very adaptable and will take other small mammals and birds as well as insects, carrion, fruit and other vegetable matter.

Its renowned adaptability has seen the fox, in recent years, move into and thrive in urban areas. Here there is less disturbance and persecution and a ready supply of food ranging from rats and mice to pigeons, hand-outs and fast food waste. Foxes do not attack cats but will take advantage of the situation if it finds one already dead.

The fox, contrary to public opinion, is a very clean animal although its strong odour may be conceived by some as unclean. It lives in family groups, in a marked territory, regularly patrolled by the dominant dog fox. Both the alpha pair make loyal parents often assisted in rearing by the non-breeding vixens in the group. The cubs are usually born underground during March and April. They stay with the group until late summer when the male cubs and some of the females will disperse to find their own territories.

EQUIPMENT AND TRANSPORT

Foxes are likely to attempt to bite anyone handling them. They may be very similar to a dog in appearance but they behave quite differently; whereas a dog will snarl and let a handler know it is going to bite, a fox will just bite with no advance warning.

The equipment needed to safely handle a fox is just like that used for a dog but it has to be used to its full purpose; any short cuts or lack of concentration will result in somebody getting bitten.

- A large net with a long handle and a padded rim can still be very useful. Added to this should be a walk-toward net which is like a high tennis net used to trap a mobile animal.
- A dog grasper with a quick release noose is the safest way of holding a fox (Fig. 23.1).
- A stout pair of gloves will offer a modicum of protection if the hands are exposed.
- The ideal tool used by many keepers, and still essential even with a caged fox, is a soft-headed broom with which the fox's head can be pinned down.
- Finally, a carrying basket made out of substantial wire mesh preferably with a crush facility to facilitate giving injections either for sedation or anaesthesia.

RESCUE AND HANDLING

If a fox can stand, and even if it has only three functional legs, it will still be very difficult to catch. It

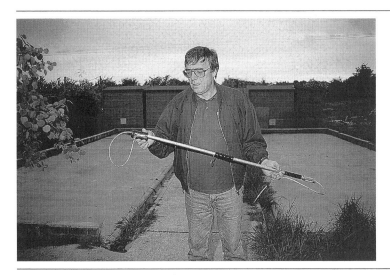

Fig. 23.1 A typical dog grasper used to initially catch a fox.

will be able to outrun even the fastest person so tactics are the sure way of capturing a casualty.

Before any attempt can be made to contain a casualty fox the carrying basket must be opened and ready. Once the fox is caught there will be no time to mess around trying to open the basket.

A mobile fox is best caught using either of the nets. The idea is to cover any escape routes and then to give the fox no opportunity to go any other way. It is worth remembering that a fox is as agile as a cat and will think nothing of scaling a 2 m fence to evade capture.

One person, with a long-handled net, should stay out of sight on the proposed escape route. The other person approaches the fox from the opposite direction. If that person also has a long-handled net it may be possible to capture the fox before it runs. If not, as it runs through the intended escape the other person, in one quick movement, brings the net down in front of the fox so that its impetus carries it into the net. The net is then held firmly on the ground.

The other person then approaches and pins he fox's neck to the ground, through the net, with the soft-handled broom. It is then possible to carefully scruff the fox through the net and pick it up. The fox and net can then be put into the carrying basket and the lid closed down. The fox is then released, the lid closed further and the net pulled out through the gap. The lid is then bolted shut.

At all times it must be stressed that the fox can and will bite through the net if it is given the opportunity.

With the walk-toward net there is less control of the fox once it has been caught. This is where the heavy gloves can be used to control the fox through the netting until it can be scruffed. It is better not to wear thick gloves when actually scruffing a fox.

Where a fox is confined, say under a shed, the dog grasper is slid over its head and closed around its neck. The fox is a fragile animal so too much pressure may cause serious injury. Just enough pressure to control it is all that is needed. With the fox under control, it is then pulled into a position where it can be scruffed. As soon as the scruff is held the grasper should be released. Do not use the grasper to pick up the fox by its neck. Once it is safely scruffed the fox can be easily put into the open basket and the lid closed.

Never ever try to just reach out and grab the scruff of a fox that is not under control. It will bite.

Generally though, scruffing a fox will make it relax rather as it does with cats. However, whenever the fox is picked up, its rump must be supported either by clutching fur over the rump (Fig. 23.2) or, when scruffed, by supporting the rump with the free hand.

No animal, especially a fox, should ever be picked up by its tail.

Throughout all these capture and handling procedures the fox remains a very frightened animal.

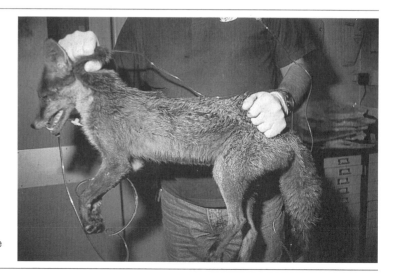

Fig. 23.2 A fox should be carried by the scruff and the rump.

Even when terrified it will still be concentrating on escape and will not hesitate to bite as this is its only means of defence. And always remember that a fox is far quicker at biting you than you can ever be in avoiding a bite. Take care.

COMMON DISEASES

Sarcoptic mange

One of the most common diseases, and one of the most obvious, that affects foxes is mange caused by the mite *Sarcoptes scabiei* (Plate 36). The mite is spread by contact.

The mite burrows into the skin and multiplies rapidly causing extensive hair loss and irritation starting at the base of the tail and hind feet and quickly spreading over the rump, back and finally to the head. With the fox scratching the irritants, tissue fluid is released forming an extensive crust of up to 1 cm thick (Plate 37). The fox may lose 50% of its bodyweight, most of its hair, its eyes and face will become encrusted and eventually the fox will die in about 4 months (Corbert & Harris, 1991).

Unfortunately the disease is usually well advanced when the affected fox is debilitated enough to be caught. However, once it is caught the disease can be easily treated (Fig. 23.3).

Initially, for the first few days, any affected fox should be given only supportive treatments such as aggressive fluid therapy, followed by liquid nutrition. A course of broad-spectrum antibiotics, long-acting amoxycillin, should be instigated together with administration of an anabolic steroid, nandrolone, either daily (Nandoral Tablets – Intervet) or every 21 days (Laurabolin – Intervet).

Once the animal is stable the treatment to control the mange can be started:

(1) Initially a subcutaneous injection or oral dose of ivermectin (Ivomec Injection for Cattle – Merial Animal Health) at 200 micrograms/kg
Or
An intramuscular injection of doramectin (Dectomax Injectable Solution for Cattle and Sheep – Pfizer) at 300 micrograms/kg
(2) The daily provision of essential fatty acids to ameliorate any allergic reactions to the mites can be supplied with Efavet™ 2 (Efanol) at 1 capsule/5 kg
(3) The ivermectin or doramectin is repeated after 2 weeks and then again, after another 2 weeks

The nandrolone and Efavet™ 2 (Efanol) should be continued throughout the fox's stay in captivity.

Zoonotic considerations

Sarcoptic mange is contagious to humans (and their dogs). In humans it is described as scabies and

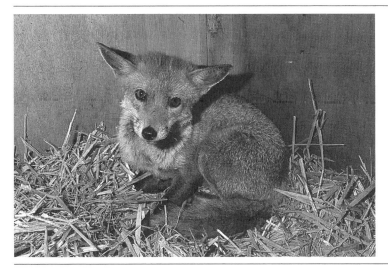

Fig. 23.3 Foxes can recover from sarcoptic mange.

should be referred to a general practitioner giving details of a possible contact source.

Dogs should not be treated but should be referred to the veterinary surgeon.

Scabies, in humans, is slow in progressing, whereas the other condition allied to sarcoptic mange rapidly spreads across the body. There appears to be, in some humans, an allergic reaction to either the dust or the mites involved. Its onset is rapid and within 2–3 days most of the torso is covered with an irritable rash. Any treatment appears to involve controlling the itching with soothing creams and proprietary antihistamines. The skin lesions usually clear spontaneously after about 3 weeks.

To avoid both of these conditions everybody handling a fox suspected of suffering from mange should wear a surgical mask, apron and gloves.

Jaundice

Most foxes that are brought in showing jaundice, a yellowing of the gums and mucous membranes, are suffering from internal haemorrhage. Only occasionally will jaundiced foxes be infected with infectious canine hepatitis or leptospirosis.

Infectious canine hepatitis (ICH)

Infectious canine hepatitis (ICH) is a disease of dogs and foxes. Most dogs are vaccinated against ICH and it has now become uncommon to see the disease in veterinary practice.

It is, however, fairly common in foxes but from which source nobody has really proven. There is a range of symptoms seen early in the disease but, as with mange, the fox has to be severely ill before it can be spotted and caught. By then the fox is usually showing jaundiced gums and mucous membranes and neurological signs.

The veterinary surgeon will require a blood sample to confirm the disease. This should be taken at triage before fluids are administered.

Antibiotics and B vitamins will assist in the treatment of the disease which is not always fatal in older animals. After the disease, foxes may develop a characteristic 'blue eye' caused by corneal oedema (Plate 38). This will usually clear.

The virus is shed in the saliva, urine and faeces of infected foxes. If a strict hygiene protocol is in place there should be no cases of cross infection between cages. However, the virus once shed is viable for up to 6 months.

Zoonotic considerations

Infectious canine hepatitis is not contagious to humans, but the clinical signs of jaundice could also be allied to leptospirosis which is contagious to humans. Strict barrier precautions should be taken with any sick fox until the veterinary surgeon has a confirmed diagnosis.

Leptospirosis

Canine leptospirosis is dangerous to humans causing Weil's disease which is potentially fatal.

In the wild leptospirosis is spread mainly in the urine of rats. In particular *Leptospira*, the Gram-negative bacteria involved, survives well in water. Foxes may contract the infection through killing and eating rats, through cuts and abrasions or contact with infected foxes. Clinical signs in foxes are usually taken as the jaundiced gums and mucous membranes. Confirmation of the disease can be by blood samples taken for laboratory testing or there is a canine antibody test kit (ImmunoComb – Biogal) which will give a guideline for the veterinary surgeon to follow through.

Any nursing of suspect animals should be under tight control and hygienic regimes. Some veterinary surgeons will regard the treatment of an infected fox as too high a risk for the staff involved. However, to some, barrier nursing and antibiotics may be feasible.

With a confirmed diagnosis the finders of the fox and anybody involved with its handling or care should be advised that if they develop any flu-like symptoms they must report to their general practitioner with details of the possible exposure. Treated early enough Weil's disease can be controlled if it is identified.

Endoparasites

Normally, as with all wild animals, a normal burden of parasites should not be a problem. However, by the time a fox is caught and brought into care it is usually seriously debilitated with a growing parasite problem. Treatment with ivermectin or doramectin, as in the mange treatments, will redress the problem.

Foxes will also harbour the tapeworm *Taenia serialis* and *T. pisiformis* as well as *Echinococcus granulosus* which can lead to hydatid disease in man. Control is with praziquantel (Droncit Injectable – Bayer) at 5.68 mg/kg.

Dental disease

Wild animals should not normally suffer with peridontal disease. Endodontic disease, however, is seen as broken teeth, especially canines are common, often exposing the pulp leaving it susceptible to invasion by bacteria and further infections. These could possibly include:

- Local infection to the jaw bone
- Systemic infection to the kidneys and heart valves
- If chronic can lead to amyloidosis and death

A fox's teeth are sharp but fragile and easily broken. To release a fox with broken teeth and pulp exposures is tantamount to abandoning it.

Before any fox is released it should receive a complete dental overhaul including root filling, extractions and general cleaning. Crowns, bridges and any cosmetic repairs are totally inappropriate.

Other conditions

Other conditions seen in fox casualties include hydrocephalus in cubs and bacterial pneumonias in adults.

COMMON INCIDENTS

It is amazing how foxes suffering from the advanced stages of a disease appear to seek out human habitation and are regularly found in sheds, garages or barns. Foxes on the roads do tend to be killed outright or else struggle off never to be found. They do seem to be less susceptible to road accidents than badgers, otters or deer. The other situation where foxes are found is when they manage to get themselves trapped.

Fences

A fox will quite often be found where it has tried to negotiate a fence but has got one leg caught in wire or chain link (Fig. 23.4). It usually has to be cut loose with fencing pliers, but it should not be immediately released because inevitably there will be some pressure necrosis leading to the need for long-term care.

Snares

Unfortunately some snares are still legal in this country (Fig. 23.5). Foxes are a regular target and

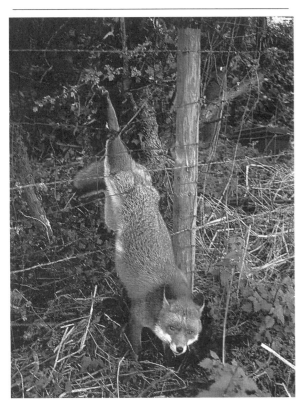

Fig. 23.4 Being caught in a fence may lead to pressure necrosis.

are often found by people out walking. Once again the snare can be cut with fencing pliers but the fox should not be released until it has been monitored for several days in case of pressure necrosis at the site of the injury.

Poisoning

It is illegal to poison foxes but it does happen. Unfortunately it is not always possible to identify the poison used so treatments, other than supportive therapy, are probably going to be ineffective.

If poisoning is a distinct possibility:

- The Wildlife Incident Unit of the Ministry of Agriculture, Fisheries and Food should be informed on freephone 0800 321 600
- If the poison is identified then the Veterinary Poisons Information Service (see Appendix 7) may be able to advise on treatments.

COMMON INJURIES

Fractures

Fractures from road traffic accidents are of the long bones of the legs, the pelvis or the spine.

Long-bone fractures can be treated as would those in a dog. The main difference is that a fox will not tolerate a leg cast if it can manage to bite it off.

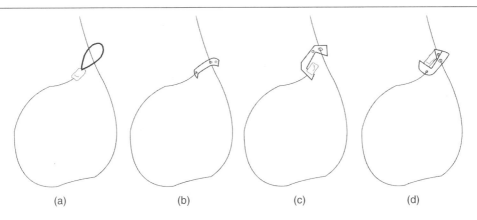

Fig. 23.5 Types of snares that are both legal and illegal, but still used. (a) Free-running (legal); (b) dual-purpose (free-running) (legal); (c) dual-purpose (self-locking) (illegal); (d) self-locking (illegal).

Even an Elizabethan collar will be ripped off and destroyed. From the outset all leg fractures, even temporary splints, should be cast in either resin or fibre-glass materials.

Pelvic fractures will usually respond to cage rest although vixens may need to be spayed before they are released if the pelvic canal is compromised.

Back in the wild, foxes will manage adequately if they have a hind leg or their tail amputated. They could not cope with the loss of a front leg, a course of action where possibly euthanasia may be the best option. A fox, even in a cage, uses its front legs to dig, without one leg it would be deprived of this essential part of its behaviour.

Bite wounds

As with other debilitating conditions, the fox with bite wounds is not going to be seen or caught until the wounds are totally infected and the animal is probably suffering from potentially life-threatening toxaemia or septicaemia. Toxaemia can be caused by toxins being released from abscesses formed at the site of the bite wounds.

Initially the fox should receive fluids coupled with:

- An intravenous infusion of a broad-spectrum antibiotic, e.g. enrofloxacin (Baytril 5% – Bayer) at 5 mg/kg daily
- Corticosteroids, e.g. methylprednisolone (Solu-Medrone V – Pharmacia & Upjohn) at 20–50 mg/kg intravenously
- Drugs to counter endotoxaemic shock

The wounds will have to be drained and treated as open abscesses.

If the tail is irreparably damaged it can be amputated with no detrimental effect on the fox's release.

Other injuries

Usually as a result of road traffic accidents, foxes have also suffered ruptured diaphragms, livers or spleens.

ADMISSION AND FIRST AID

At triage it is generally a safe exercise to muzzle the fox but be very aware that any bleeding in the mouth or vomiting could be life-threatening.

Intravenous fluids and corticosteroids can be simply administered through the cephalic veins or lateral saphenous veins. The latter may be preferable as even the most debilitated fox will chew through its giving set in a matter of minutes. For this reason a fox should be given as much fluid as possible while it is being controlled and observed. Once it is in a recovery cage it will destroy the drip.

A very excited or unmanageable fox can be sedated using diazepam at 1 mg/kg given intravenously or intramuscularly.

CAGING

Foxes are very destructive and will constantly try to dig or bite their way out of any cages. Wooden cages are not really suitable. Solid kennels with barred gates are preferable. The use of wire mesh is not recommended as foxes will often fracture their canine teeth in their effort to escape. However, in the presence of humans the foxes will usually lie undisturbed. They will become active, at night, when they are left alone.

Foxes do not need bedding but plain newspaper is ideal for the bottom of their cages. They will tip food and water bowls which should preferably be stainless steel and spill proof (Hagen Non-Spill – Rolf C Hagen).

Old logs will provide something to gnaw which will not damage their teeth.

Once out of cage care and prior to release the foxes should be kept separately in solid pens with barred gates. A hut will provide shelter. No bedding other than a raised platform is necessary.

FEEDING

In the wild the preferred diet of foxes is whole animals. In captivity these can be provided by buying frozen rabbits, chicks, mice or rats. Clean, fresh road kills of all species except hedgehogs will also be readily taken. If this diet is not available then any good-quality dog or cat food is adequate in the short term.

RELEASE

Adult foxes are strictly territorial and should be released exactly where they were found. If there is any doubt as to the exact location the author has known foxes travel 10 miles to get back to their territory. So just releasing in a suitable area near to where they were found would seem to be acceptable.

Obviously some areas with gamekeepers are going to be unsuitable for returning foxes. To relocate them to a safer area, try to pick the outskirts of a large town with a known fox population, like London or Bristol. Here a release pen with a shelter should be erected where the fox can be kept for a few weeks. After that the door can be opened surreptitiously and the fox allowed to make its own way out. Food and water will continue to be put in the pen so that the fox can return if it needs to.

Tame foxes, blind foxes and toothless foxes should not be released.

LEGAL IMPLICATIONS

The fox enjoys some protection against cruelty under the Protection of Animals Act 1911 and the Wild Mammals (Protection) Act 1996.

Unfortunately it can still be hunted with dogs, snared or shot. But this may change in the future.

24
Mustelids

Species seen regularly:
Weasel (*Mustela nivalis*), stoat (*Mustela erminea*), mink (*Mustela vison*), badger (*Meles meles*), otter (*Lutra lutra*) and occasionally polecat (*Mustela putorius*) and pine marten (*Martes martes*).

Domestic species:
Ferret (*Mustela furo*) and polecat-ferret.

NATURAL HISTORY

The mustelids are an advanced group of carnivorous mammals noticeable by their long, sinewy bodies. It is only the badger in this country, that has a more rotund shape.

The weasel, stoat, polecat and pine marten hunt and take all species of small mammal, bird, amphibian and reptile. The otter and, to some degree, the mink subsist on a diet of fish and aquatic crustaceans. Both species will also readily take frogs and small birds and mammals.

The badger, the largest and most numerous of Britain's mustelids, is an extremely powerful animal with a fairly omnivorous diet consisting mostly of earthworms and vegetable matter in drier weather conditions.

The polecat and pine marten are very rarely offered for rehabilitation whereas the scarce otter is becoming a more frequent casualty as it recolonises its former haunts in inland Britain.

The weasel and the stoat are occasionally casualties while the badger is very often in need of rescue and treatment.

The domestic ferret has evolved from wild polecat stock. It is used to hunt rabbits and frequently escapes from captivity. It has generally failed to establish a viable feral community as escaped ferrets are usually easily found, picked up and taken to rescue centres.

The polecat-ferret has similar, if somewhat paler markings than the truly wild polecat and it can usually be approached and picked up. The wild polecat is a much finer specimen and would not take kindly to being picked up. Its stronghold is in Wales but gradually it too is recolonising, in its case the West Midlands.

EQUIPMENT AND TRANSPORT

All species of mustelid have a very powerful bite. To handle the smaller species, the weasel and the stoat, thick welders' gloves are just about bite-proof.

The large species will easily penetrate thick gloves and should only be handled with the aid of a dog grasper. Otters should be caught with a net with a padded rim so that they cannot damage their teeth.

A soft-headed broom is always useful in controlling all the larger species, except otters may be able to writhe out of its control.

Similarly, containers to carry these animals must be robust and constructed of heavy gauge wire. Small baskets with 10 mm mesh are suitable for weasels and stoats. For the other species, especially badgers and otters, the need is for the really heavy-gauge baskets made especially for badgers. They should also have a crush facility in order to be able to inject the animal without opening the basket. An otter may be difficult to 'crush' in a basket designed

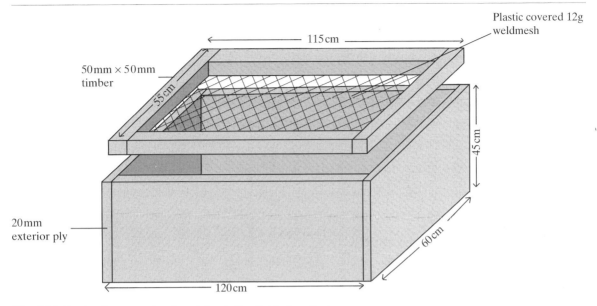

Fig. 24.1 Design for a wooden 'crush basket' suitable for otters.

for badgers but a 'vertical crush' basket can be made from timber (Fig. 24.1).

Apart from the power of these animals, many of them have the ability to emit obnoxious smelling liquids when captured. A sound ploy is to put a polythene sheet under the basket as it is transported in a car or van. The skunk (*Mephitis mephitis*), though not British, is also a mustelid and gives you some idea of the power of these protective scents.

RESCUE AND HANDLING

The badger is the mustelid most often in need of rescue (Stocker, 1994a), but as the numbers of otters increase they too are needing rescuing, especially in Scotland and Shetland. The other smaller species sometimes get into trouble but only those that are disabled are able to be caught.

All the species are dangerous but the badger and otter do possess the most serious bites, which must be avoided at all costs.

The road traffic victim that remains at the scene of an accident is usually seriously injured or unconscious. Surprisingly it will still have the ability to bite at lightning speed. This is where the broom comes in handy. First, as always, set down and open the carrying basket. The soft head of the broom is touched to the animal's head. If the animal does not react then the broom is used to *securely* pin the neck and head to the ground. Then, tentatively, an attempt can be made to scruff the animal. Badgers have surprisingly little scruff available so attempts at scruffing may be unsuccessful. If scruffing is unsuccessful then the dog grasper must be used. If a scruff can be held and the badger does not react, release the broom and with the free hand clutch a patch of skin and hair over the rump and lift the animal at arm's length. Put it immediately into the basket, release it quickly and shut the lid.

Otters have a surprising amount of loose skin around the scruff and should be securely scruffed with two hands (Fig. 24.2).

Sometimes a badger or otter will revive half-way through the procedure and before it is safely in the basket. Should the animal struggle free then do not attempt to re-catch the animal by hand but rather start again this time using the dog grasper or a padded net for an otter.

If there is any doubt about being able to control the casualty then do not hesitate to use the dog grasper. With badgers or otters the grasper is slid over the neck and over one front leg. The noose is

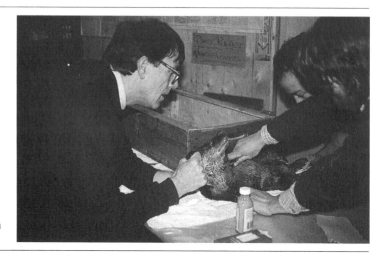

Fig. 24.2 An otter can be scruffed with both hands.

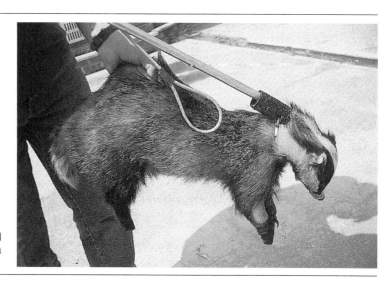

Fig. 24.3 Badgers are robust and strong. They should be picked up with a grasper and support of the rump.

slid forward to just behind the front leg, if possible, and pulled closed. These animals are powerful so the grasper should be closed as tightly as possible. With the grasper held tight in one hand, the free hand is used to pick up the animal by the rump, once again at arm's length. It should not be lifted just with the grasper (Fig. 24.3). The animal is then put into the basket, the lid closed on the grasper, the grasper released, withdrawn and the basket bolted shut.

Never pick up an animal by its tail which could be permanently damaged.

Badgers in particular are not as agile as the other mustelids and regularly fall into situations where they cannot get out. These have been dry wells, dry swimming pools, corn cellars and slurry pits (Fig. 24.4). Provided the badger has only been trapped during the previous night and is not injured, it can simply be rescued and immediately released.

The mink, polecat and pine marten should also be handled with a dog grasper. They are much more fragile than the larger species and should be handled more sympathetically. The noose on the grasper is slid behind but up against the front legs. It is important not to pull too strongly but simply and quickly lift the animal, on the grasper, and deposit it in the carrying basket.

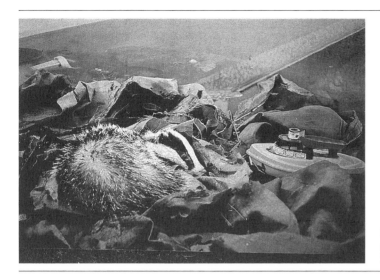

Fig. 24.4 Badgers will often fall into pits and not be able to climb out. This one fell into a dry swimming pool.

The weasel and stoat are too small for handling with a grasper, but stout gloves give adequate protection.

Once in captivity all these mustelids, especially the otter, are difficult to muzzle before any procedures are even attempted. As always, an animal with bleeding in the mouth or in danger of vomiting should not be muzzled. Diazepam at 1 mg/kg can be used to quieten the animal for first-aid procedures.

Badgers, with their short snouts, can be muzzled but will attempt to rip off any muzzle with their long front claws. As they are extremely dangerous animals they should be fitted with two muzzles, one of which should be a cotton open weave bandage (Vet W.o.W – Millpledge Pharmaceuticals) tied tightly. Badgers will not use their long claws in attack.

COMMON DISEASES

Most of the mustelid species are comparatively free of recognisable diseases. Any that may be suspected should always be referred to the veterinary surgeon for diagnosis and treatment.

Dental disease

Badgers, in particular, often show teeth that have suffered trauma, wear and disease. Pulp exposures in the canine teeth are common and should be treated before an animal is released. Otters also show traumatised teeth and all the other mustelid species should receive a complete dental overhaul before they are released.

Animals with four canines extracted should not be released and otters, which have to catch fish, should not be released if their canines are shortened after fractures and dental treatment.

Parasites

Internal

Apart from the normal burdens of ectoparasites the only notable nematode is *Skrjabingylus nasicola* which can infest the nasal cavity of most species. Control of nematodes is with ivermectin or doramectin.

External

Fleas and lice can cause major problems to badgers. Heavy infestation can be controlled with pyrethrum-based flea powders. The veterinary surgeon will be able to advise if there is a danger of anaemia in the affected animals and prescribe remedial treatments.

Bovine tuberculosis

Very much a disease plagued with controversy, bovine tuberculosis can infect both badgers and

Table 24.1 Estimated time periods of delayed implantation seen in some mustelids.

	Pine marten	Stoat	Mink	Badger
Mating	July–August	May–July	March	February–Autumn
Approximate date of implantation (beginning of gestation)	February–March	March–April	April	Late December–early January
Length of gestation	30 days	4 weeks	28 days	7 weeks
Probable month for parturition	March–April	April–May	May	February

domestic cattle. It is centred around the southwest of England in Gloucestershire, north Avon, Cornwall and sometimes in Devon. In these areas it is thought that up to 20% of badgers may be infected (Neal, 1977).

Common effects of the disease are tuberculous pneumonia and nephritis with lesions; often found are acute pleurisy, pericarditis, hepatitis, encephalitis, arthritis, osteomyelitis and general enlargement of the lymph nodes (Gallagher & Nelson, 1979).

In advanced stages of the disease changes in behaviour have been noted and a tendency to move into the environment of humans, often settling into barns and outhouses.

It is important to establish whether badgers in an area are likely to be infected with bovine tuberculosis. The veterinary surgeon will be able to advise and give direction on how to deal with suspect casualties. The basic principles are to take all precautions as the disease can be spread by aerosols from an infected animal, in urine and with discharges from wounds (Lewis, 1998). It is thought the disease is passed to other badgers through bites or respiratory aerosols.

Any staff likely to be involved in sensitive areas should ensure that their BCG vaccination is in place.

Aleutian disease

Some mustelids, notably mink and ferrets, are recorded as susceptible to the parvovirus Aleutian disease. Other species, particularly polecats, may be at risk.

All mink should be serologically tested on admittance and if registering positive, should be humanely destroyed. Quarantine in the intervening period is crucial. In this country it is illegal to release a mink and a licence is needed to keep one in captivity. Mink casualties may be taken by zoos as long as the animals have a certificate indicating a negative result for Aleutian disease.

There may be no symptoms if an animal is positive for Aleutian disease, but the disease itself can be very serious causing recurrent fevers, weight loss, thyroiditis, posterior paralysis and then death (Oxenham, 1991). There is no specific treatment so it is essential that the disease is not passed to other mustelids.

Delayed implantation

Some species of mustelid, namely badgers, pine martens, stoats and mink, practise 'delayed implantation'. With this phenomenon, which is still not fully understood, the animals can mate and fertilisation take place at almost any time of the year. However, the blastocysts on reaching the uterus do not implant in the usual way. Instead they remain free within the uterus before becoming embedded in the uterine wall, the animal effectively becoming pregnant for the normal time and giving birth a short while afterwards.

This phenomenon particularly affects rehabilitation efforts in that any of these species could be fertilised long before any gestation takes place, and may be pregnant even though it has been in captivity for up to 10 months (Table 24.1). The young may then be born even if the female has had no access to males of her species while in captivity. Every effort should be made to facilitate her to bring up her young as naturally and undisturbed as possible. Release should be as a group, into a new territory, once the young are grown.

Pneumonia

Many cases of pneumonia have been recorded in otters. Bacterial pneumonia or pleuropneumonia have both been reported in wild and captive animals (J.C.M. Lewis, pers. comm.).

COMMON INCIDENTS

Road traffic accidents

By far the most common cause of unnatural mortality in badgers, otters and polecats is being involved in a collision with motor vehicles. It is estimated that 20% of Britain's badger population are killed on the roads every year and 80% of known deaths of otters and polecats are also on the road. Possibly other mustelids, like pine martens, mink, weasels and stoats, also lose vast numbers to motor vehicles.

The smaller animals are probably always killed outright but some badgers and otters do survive the impact. On many occasions the injured animal will crawl off never to be found again, but many live casualties are left on the road, are rescued and brought in for treatment.

Bitten or ousted badgers

Just as diseased badgers will seek human surroundings so do many badgers that have been involved in fights or seem to have lost their place in the badger colony. The latter seem to be old badgers often with chronic dental problems and a general loss of condition, together with typical but extensive bite wounds over their rumps (Plate 39).

Although rescued badgers should be released where they were found, these old badgers should not be released. After their teeth have been sorted out and they have gained condition they may well be kept in a semi-captive colony.

If these badgers are young and fit they can be introduced to similar badgers and released via an artificial sett.

Vagrant badgers

Similarly, badgers are sometimes found in the centre of large towns where there is no recognised population of badgers. They may be ousted from a colony or simply lost but whatever the reason for their predicament they cannot be released where they were found. These too will have to be released through an adopted colony and an artificial sett.

Orphaned badgers

Other badgers regularly found in strange circumstances are freshly weaned cubs that appear to have strayed away from their home territory. There is no way of knowing where their home territory is and they would be in serious danger from other badgers if they were released in the wrong area. Orphaned badgers should also be included in a group release through an artificial sett.

Snares, netting and other hazards to badgers

Some snares are still legal for use in trapping some animals, like foxes and rabbits. They are illegal for use to trap badgers but they are generally indiscriminate and badgers regularly get caught in them.

A badger caught in a snare will struggle violently fraying the snare so that it locks tight when, in fact, it should be free running. It is probably not possible to safely relieve a badger of the snare without anaesthetic. Because of this trapped badgers should be taken, complete with snare still attached, to a treatment facility.

Similarly, badgers have been found trapped in football nets, tennis nets and pig fencing. They all have to be anaesthetised to have the offending material removed (Fig. 24.5).

Anaesthesia can be with isoflurane and oxygen via a face mask but if the badger is lively and dangerous then combinations of medetomidine (Domitor – Pfizer) at 100 micrograms/kg and ketamine at 5–7.5 mg/kg injected intramuscularly will relax the animal. Profound respiratory depression is a hazard the veterinary surgeon should be aware of. Atipamezole (Antisedan – Pfizer) is the antagonist to reverse medetomidine.

With all of these types of entanglement there is a distinct likelihood that pressure necrosis will become evident in the area from where the snare has been removed. Because of this any affected animal should be closely monitored for 7 days.

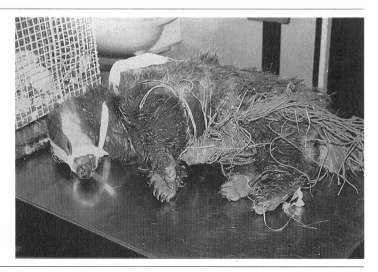

Fig. 24.5 Badgers trapped in netting will need to be anaesthetised to be safely extracted.

Cat attacks

The domestic cat is a prime predator and it will even attack smaller, usually juvenile or infant weasels and stoats. In fact they often present their owners with live weasel or stoat kittens.

Treated with a course of long-acting antibiotics to counter the bacteria inflicted by the cat, these tiny mustelids are simple to rear and release (see page 257). They are also easily tamed which would prohibit their release and so precautions to avoid taming must be taken.

COMMON INJURIES

Fractures

Badgers and otters that survive road traffic accidents may well receive fractures. However, because of the hefty make-up of these animals, fractures are not as common as they might be. Also this hefty make-up and muscular frame sometimes make the fractures hard to detect through palpation. Usually a casualty is reported to not be using one or two back legs. X-rays will pinpoint the fractures and give the veterinary surgeon a starting point in trying to treat them.

The long bones of the legs, the jaw and the skull have all been recorded as susceptible to fractures. Of course spinal or pelvic fractures can also occur

in serious accidents. It is usually the leg bones that are fractured and being difficult to immobilise with casting, the veterinary surgeon will probably have to resort to some type of mechanical fixation.

However, the bones of these animals have evolved for their specific lifestyles and are quite unusual compared with cats or dogs. Reference to a skeleton, or at least a diagram, does help (Fig. 24.6).

With fractures analgesia is going to assist the healing process. We have records of the use of flunixin, carprofen and, if there is no head trauma, buprenorphine with no ill effect.

In cases of paralysis or pelvic fracture, where there is a likelihood of recovery, then the animal's bladder should be checked at least twice daily and expressed if it is not emptying naturally.

Amputations

Badgers are notorious in having fractures that do not heal – non-unions. Sometimes amputation is the only remedy. Each animal requiring an amputation should be assessed of its suitability to cope in captivity.

All the mustelids would fail in the wild if they were to lose any leg. The hunting species would be at a distinct disadvantage and a badger without a front leg could not dig for food and without a hind leg would find it difficult to negotiate backwards out of tunnels.

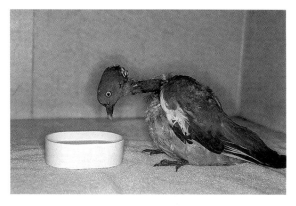

Plate 25 The wood pigeon, even after major suturing of neck wounds, is a very powerful bird.

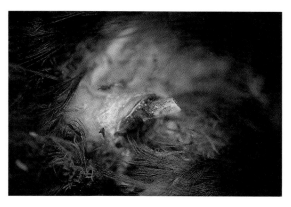

Plate 26 Casualty corvids often have exposed, devitalised bone fragments.

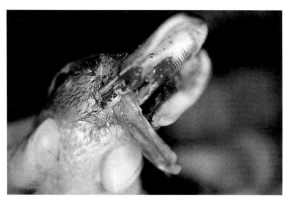

Plate 27a

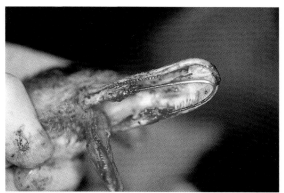

Plate 27b

Plate 27 The PKP method of fixing a prosthetic bottom beak to a duck (see also Plate 17). (a) The lower jaw has broken off just in front of the commisure of the beak. (b) A Kirschner wire is used as scaffold. (c) Suturing of the prosthesis to the soft tissue and skin completes the procedure.

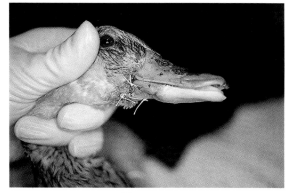

Plate 27c

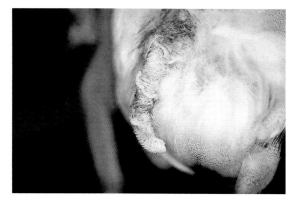

Plate 28 Prolapsed penis of a mallard drake.

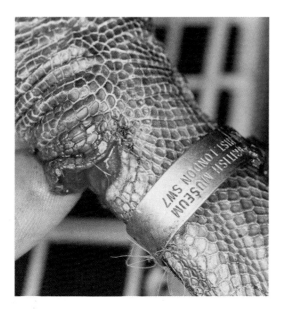

Plate 29 How a metal ring can slide up into the hock joint.

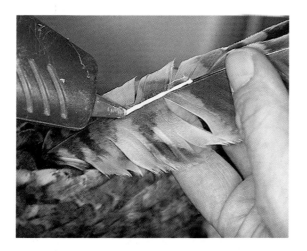

Plate 31 Hot gluing a bent feather on a tawny owl.

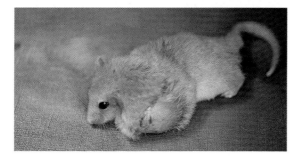

Plate 33 The hazel dormouse may have abscesses.

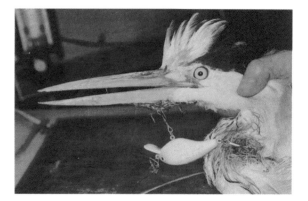

Plate 30 The beak of a heron can be a dangerous weapon.

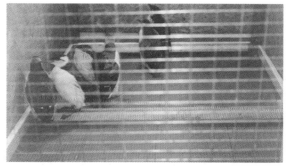

Plate 32 Washed birds are placed in a recovery area with overhead heat lamps (not shown).

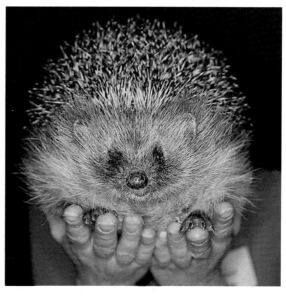

Plate 34 Hedgehogs may become inflated with balloon syndrome.

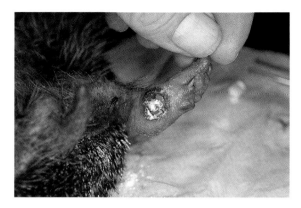

Plate 35 Crushed foot disease is another hedgehog phenomenon.

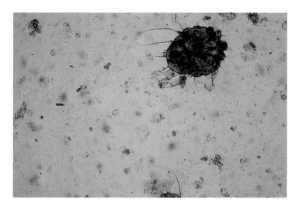

Plate 36 The mange mite *Sarcoptes scabiei* seen under the microscope.

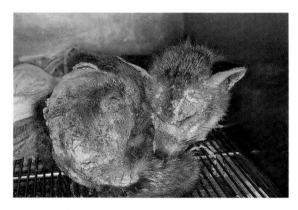

Plate 37 Sarcoptic mange will eventually kill a fox unless it is treated.

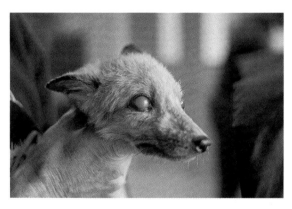

Plate 38 Infectious canine hepatitis (ICH) may leave a characteristic 'blue eye' (Photo: JCM Lewis).

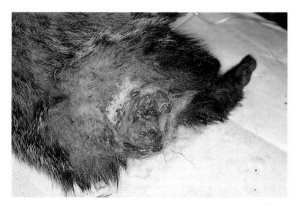

Plate 39 Typically badgers will inflict bite wounds to the rump area.

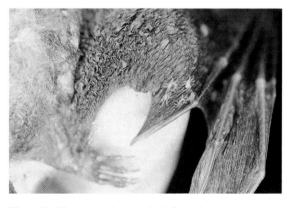

Plate 40 Many bats have mite infestation.

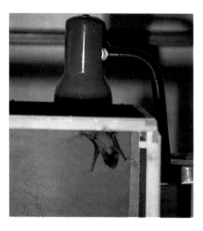

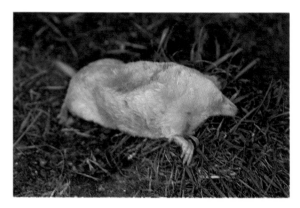

Plate 41 A butterfly cage, with an overhead heat source, makes ideal housing for bat casualties.

Plate 42 Moles are of various colours but are all the same species.

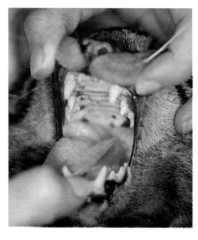

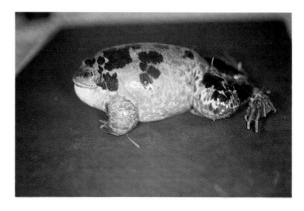

Plate 43 Wildcats, like all mammals, should have remedial dental work carried out especially after jaw injuries.

Plate 44 Frogs inflated with air can have it aspirated with a needle, syringe and three-way tap.

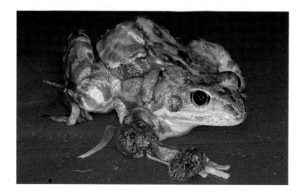

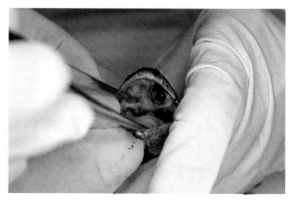

Plate 45 Frogs can have lacerations, received in garden accidents, sutured.

Plate 46 Frogs can sometimes adapt to disability.

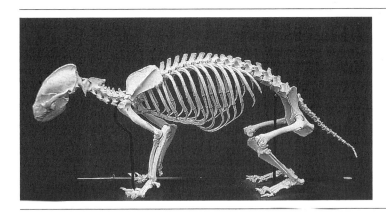

Fig. 24.6 Reference to a mounted skeleton of a badger will assist the veterinary surgeon with orthopaedic anomalies.

The hunting species could be kept in captivity but a badger has to dig and could not cope living on a solid base in a cage or pen.

Bite wounds

Badgers often fight with each other inflicting extensive but shallow bite wounds on each others' rumps above the tail (Plate 39). They will also bite around the head and neck. This is normal badger behaviour and usually, metaphorically, ends in the badgers shaking hands and returning to the same sett (S. Harris, pers. comm.).

Badgers are sometimes weakened by the skirmishes and ensuing infection and are found and taken into care. In the summer the wounds are often full of maggots. In these cases dusting with Negasunt (Bayer) will kill the maggots with apparently no ill effect on the badger. The wounds can then be flushed of debris and dead maggots and doused daily with Dermisol Multicleanse Solution (Pfizer). A course of broad-spectrum antibiotic will assist the healing.

It is debatable whether these badgers should be returned to their original territory. The author knows of one case where a female was twice rescued with bite wounds but then went on to become one of the breeding sows of her sett. Many badger casualties, for reasons other than bite wounds, have scars on their rumps from previous skirmishes. These bites seem to be just one facet of the badger group lifestyle that we do not fully understand.

Otters may show wounds inflicted by conspecifics around the anogenital region and the head.

Concussion

Badgers, in particular, are often found unconscious after being hit by a car or sometimes a train. There may be no apparent injuries but obviously concussion is a possibility. Treated as head trauma cases, these animals can be concussed for several days and will need to be maintained on carefully managed fluids. Most will, however, make speedy recoveries.

Internal injuries

Obviously with the sort of trauma these casualties experience, there are going to be various injuries to the internal organs. On post-mortem, ruptured spleens, livers or diaphragms are fairly common.

It is very much up to the veterinary surgeon to establish whether there are internal injuries and decide which course of action to take.

ADMISSION AND FIRST AID

All the mustelids, no matter how awkward, must be given fluids on admission. They will all bite so every precaution must be taken to prevent injury to staff.

In observing vital life signs it is worth noting that beneath the badger's tail is a subcaudal scent gland that has the appearance of a fundamental orifice. It has been known for operatives to try to take core temperature readings here. The rectum is just below the gland.

Badgers are the most common mustelid casualty and when being intravenously infused do not tend to bite through the giving set as do foxes.

Otters are subject to post-capture myopathies and benefit from infusion of Hartmann's solution and administration of vitamin E and selenium (Dystosel – Intervet).

CAGING

In intensive care the mustelid species must be kept in strong metal cages, preferably with dividers to facilitate easier cleaning. Badgers are extremely powerful and really warrant the use of stainless steel kennels such as those manufactured by Shorline. Otters, preferably, should be kept in brick kennels where they cannot damage their teeth on wire or bars.

Inside a weasel cage a small plastic aquarium with a trapdoor in the lid is an ideal nest box. The trapdoor can be closed with the weasel inside to move the animal as it will be too fast to catch any other way.

Once they have recovered all the species should be kept outside to acclimatise to the weather. All these animals can climb so any pens must be covered or have an unclimbable overhang and preferably have the sides of the pen sunk 0.75 m into the ground to stop them digging out. Otters and mink should be given facilities to swim after treatments have been concluded and badgers should be allowed to dig, but not too deeply or else they will excavate a whole sett in no time at all.

FEEDING

All the mustelid species are carnivorous and should be fed on whole animals such as day-old chicks, mice or rats. Otters should be given whole large fish, especially trout. A white fish diet will need a thiamine supplement with Fish Eaters Tablets (Mazuri Zoo Foods) secreted in the fish.

Any casualties that seem reluctant to start feeding or are not strong enough to feed themselves can sometimes be tempted with vanilla-flavoured Ensure (Abbott Laboratories). It can even be fed with a 50 ml syringe to animals that are particularly weak (Plate 10).

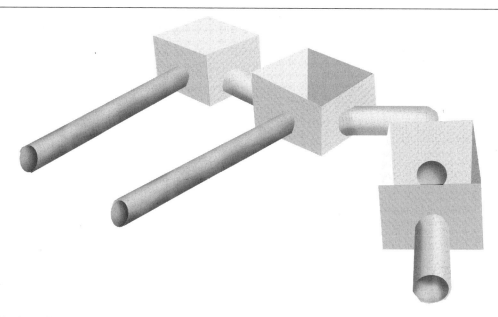

Fig. 24.7 An artificial sett based on the design of Naylor pipework.

RELEASE

The golden rule with all these species is to return them to exactly where they were found. They will recognise that area and can simply be let free, with no other provision other than it being a safe time of day or night, depending on the species.

Mink, of course, should not be released (Wildlife and Countryside Act 1981). Neither should ferrets, which are domestic animals. They should be found a suitable home.

Badgers are often found in unsuitable locations, lost or ousted. These can be relocated after first finding a suitable area that is free from any resident badgers. Local foresters or badger groups will be able to advise on any vacant territories.

Because of bovine tuberculosis it is not advisable to relocate badgers from the southwest to any other parts of Britain. The current Brock test to diagnose bovine tuberculosis in badgers is particularly unreliable and can throw up false negatives or false positives.

It is quite an involved procedure to relocate badgers starting with introducing the individuals and getting them living together as a group. In a suitable area an artificial badgers' sett is then constructed where it can be monitored but where it is away from the public glaze. Referring to the local badger group will get assistance in the sett's construction and monitoring.

The use of electric fences is advocated to keep the badgers enclosed in the artificial sett for a period but there are doubts about their humane use. Our method of confinement would be a wire fence that can be removed after a week or two. The badgers will escape long before that but if familiar food is always available they may adopt the sett. However, normally they choose to live elsewhere and will dig their own sett in the vicinity. The artificial sett will nevertheless remain suitable and even attractive with its supply of hay and fresh food (Fig. 24.7).

LEGAL IMPLICATIONS

All the mustelid species are protected against cruelty by the Protection of Animals Act 1911 for captive animals and the Wild Mammals (Protection) Act 1996.

Badgers benefit from the more blanket protection of the Protection of Badgers Act 1992 which prohibits killing, taking, disturbing or possessing a healthy badger. Legislation, though, allows for the possession or humane killing of a sick or injured badger. The legislation was innovative in that the badger sett is also protected, the first time that a wild mammal had received this type of cover.

Mink can only be held with a licence under the Destructive Imported Animals Act 1932. The release or escape of mink is prohibited by Schedule 9 of the Wildlife and Countryside Act 1981.

25
Deer

Species seen regularly:

Fallow deer (*Dama dama*), roe deer (*Capreolus capreolus*), muntjac (*Muntiacus reevesi*) and Chinese water deer (*Hydropotes inermis*).

Species seen occasionally:

Red deer (*Cervus elaphus*) and sika deer (*Cervus nippon*).

NATURAL HISTORY

Only the red deer and roe deer are true natives of Britain. Fallow deer were introduced during the Roman occupation, whereas muntjac and Chinese water deer only established a feral population in the early part of the twentieth century. The sika is very much a deer of parks and collections, but escapees do occur especially after high winds bring down fences.

The red, fallow and sika deer are all deer that form herds whereas the roe, muntjac and Chinese water deer tend to be either solitary or in pairs.

They all have a rutting season in late summer or autumn except muntjac who have no defined season and appear to practise opportunistic rutting at any time of the year. Consequently, all the other species give birth to their young in the summer months, while muntjac will give birth at any time of the year and even in the dead of winter.

All the male deer, except Chinese water deer, grow antlers each year after the previous year's have been shed. While they are growing they are covered in 'velvet' which is highly vascular and bleeds copiously if it is damaged.

Muntjac bucks and Chinese water deer have elongated upper canine teeth which protrude, below the upper lips in a muntjac and below the bottom jaw in a Chinese water deer (Fig. 25.1).

Terminology to describe the various sexes of the species is:

- A red deer male is a stag; a female a hind; the young are calves
- In all the other species the male is a buck; the female a doe; the young are fawns; and a male who does not grow antlers is a hummel

The red deer is mostly found in remote areas of wilderness such as the Scottish Highlands and high moorland in England. It rarely, if ever, is presented for rehabilitation. The fallow deer and roe deer are widespread being especially numerous locally in deciduous woodland. Muntjac are becoming more numerous but seem now to be restricted to ten core counties in the south and east of England where they are often found in or around human habitation especially in gardens. Chinese water deer have established a small stable feral population in south Bedfordshire and north Buckinghamshire.

EQUIPMENT AND TRANSPORT

All deer are large, or reasonably large, and require suitable equipment in order to catch them, transport them and control them while at a medical facility or rehabilitation centre.

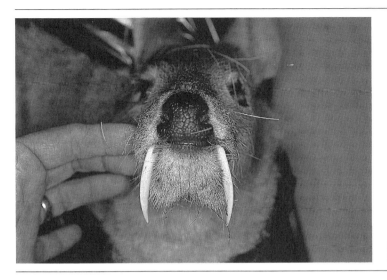

Fig. 25.1 The tusks of a Chinese water deer can be dangerous.

Rescue and capture

The equipment needed to rescue and capture all types of deer, except red deer, includes long-handled large nets, walk-toward nets and, possibly, for larger mobile deer such as fallow, the facility to sedate an animal with a tranquilliser dart.

Red deer will definitely need tranquillising but will need a horse box for transporting. The veterinary surgeon should be summoned to decide the course of action and whether there is a possibility of treatment at a veterinary equine facility.

Carrying

Small deer like muntjac, Chinese water deer and roe deer can usually be carried by one person if they are not too lively. As soon as possible, however, they should be masked with a cloth mask, a range of which can be made to a pattern copied from the old Nature Conservancy Council publication *The Capture and Handling of Deer* (Rudge, 1984) (Fig. 25.2). Non-adhesive cohesive bandage, e.g. Co-Flex (Millpledge Pharmaceuticals), can also be used to blindfold a deer to keep it calm.

Muntjac and Chinese water deer should be put into carriers, either a large pet carrier or a small wooden box especially designed for carrying small deer (Fig. 25.3). Hay on the bottom of each will assist the deer in maintaining a foothold.

Fallow and roe deer should be masked over the eyes and can be safely carried strapped to a stretcher. If these animals can be caught they are probably suffering from fractures and bruising and to move one without a stretcher is probably inflicting unnecessary suffering.

In care

Muntjac and Chinese water deer do appear to be the most difficult to handle once they are at a medical facility. In order to calm them and provide first aid, a harness which allows access to every part of the casualty has been designed (Stocker, 1996). It is simply made from a stretcher fixed to the top of a medical trolley with four holes cut to take the legs. Two Velcro straps secure the deer.

While suspended each leg can be examined and treated if necessary. An intravenous infusion can be introduced to either of the legs and an oxygen mask, if required, can be easily put over the muzzle. Deer often need suction to clear the saliva or, in a casualty, blood from their mouths. Notably deer may produce copious amounts of saliva during anaesthesia. Atropine is not effective so suction should be always available. Being suspended in the trolley, deer will even tolerate this stressful procedure which can be carried out without undue restraint and discomfort to the deer (Fig. 25.4).

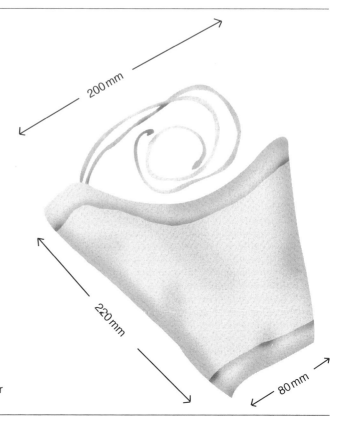

Fig. 25.2 Pattern for cloth masks suitable for various deer species (after Rudge, 1984).

Roe deer can be comfortably accommodated in a slightly larger trolley. Fallow deer adults are really too large to be lifted up and into a trolley. These can be safely treated, still on a stretcher, but at floor level.

RESCUE AND HANDLING

With deer, it is important to establish whether one actually needs rescuing or whether it should be left well alone.

One situation that is frustrating to those involved in wildlife rescue is when a fawn is found sitting quietly in a sheltered spot and is picked up. Female deer will leave their very young fawns, for most of the day and night, in secluded spots. They will only return to suckle. This is perfectly normal so young deer found sitting quietly should be left alone and the scene vacated as quietly as possible.

When a fawn is picked up it can still be returned, up to 48 hours later, to the spot where it was found. A watch should be kept from a considerable distance, preferably from a car, just to make sure the female does return.

The other situation when to leave well alone is when a fit adult deer, especially a muntjac, is seen in the garden. It will have managed to get into the garden and will manage to get out if left alone until nightfall. Attempts to catch it will usually result in the animal or somebody getting injured.

Fallow deer

Fallow deer are probably going to be the largest of the deer needing rescue. They are often injured either by road traffic accidents or getting trapped in fences. The road traffic victim will either make off at uncatchable speed or be so severely injured that it cannot move more than just a few metres.

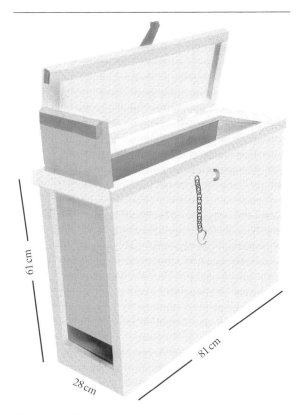

Fig. 25.3 Diagram of wooden crate suitable for transporting small deer.

Even to rescue a fallow deer that cannot move will take two people. The approach is to throw a blanket over the deer's head, then one person will hold the head and neck while the other controls the hindquarters. A deer with antlers is easier to control as sound antlers make ideal handles for controlling the head and controlling them stops them being used to injure anybody.

With the blanket over the head the fallow can then be rolled or lifted on to a stretcher and strapped down. It is not practical to try to lift a large deer without a stretcher. All deer should be maintained on their keels or alternatively lying on their right-hand side. These deer can be kept and handled on the stretcher throughout their transport to, and during initial treatments at, the medical facility.

Fallow deer caught in fences are usually much livelier than the road traffic victim and can be very difficult to handle. A deer caught by its antlers that has no injuries can have the wire cut away from the antlers and then be let free. However, any deer caught by the legs will have to be held and taken for treatment. They also have to be cut free but then have to be strapped to the stretcher for carrying. They are not going to be willing participants in this and should really be sedated before they are even cut free. A blanket over the head will help calm an animal as will one of the masks. Sedation can be with diazepam injected at 1 mg/kg intramuscularly; this is the only way to safely handle a large fallow deer.

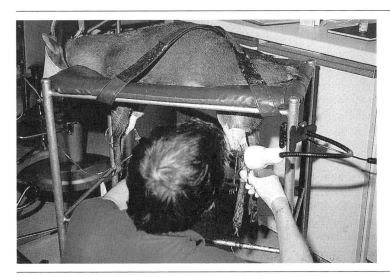

Fig. 25.4 A trolley/harness will greatly assist in the handling of small deer.

Any fallow deer that cannot be approached but needs capturing will need the services of someone with a rifle or blow pipe that fires tranquillising darts. A range of injectable anaesthetics are available to veterinary surgeons for use in this type of equipment and can be effective at the occasional times when capture is the only option.

Roe deer

Roe deer should be rescued and treated with similar methods to those used in fallow deer. The roe is smaller and easier to handle though the buck's antlers can be wickedly sharp.

Muntjac

Muntjac are increasingly common casualties in the counties north, east and west of London. Road traffic accidents are responsible for most of the casualties although the incidences of getting trapped in fences or attacked by dogs are on the increase.

The victims of road traffic accidents will usually be held or remain in the locality until a rescue team arrives. Some do manage to make off and can usually never be found. A muntjac that has been held or cannot move after an accident can be masked, carefully lifted and laid in the carrying box.

Muntjac, however, can be very lively and being very agile and strong can present problems to capture even if they have fractures to one or more legs. A mobile muntjac can often be intercepted and caught with a long-handled large net. Once caught they will scream but one person can usually manage to control them and get them into the carrying box.

Sometimes the muntjac cannot be approached and will flee at the first opportunity. With these casualties a strategy involving the use of walk-toward nets can usually be arranged. Basically the nets are put up across a possible escape route. A catcher hides nearby (Fig. 25.5). The deer is then panicked to run into the nets. If it is allowed to dawdle it may notice the nets and veer off to one side. The chasers should run at it shouting and make it run towards the nets. Once it hits the nets, it should become entangled enabling the catcher to get an initial hold of it. The chasers, by then, will be able to assist in getting the deer untangled and into the carrying box.

Usually one person can carry a muntjac by holding it under one arm around its body while the free hand controls the head. Do not try to control the legs. They will kick with their legs and having sharp hooves can tear clothing and injure people. A buck will also throw up its antlers, hence the reason for holding the head. The secret is to get it into the carrying box as quickly and quietly as possible.

At the medical facility the muntjac is put into the deer harness-cum-trolley. In here it cannot cause damage to either itself or anybody treating it. Its legs will be hanging free, and can be treated, stabilised, if fractures are present, sutured or held for intravenous cannulation. It can be maintained in the harness until put into an intensive care unit.

Without a harness two, three or four people are going to be needed just for first-aid procedures. Diazepam will help but after the third or fourth intravenous cannula has been kicked out even a makeshift harness will save much time and aggravation.

Muntjac are also regularly caught in fences or, peculiar to them, in between the bars of wrought iron gates. They usually have to be cut free, put into the carrying box and must be taken into care for treatment and monitoring.

Chinese water deer

These are somewhat irregular casualties but are usually road traffic accident victims. They are slightly larger than muntjac but rescue, transport and handling are all very similar.

Hobbling

Although hobbling, that is strapping a casualty deer's legs together, has been tried and advocated, it is now deemed unnecessary and can, in fact, be damaging to the delicate structure of a deer's legs.

COMMON DISEASES

Post-capture myopathy

Post-capture myopathy or exertional rhabdomyolysis is a necrosis of skeletal and cardiac muscle

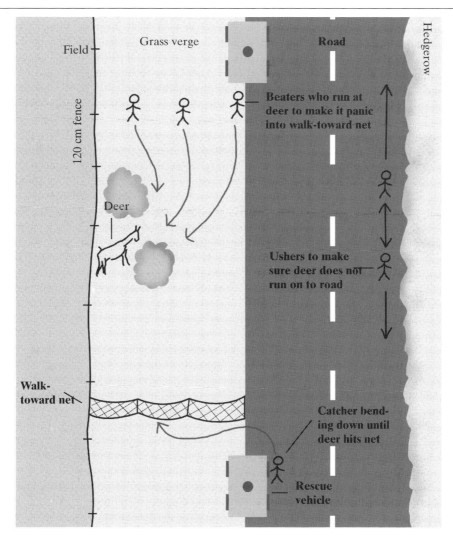

Fig. 25.5 The strategy of catching a small deer, e.g. muntjac, with walk-toward nets.

which occurs after stressful physical exertion (Barlow, 1986). Catching and handling deer is stressful and tiring for the animals so deer are particularly susceptible to post-capture myopathy, especially if they have been chased.

It is fair to assume that any wild deer taken into care is a candidate for capture myopathy for up to 4 weeks after capture. Symptoms include torticollis, depression, convulsions with a high fever. Death is almost always the outcome after symptoms become apparent.

Prevention can be helped by handling the deer sympathetically and keeping it in quiet, darkened outhouses. Drugs allied to treatment for shock such as fluids, corticosteroids, vitamin E, selenium and sedatives can help allay the onset of the condition.

Internal parasites

All deer will show a burden of endoparasites which generally should not pose problems. However, the stress and trauma a deer experiences in being injured, rescued, treated and confined can predispose to an overburden of parasites.

Treatment with ivermectin (Ivomec Injection for Cattle – Merial Animal Health) at twice the normal dose, i.e. 400 micrograms/kg given subcutaneously, is usually effective.

Lyme disease

Caused by the spirochaete *Borrelia burghdorferi*, Lyme disease is transmitted by ticks, particularly ticks of the deer, and *Ixodes ricinus*, also known as the sheep tick.

The disease is a zoonosis and can cause serious disease and even death in humans. Luckily the deer casualties that we see do not seem to carry many ticks. However, a tick can climb on to a person and lock its bite into the skin without the person feeling a thing. If one is found it should be removed making sure the barbed proboscis, the hypostome, is completely removed. To remove a tick it can be anaesthetised with local anaesthetic and pulled out. Alternatively a proprietary tick remover such as the O'Tom Hook will make its removal much easier.

Any skin reaction or swelling (a typical Lyme disease reaction is a circular area of reddened skin) should be referred to a general practitioner giving details of the fear of Lyme disease. Antibiotics can treat the disease in its early stages.

Arthritis

One of the more lasting effects of Lyme disease in humans involves the onset of arthritis. There seem to be no records of Lyme disease affecting deer and bringing on arthritis.

However, we are seeing a large number of muntjac casualties with chronic arthritis of the limb joints. The probable source of this, apparently endemic, arthritis could be the joints themselves. Muntjac leg joints are prone to luxation which in itself can lead to arthritis even in young animals. In some cases the arthritis is so far advanced that the muntjac cannot walk (Fig. 25.6). In cases like this or in trauma cases, where joints on separate legs are damaged, the question of euthanasia must be considered.

COMMON INJURIES

Fractures and luxations

Leg fractures and luxations

Deer are very susceptible to major leg damage especially fractures. Below the elbows and the stifles there is very little soft tissue covering the bones whereas the humeri and femurs often have thick muscle cover which gives them some protection. In road traffic accidents, which are the main cause of injury to deer, the legs are frequently fractured as are the pelvis and the spine. The leg fractures are often compound and should, if possible, be temporarily splinted at the scene of any incident. In triage and first aid any compound fractures should be irrigated with sterile saline and, along with any closed fractures, should be aligned and immobilised until the veterinary surgeon decides on a course of management.

It is possible to provide a temporary reduction in a conscious deer. It will soon let you know, by kicking, if the procedure is at all painful. The temporary reduction should be immobilised with a synthetic casting tape laid over two stirrups of 2.5 cm adhesive tape. A Robert Jones bandage or any padding usually results in the cast falling off. Obviously with a synthetic cast an oscillating saw is going to be needed to remove it.

Any open fractures should be cleaned and covered with a moist dressing such as paraffin-tulle (Grassolind – Millpledge Pharmaceuticals) or a hydrogel dressing (Bio Dres Wound Dressing – BK Veterinary Products) before being cast.

Immobilisation of most fractures will result in no more damage to tissues before the veterinary surgeon intervenes. Most will await the veterinary surgeon's attention but Monteggia fractures, where there is a fracture of the ulna and a dislocation of the head of the radius, can deteriorate if not attended to immediately (see Fig. 7.3).

Stabilisation of leg fractures by the veterinary surgeon can be by all methods including intramedullary pinning and the use of external fixations. Casts can tend to slip or cause pressure sores and should be avoided as the chosen course of treatment.

Often fractures are accompanied by compound dislocation of joints and epiphyses with many of

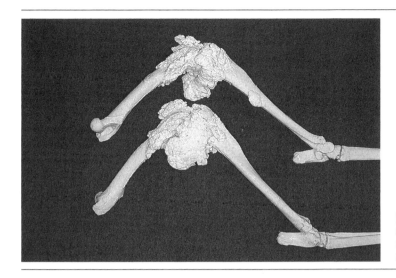

Fig. 25.6 Many muntjac are being seen with arthritic lesions. This female muntjac could not move either of her stifle joints.

the ligaments involved being shattered and irreparable. Initially again these should be cleaned, reduced, dressed and cast with resin plaster until the veterinary surgeon can attend. Treatment may involve arthrodesis of the joint or amputation, both of which can lead to problems for released animals.

Amputation of legs

A male deer has to be able to combat other male deer. With a leg amputated it would be at a distinct disadvantage. It may realise this and not get involved in rutting head-to-heads but there is no guarantee this would be the case. It should not be released.

However, keeping it in captivity can cause as many problems. One or more bucks will lead to fighting in the rutting season and with fallow or roe deer a captive buck can become a very dangerous animal during the rut.

Castration will usually calm an animal's instincts but in deer this would cause a drop in the level of testosterone. Without a fluctuation in testosterone the antlers will not shed with the following year's growth erupting underneath them every year. Castrated bucks end up with massive deformity of their antlers known as 'perruques'. Perruques are especially problematic in roe deer.

Generally the prognosis for deer buck casualties should be made with all these points taken into consideration.

Female deer with amputated legs are less of a problem in captivity. With a hind leg missing they usually cope very well but sometimes the lack of a front leg causes major problems resulting in humane euthanasia.

Pelvis or spinal fractures

Fractures of the pelvis or spine can be evaluated by the veterinary surgeon. Does with constriction of the birth canal after a pelvis fracture should be spayed before release. In fact many muntjac does will already be pregnant and may require a caesarian section. X-rays will identify a fetus.

Jaw fractures

Correct alignment of fractured jaws are crucial in deer because their method of feeding involves crushing and re-crushing food between their molars. Reduction and stabilisation of a deer's jaw should be coordinated from the inside of the mouth ensuring that the teeth are correctly aligned.

Skull fractures

Major skull fractures involving the cranial cavity can occur but are not very common. More common is the situation where a muntjac buck will have fractured the stem of an antler. The fracture will usually be below the pedicle in the stem which is part of the skull (Fig. 25.7). It can be stabilised by binding it with 2.5 cm resin casting tape (Vet Glas – Millpledge Pharmaceuticals) to the opposing stem. Both stems are sometimes fractured and can be cast in the same way but supported with tape under the jaw.

Sometimes, in growing antlers, the velvet covering is torn and bleeding. Any tears can be cleaned with sterile saline and be sutured.

Analgesia

Analgesia can be provided with carprofen, flunixin and, if there is no head trauma, buprenorphine.

Dog bite wounds

As small deer, especially muntjac, venture nearer to human activity they increasingly become the victims of attack by dogs. They are also, on occasion, mauled by fox hounds. The wounds are usually extensive and deep involving the muscle mass around the hindquarters. If the deer is cornered then bites to the abdomen, neck and head are common. Fawns are often picked up by the head resulting in fractured skulls and fatal brain damage.

Initially, on admittance, the wounds are only dressed with Intrasite Gel (Smith & Nephew) after any haemorrhage has been stemmed. Antibiotics are started with long-acting amoxycillin, to counter *Pasteurella multocida* a bacteria common in dogs' mouths, and metronidazole to cope with anaerobic bacteria.

The wounds themselves can be dealt with after 24 hours when the deer should be stable enough for sedation or anaesthetic.

Ligature or scrape wounds

Both of these wounds are caused when a deer gets stuck in a fence or wrought iron gate. In the former the ligature may well have severed blood vessels, ligaments, tendons and nerves below the wound. It is worth trying to get the wound to heal with regular dressings of a hydrogel such as Bio Dres Wound Dressing (BK Veterinary Products). Any joint involved, usually the hind fetlock, will usually need to be arthrodised but the deer will still be able to use it. Preparation H (Whitehall Laboratories) will help maintain circulation.

Where all the blood supply has been destroyed any tissue beyond the wound will die off. The leg would then need amputation, usually mid-femur amputation is a more manageable disability for the deer.

When a deer has been trapped between the bars of a wrought iron gate there will be skin lesions where the fur has been rubbed away. Provided that there are no internal injuries, the skin lesions

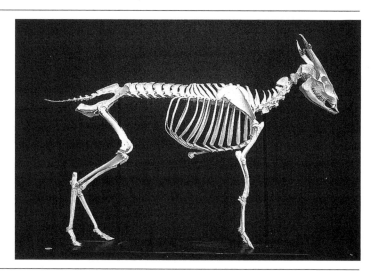

Fig. 25.7 A muntjac skeleton shows the fragile bones that are so susceptible to traffic damage.

will dry and eventually heal completely. Initially treating with Dermisol Multicleanse Solution (Pfizer) will assist with debridement and support healing.

ADMISSION AND FIRST AID

Triage in theory is a rapid, initial examination. In deer, though not so rapid, the initial examination should, if possible, evaluate the animal's potential for release, or at least captivity. Often discussion or a second opinion helps make the decision whether to treat the deer or whether it is never likely to recover full mobility.

In these situations some criteria are a direct indicator of euthanasia as the only option and can save a lot of pointless stress trying to stabilise the deer. Signs of a deer with no foreseeable future could be:

• Fractured spine
• The loss of two or more legs
• The loss of just one leg in a male deer
• Predisposition to arthritis in more than one leg
• Chronic arthritis in more than one leg
• Irreparable jaw damage
• Blindness

However, on a more positive note, most deer casualties are not suffering from severe disabilities or injuries like these. Most of them can be treated with a good chance that they will make a full recovery and can be released.

On admittance all deer should be infused intravenously with fluids and methylprednisolone. Methylpredisolone may cause a pregnant deer to abort but it is so important in countering shock that many firmly believe it must be used for these deer casualties. Fallow deer are easiest to deal with still strapped to their stretchers and on the floor; muntjac, roe and Chinese water deer are definitely much easier to treat suspended in a trolley harness.

Muntjac have particularly tough skin making it impossible to insert a cannula without first cutting down to the vein, usually the cephalic or lateral saphenous. Using rat-toothed forceps and a No. 11 scalpel blade the veins are reasonably large and easily accessed by a 20g (32mm) catheter. All species require this size of catheter except fallow deer where 18g (51mm) catheters are more appropriate.

As well as fluids, all deer will benefit from vitamin E compounds with selenium (Dystosel – Intervet) given intramuscularly at 1ml for muntjac and up to 3ml for fallow deer. Broad-spectrum antibiotics, normally long-acting amoxycillin, should be provided as shock is inevitably present.

Fractures should be cleaned and temporarily stabilised. Dog bite wounds are dressed with Intrasite Gel (Smith & Nephew) and held with loose sutures to maintain the integrity and shape of the skin. Ligature wounds are cleaned with Dermisol Multicleanse Solution (Pfizer).

Euthanasia, should it be necessary, should be with barbiturates given intravenously. There is no need for shooting or captive bolt pistols. Drugs are far less traumatic.

CAGING

Deer are the animals that should never be kept in cages or kennels. They do need solitude especially away from people. Preferably they should be kept in sheds isolated from the hubbub of general practice or a rescue centre.

Small deer are best suited to sheds with a floor area no larger than 1.8m × 1.2m. Fallow or roe deer would need 2.4m × 1.8m. The roof should be no higher than 1.8m. Do not be tempted to provide larger areas for the deer as given more space they are more likely to injure themselves and their handlers. Most sheds have uprights that are proud in the shed area. These are better rounded off or the shed lined with stockboarding from floor to ceiling (Fig. 25.8).

Lighting should be with red bulbs which in theory should be invisible to the deer who are colour blind. The red light left on all the time enables people to see in the shed without having to click a switch. The quieter the better for deer.

Hay can be laid quite deeply both for bedding and eating. Sometimes a deer may not be able to stand up for some time. It is a good idea to have some sort of draining floor to keep the animal dry. At The Wildlife Hospital Trust (St Tiggywinkles) deer sheds are on concrete bases with calf mats overlaying the cold stone, then hay. In some of

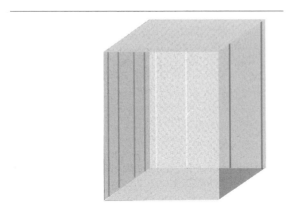

Stockboarding (Floor to ceiling)

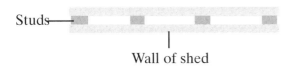

Studs

Wall of shed

Fig. 25.8 Suggestion for a deer shed lined with stockboarding.

the sheds built-up drainage floors have been made based on industrial matting. These keep those prone deer dry and can be removed and washed at regular intervals.

In winter, and for shocked deer, heat lamps are provided. In summer the sheds have to be ventilated in case they overheat in sunlight.

After deer have finished treatment in their sheds they are either released or else kept in large paddocks with other deer until they are fit for release. The deer paddocks are fenced with a 2 m high deer fence which is sprung so that if a deer runs into it, it will simply bounce off.

Various huts and hutches are put around the paddock to serve as shelters and an automatic drinking water system is provided because deer, especially fallow, drink copious amounts of water. Mineral block should be provided under rainproof shelters.

FEEDING

Naturally deer are either grazers or browsers. In captivity it is possible to allow some access to grass

for grazing and browse can be cut from local hedgerows. It is difficult to provide enough fodder naturally so deer can be offered a range of artificially prepared foods.

The diet provided is coarse goat mix, available from most agricultural merchants, as an addition to the deer's hay. Alfalfa can be provided for more roughage, high protein and calcium, and browsers pellets (Mazuri Zoo Foods) offer more nutrition to a deer that needs building up. A deer that is receiving antibiotic therapy will need a pro-biotic additive to its feed. Vetrumex (Willows Francis Veterinary) is suitable.

Some deer, especially roe, are reluctant to feed in captivity. In not feeding they very quickly lose weight and condition with rumenal stasis accelerating the decline. There are two ways of dealing with this:

(1) The deer can be infused with peripheral nutrition through its intravenous cannula sites. Nutriflex Lipid Peri (B Braun Medical) has been very successfully employed in restoring condition to debilitated deer or those recovering from surgery. It is infused at slightly less than a maintenance rate, i.e. 30 ml/kg daily for 48 hours.
(2) The other method is to remove the rumenal contents of a deer killed by trauma, say a road traffic victim, and to freeze it in polythene bags. This can then be defrosted and fed by stomach tube into the rumen of a debilitated deer. The gut flora from the dead deer should immediately start to ferment and kick-start the rumenal processes.

Fruit

It is not a good idea to feed deer on fruit as they may prefer this to a more balanced diet and can rapidly lose condition and develop fermentation bloat. Similarly greens and carrots are not particularly suitable. Tit bits occasionally may help in getting a new patient to feed.

RELEASE

Taking animals out to release is a bit more hectic than bringing in a weakened casualty. Deer, in particular, if they are fit for release will be full of energy, strength and an unswerving instinct to escape.

If deer are maintained in paddocks prior to release they may need to be restrained with tranquilliser darts before they can be handled and transported. Muntjac, roe and Chinese water deer can all be safely accommodated in carrying boxes. Fallow deer, however, will need a small box trailer to carry them to a release site.

All deer should be released where they were originally found. Muntjac, however, are sometimes found in gardens and obviously should not be released there. They can only be released by a licensed person within 1 km of where they were found. A piece of woodland or open area in the vicinity would be suitable.

LEGAL IMPLICATIONS

Wild deer have some protection against cruelty with the Wild Mammals (Protection) Act 1996. In captivity they are protected by the Protection of Animals Act 1911.

The other legislation that affects deer rehabilitation is that muntjac are now included on Schedule 9 of the Wildlife and Countryside Act 1981. This means that it is an offence to release a muntjac or allow one to escape.

There are provisions for rehabilitators who can apply for a licence to release muntjac in the ten core counties and within 1 km of where they were found. Many rehabilitators have this dispensation so any treated muntjac should be released through their auspices.

The use of tranquilliser darts is through a special rifle or a blow pipe. These weapons are covered by firearms legislation and need a licence from the local police. They no longer need an additional Home Office Licence.

26
Bats

Species seen:

Barbastelle	*Barbastella barbastellus*
Serotine	*Eptesicus serotinus*
Bechstein's	*Myotis bechsteini*
Brandt's	*Myotis brandti*
Daubenton's	*Myotis daubentoni*
Whiskered	*Myotis mystacinus*
Natterer's	*Myotis nattereri*
Leisler's	*Nyctalus leisleri*
Noctule	*Nyctalus noctula*
Pipistrelle	*Pipistrellus pipistrellus*
Brown long-eared	*Plecotus auritus*
Grey long-eared	*Plecotus austriacus*
Greater Horseshoe	*Rhinolophus ferrume-quinum*
Lesser Horseshoe	*Rhinolophus hipposideros*

On rare occasions vagrants from Europe or America are found in this country and other species are being added to the British list as they are identified.

As identification of most bats is particularly difficult, a good reference guide is essential (see Corbet and Harris (1991) and Stebbings (1993)).

NATURAL HISTORY

Bats are the only mammals capable of sustained flight. The wing of a bat extends to an elongated hand with a flexible membrane of skin stretched from the body to the tips of the fingers and tail. The thumb or first finger is exposed with a sharp claw that enables the bat to cling to or climb trees, walls and roof linings (Fig. 26.1).

Bats have small eyes but locate their surroundings and prey with echo-location techniques similar to a ship's sonar navigation system. A bat may have modified ears and noseleaves to facilitate the echo-location capability.

One other natural ability that would affect their care is that when bats are resting they can become torpid and adjust their body temperature near to the ambient temperature of their surroundings; they are heterothermic.

Further than this they are one of the few British mammals to fully hibernate. Usually this is in secluded sites where there are not great temperature fluctuations and there is a degree of humidity.

Bats are generally long lived with records of 20 years or more.

EQUIPMENT AND TRANSPORT

Bats needing to be taken into care are not flying so there is no need for a net. However, even with a net, the bat's echo-location would enable it to avoid being caught if it were flying.

The equipment needed for bats includes a pair of light leather gloves, to avoid getting bitten, and any sort of small container for containing them. Bats can squeeze through the smallest of holes so any container must be escape-proof.

Hagen produce a range of small plastic 'small pals pens' with slotted plastic lids. The smallest model (H351) will contain any bat. The only provision for bats is to drape some quilted kitchen paper towel over the inside walls to allow the bat to climb and hang on.

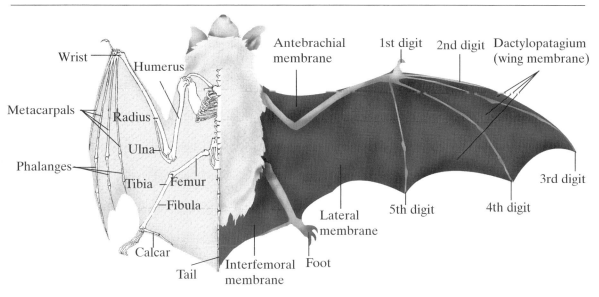

Fig. 26.1 Expanded bat wing showing skeletal structure.

Bats are very small so magnifying optical aids such as surgeon's loupes or magnifying head bands are going to help with smaller injuries (Fig. 26.2).

RESCUE AND HANDLING

A bat that needs rescuing can usually be simply picked up or, as many are spotted clinging to walls, picked off.

Some species are extremely small and can be easily injured unless care is taken in handling them. Generally they should be laid across the fingers with the thumb firmly but gently holding them down (Fig. 26.3).

If they are not torpid they can be noisily aggressive and make to bite. The wearing of light gloves will prevent their tiny teeth causing any injury. Without gloves the smaller species may or may not be able to penetrate the skin but the larger bats, the noctule and the serotine, have quite a powerful bite.

Whatever container they are carried in, a lining of quilted paper towel will give them a secure way of steadying themselves and scurrying out of the light.

DISEASES

Bats are, like other wild animals, reasonably resistant to disease. However, any bat brought into care could be suffering from a disease not yet described in that particular species. The one disease that has carried a lot of publicity in recent years is rabies. It is a well-known fact that bats in other countries are infected with rabies and cases of people developing rabies after being bitten by bats are not uncommon in some countries.

Rabies

In this country in a 10-year survey of bats by the Rabies Research and Diagnostic Unit at the Central Veterinary Laboratory, 1882 bats of 23 species were screened for the rabies antigen (Whitby *et al.*, 1996). All were found to be negative. The Central Veterinary Laboratory are still seeking bat carcasses (Appendix 5).

However, in June 1996 a Daubenton's bat was rescued at Newhaven in Sussex showing unusual behaviour. Rather than the normal threat and bite behaviour, this bat was overly aggressive attacking everything it could and biting the rescuer on many

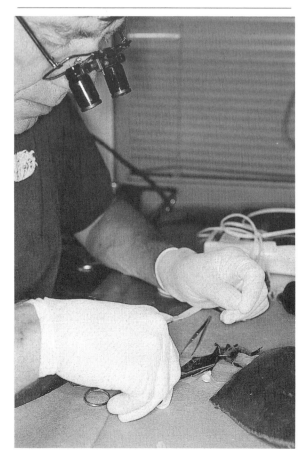

Fig. 26.2 Bat injuries are often so tiny that the use of surgeon's loupes help identify specific defects.

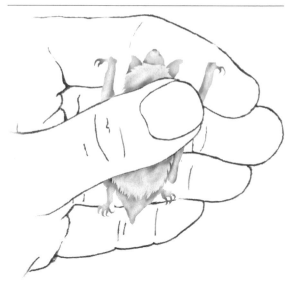

Fig. 26.3 How to hold a bat firmly but gently.

occasions. The bat appeared to be fitting and was put down. At the Central Veterinary Laboratory the polymerase chain reaction (PCR) tests (a process whereby small amounts of DNA may be amplified) proved positive for European Bat Lyssavirus type 2 (EBL 2). The finder received post-exposure prophylaxis from the moment the bat was thought to be infected. She had suffered no ill effects from her encounter. This type of rabies is different from the sylvatic rabies that infects other mammals such as dogs, cats and foxes. EBL2 has not been recorded from any wild or domestic animal other than a bat.

The likelihood of another rabid bat occurring in Britain is remote but still a possibility. This particular Daubenton's bat may have been British or

it may have arrived from mainland Europe on a ship or by flying across the English Channel. Nobody knows for sure but anybody handling bats should be particularly vigilant.

The Bat Conservation Trust have published guidelines that apply to rehabilitators and veterinary staff as well as licensed bat workers, all of whom would possibly handle sick or injured bats. The full guidelines and recommended procedures can be found in Appendix 1.

Ectoparasites

Bats will carry a range of host-specific ectoparasites including fleas, mites (Plate 40), ticks, a bug (*Cimex pipistrelli*) and on horseshoe bats the nycteribiid fly (*Phthiridium biarticulatum*).

Insects can be safely removed using WHISKAS exelpet (Pedigree Masterfoods) flea powder. This should be dusted into the fur with a small dry paintbrush. Stronger insect repellents may well be toxic to bats. Mites can be picked off with a small paintbrush dipped in water. A systemic acaricide such as ivermectin (Ivomec Injection for Cattle – Merial Animal Health) mixed 1:99 with propylene glycol can be administered subcutaneously or orally at 0.02 ml/10 g.

Sticky wing

Sometimes when a bat is in captivity and not using its wings regularly, the interior of the folds of the wing may become sticky and odorous. This may be a mixture of bacteria and yeasts. It should be washed off with a warm salt solution.

Wing membrane necrosis

Nobody knows for sure what causes wing membrane necrosis wherein the membranes dry, crack and flake away. The necrosis will also travel into neighbouring bone. The cause may be bacterial or fungal. It may be caused by trauma or through a lack of humidity.

Systemic antibiotics have been tried as a treatment but the results have been erratic. The most success appears to be by massaging E45 (Crookes) cream into the membranes.

Whatever the attempted remedy any course of treatment is going to take a long time.

Hair loss

Many young bats and long-term captives seem to develop patches where their fur will be missing. Pipistrelles are particularly prone to this complaint. Once again there has been no specific definition of a cause. Perhaps it may be traumatic where a bat rubs itself on a water bowl or is sucked by a contemporary. It may even be dietary or caused by excess handling.

Generally the condition will recede if the bat is not handled and kept on its own. The administration (orally) of essential fatty acids (EfaCoat Oil – Schering-Plough Animal Health) may be of use with this condition and that of wing membrane necrosis. There are very few records of any attempts at treatment and as this is a very common condition a solution will assist many bats being returned to the wild.

Subcutaneous emphysema

No definitive cause can be found for this condition wherein the bat is found with areas of its body inflated with air. The remedy is simple but effective:

- The skin over the swelling is cleaned and swabbed with surgical spirit

- Using an insulin syringe the air is aspirated
- A course of broad-spectrum antibiotics is started
- Swellings may reappear and will have to, again, be aspirated

The condition will generally resolve.

COMMON INCIDENTS

Cats

The most common incident affecting bats is being caught by a cat. Usually live bats are rescued from cats by the pet owner and taken to a rescue centre. Sometimes a cat will become a regular stalker of a bat colony causing deaths and injuries on a daily basis.

Vagrants

Bats will be found during the day clinging to outside walls or just lying on the ground. They are probably trauma victims but no definite reason for their debility can be found. Normally they are dehydrated and consequently in shock. Once they are stabilised and fit for release they should be returned to the area where they were found.

Orphans

Baby bats are sometimes left in a nursery while their mothers are out hunting. They can also cling to their mother and join her on flying trips. Whatever happens destitute baby bats are regularly encountered and rescued.

Rather than just adopting an orphan, attempts should be made to get it back to its roost. Just putting an orphan into a known roost does not seem to work. The babies are invariably found dead. The solution is to give the mother a chance to recover her youngster which can be rescued if she does not appear.

A very simple device is a wooden baby bat hanger. A piece of untreated sawn timber approximately 500 mm × 200 mm is mounted vertically on an upright post, a 50 mm fence post set up in some soft ground. Provided the weather is fine, just before dusk the baby bat is encouraged to cling vertically to the board. If it is near to the colony, as the bats leave to feed the baby bat should call.

Hopefully its mother will hear the call and will come to the board to collect her youngster (Fig. 26.4). An hour after dusk, if its mother has not returned, the baby can be removed and taken into care.

OTHER INCIDENTS

Sometimes bats are involved in bizarre incidents that could never be expected. Here are two cases which illustrate the nature of these incidents.

(1) A cottage was struck by lightning and a part of the roof destroyed. In the roof was a colony of bats; some were killed by the lightning while others received major injuries.
(2) A nursery of noctule bats in an old woodpecker hole was found after the tree containing it had been felled. The woodpecker nest cavity had to be sawn open to remove the nine babies. Some were already dead and some died later, all from fractured skulls. The remaining babies were reared and released (Fig. 26.5).

COMMON INJURIES

Anaesthesia

Sometimes it is hard to imagine, but a tiny animal, like a bat, will have a complete nervous system and will consequently be able to feel pain and discomfort from the tiniest defect. It is, therefore, not going to lie still for any treatment procedure. In the past, some people induced torpor by putting the bat in a refrigerator before any treatments. The torpor may still the bat but has no analgesic properties.

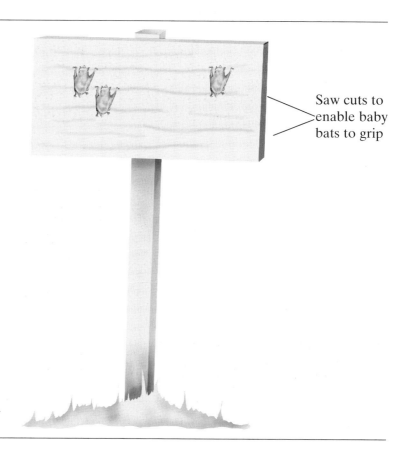

Saw cuts to enable baby bats to grip

Fig. 26.4 Design for wooden hanger for re-uniting orphan bats.

This is tantamount to cruelty and should *never* be considered.

The anaesthetic of choice for a bat would be isoflurane, with a high flow rate of oxygen, administered through a face mask fashioned out of a syringe case or rubber tube (Fig. 26.6). Being small, any bat under anaesthetic is going to rapidly lose heat. A heated table or heat mat is essential. The oxygen should be continued for some time after the anaesthetic is switched off.

ANALGESICS

A fracture in a bat's wing is going to be painful. It may be possible to administer small enough amounts of analgesics if they are diluted in Water for Injection. Flunixin, carprofen and buprenorphine could be useful. If this is not possible then frequent applications of a topical local anaesthetic, included in a teething gel sold in pharmacies for use in babies, may bring some relief.

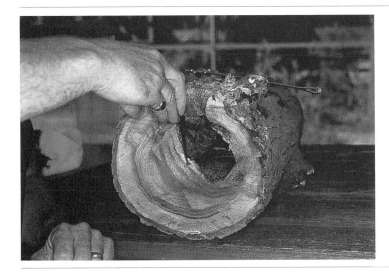

Fig. 26.5 A woodpecker hole used as a nursery by several female noctule bats.

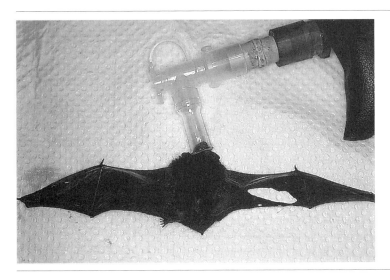

Fig. 26.6 Bats can be given gaseous anaesthesia through a face mask made out of a plastic tube.

Wing tears

Tears to the membranes of the wings are very common. They range in size from pinhead to the complete membrane torn off between fingers or body and fingers.

Small tears will resolve themselves. Bats, however, can often still fly adequately even with tears in the wing. It is worth trying to get them to fly before trying remedial treatments. Major tears can be sutured with a 7/0 swaged-on absorbable suture but it is very difficult to get the tear edges into apposition. Similarly using tissue glue (Vetbond – 3M) is another option but again it is nearly impossible to get the edges of the defect to meet.

One technique allows the debriding of the tear leaving fresh incised edges that are more likely to heal. The technique (Fig. 26.7) has to be carried out with the bat under anaesthetic:

(1) A strip of clear microperforated tape (Omnifilm – Millpledge Pharmaceuticals) is laid adhesive side upwards on the table.
(2) At the edges of the defect, where the membrane has rolled up, it is unfurled until the tear edge is exposed.
(3) The first edge is laid along the adhesive tape and is kept unfurled and pressed completely flat on the adhesive.
(4) The opposite edge is unfurled and laid next to the first edge but overlapping.
(5) Tissue glue is then applied under this overlapping edge and the two sides held together.
(6) The edges are then cleaned and swabbed with surgical spirit.
(7) When the area is dry a No. 15 scalpel blade is run down the centre of the overlapping edge making an identical incision along both edges. The tape underneath should not be cut as it keeps both edges in apposition.
(8) Removing the loose edge, permeable clear wound dressing (Opsite Flexi-grid – Smith & Nephew or Tegaderm – 3M) is laid over the incision and firmly attached.
(9) The bat is turned over, the adhesive tape is removed along with the second debrided edge of the first area of membrane.
(10) Another strip of permeable clear wound dressing is laid over the back of the join, the bat turned over and the join pushed home.
(11) A course of broad-spectrum antibiotics is started.
(12) After 10 days the join should be healed and the tape can be removed.

Fractures

Any fractures suffered by a bat will usually be of the wing bones. Holding the bat up to a light source and extending each wing will highlight most fractures as well as any bleeding into the tissues.

Many fractures, however, are going to be open fractures usually of the humerus or radius – the ulna is insignificant and not normally a problem. Fractures or, more often, amputations of the fingers (metacarpals and phalanges) regularly coincide with major tears of the wing membranes. Open fractures can be thoroughly cleaned with sterile saline. The skin sheath can usually be withdrawn to allow the exposed bone to be reduced and covered.

Stabilisation of fractures in a bat's wing requires a large degree of innovation including the following.

Splinting

Splinting can be achieved with small lengths of adhesive tape folded over the edge of the wing excluding the joints. The usual problem with this very simple technique is that the bat will often chew at the tape and eventually pull it off.

More stable splints have been fashioned from small strips of Vet-Lite (Runlite) which can be easily moulded after being doused in hot water.

The joints are avoided with splints for the same reason they are avoided in birds. Any ankylosis could well impede a bat's manoeuvrability in hunting.

Tissue glue stabilisation

Another method of stabilising compound fractures of the humerus and radius is with tissue glue (Vetbond – 3M) (Lollar & Schmidt-French, 1998).

With a humerus fracture, the wound is cleaned and the bones reinstated under the skin. A

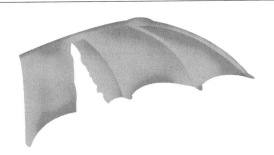

Tear

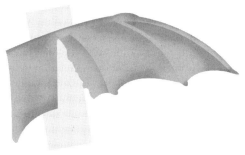

First edge of tear is stuck to adhesive side of clear microperforated tape.

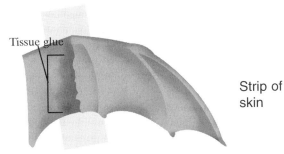

Tissue glue

Pull second edge of tear on to tissue glue along first edge.

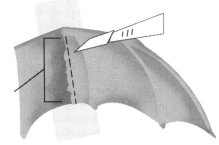

Strip of skin

With scalpel cut through both layers of membrane but not through tape.

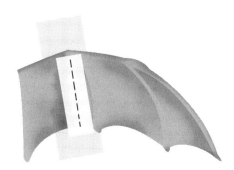

Remove strip of skin. Put strip of wound dressing over front cut and press firmly down. Turn wing over.

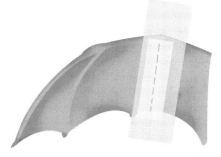

Remove original strip of adhesive tape with other strip of skin. Cover back of cut with strip of wound dressing.

Fig. 26.7 Suggested method of aligning major wing tears in a bat.

few drops of tissue adhesive are placed, not poured, on to the dorsal surface of the wing membranes on each side of the defect. No adhesive is allowed on the wound itself. Then quickly but gently the wing is closed in a natural position by pressing the forearm against the humerus and the humerus against the body (Fig. 26.8). Over the following 4–6 weeks, do not let the bat try to fly. Any pieces of adhesive that have worked loose should be removed and replaced, on a daily basis, with fresh tissue glue.

Fracture of humerus

Fracture of radius

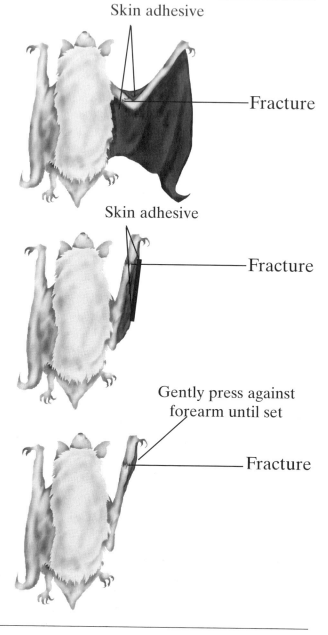

Fig. 26.8 Tissue glue stabilisation of bat wing fractures (after Lollar & Schmidt-French, 1998).

Similarly, compound fractures of the radius can be stabilised by running a continuous line of tissue adhesive along the entire length of the dorsal side of the outermost fingers. The outer finger is then pressed up against the damaged radius in a natural position. Once the adhesive has hardened the daily protocol of adhesive replacement will continue for 4–6 weeks.

Intramedullary pinning

The intramedullary cavity of both the humerus and radius is minute. However intramedullary pins have been fashioned out of fine gauge (26 g, 27 g, 30 g) hypodermic needles or the inserts from spinal needles. Their success in varied but most fail through osteomyelitis or an inadequate blood circulation and healing capability. Antibiotics should be targeted at skeletal infection. Lincomycin (Lincocin Aquadrops – Pharmacia & Upjohn) or clindamycin (Antirobe Capsules – Pharmacia & Upjohn) have been found effective, but lincomycin may lead to diarrhoea.

External fixation

This would be the treatment of choice but all depends on the thickness of the fractured bone. Hypodermic needles of 30 g are the only transverse pins that would be small enough to pass through the bones of most bats. However, if it is possible then they can be held rigid with cross struts of Hydroplastic (TAK systems).

Amputation

Bats can survive in captivity after the amputation of a wing or part of a wing. They will need both thumbs to be able to walk and climb and euthanasia should be considered if that is not possible.

TRIAGE AND FIRST AID

The structure of a bat and the extent of its injuries can easily be seen as soon as it is admitted. Often portions of the wings are missing prohibiting any chance of release. The assessment at triage is going to be: will the bat be releasable and if not can it be comfortably maintained in captivity.

Fluid administration

All newly admitted bats should receive warmed subcutaneous fluids, preferably Hartmann's solution laced with 10% Duphalyte (Fort Dodge Animal Health).

The fluids can be administered in insulin syringes beneath the skin over the back. Dose rates vary from 0.3 ml for a pipistrelle to 0.8 ml for a serotine bat. This can be repeated every 12 hours.

Bats often do not start drinking on their own; they can be encouraged with Lectade (Pfizer) from a small paintbrush or pipette.

Antibiotics

Antibiotics to treat attacks by cats, and the resultant *Pasteurella multocida*, should be amoxycillin, preferably reconstituted oral drops, given at 40–50 mg/kg twice daily. At these tiny amounts the dose can be taken as the smallest drops possible. Clamoxyl Palatable Drops (Pfizer) have the longest reconstituted life of 14 days.

Amoxycillin is also suitable as the broad-spectrum antibiotic for bats in shock or with skin wounds.

EUTHANASIA

By far the most effective, least traumatic method of euthanasia for bats is to anaesthetise them first with gaseous anaesthetic and then administer an overdose of barbiturates intracardiac or intraperitoneally (Stocker, 1997).

CAGING

The simplest form of caging for bats, and the easiest to keep clean, are the plastic Small Pals Pens made by Rolf C Hagen and sold in most pet stores. Quilted kitchen paper towel can be draped down the insides for the bats to cling to and to hide under.

Radiant warmth can be provided with a red light bulb in a small flexible table lamp.

A slightly more expensive container is a cage designed for bugs or breeding butterflies. Its sides are made of stretched taut fine nylon mesh. This enables the bats to easily climb as they prefer to roost at the highest point possible. Again radiant warmth can be provided with a red light bulb (Plate 41).

A larger container could be a small two-compartment rabbit hutch with the wire mesh replaced with finer mesh. The walls and ceiling should be covered with fine nylon mesh enabling the bats to climb and roost in the closed compartment.

Bats that are for release should be given the space to exercise and fly and demonstrate their ability to catch insects.

Based on the dimensions given in the Nature Conservancy Council's (now English Nature) publication *The Bat Workers' Guide* (Mitchell-Jones, 1987), The Wildlife Hospital Trust (St Tiggywinkles) has constructed a bat flight cage where insects can be attracted and bats can be allowed to roost and fly; it can even be used as a release facility. The dimensions are 4.9 m × 2.5 m × 2 m covered on three sides with $\frac{1}{4}$ inch galvanised mesh. The base is concrete to allow grounded bats to be seen easily. Bat boxes, feeding stations (for mealworms and waxworms) and water fountains are set in various places. The nest boxes can be warmed electrically if it is thought necessary. In the centre of the flight cage is an ultra-violet fluorescent lamp that attracts insects for the bats to hunt.

FEEDING

Bats naturally hunt and eat flying insects. In captivity it is obviously not possible to provide a natural diet but alternatives are available.

Mealworms

Mealworms (*Tenebrio molitor*) are the standard fall-back to feed bats. Initially it may be necessary to cut the heads off the mealworms and squeeze some of the insides on to a bat's mouth to get it interested.

Eventually the bats can be trained to take headless mealworms from a dish. Once they have mastered this task then the mealworms can be left whole. The only trouble is that they are highly mobile and can escape. The secret is to put them in a straight-sided dish such as a ramekin. One thing to beware of is that vagrant mealworms have been known to attack small bats like pipistrelles.

Mealworms are good feed for bats but are lacking in some minerals. Dusting them with multi-vitamins does not provide the additives bats need. However, there are products that will be absorbed by the mealworms and provide the necessary supplements. Mealworm Diet Calci – Paste (IZUG) is suitable.

Waxworms

The larvae of the waxworm *Galleria mellonella* have a softer outer skin than mealworms and are not as mobile. They are suitable for smaller bats and youngsters. They too should be supplemented with Nutrobal (Vetark Animal Health) or Mealworm Diet Plus (Mcdivct).

Maggots

Bats will take blow-fly maggots, the gentles sold in angling shops. The stipulation must be that they are cleaned. That is to say that they have been starved so that the toxic contents of their gut will have passed through.

Table 26.1 Average weights of British bats.

Species	Weight
Pipistrelle	4–7 g
Whiskered	4–8 g
Lesser Horseshoe	5–7 g
Brown long-eared	6–12 g
Daubenton's	6–12 g
Natterer's	6–12 g
Barbastelle	6–13 g
Bechstein's	7–13 g
Grey long-eared	7–14 g
Leisler's	11–20 g
Serotine	15–35 g
Greater Horseshoe	16–31 g
Noctule	18–45 g

There are going to be differences pre-hibernation, during hibernation and post-hibernation.

Obesity

Bats, especially the larger species, can overeat and put on too much weight. Obese bats can lose the ability to fly and will need to be put on a diet.

Weighing a bat every day will give an indication of its well-being and will highlight any increases in weight. A chart of average weights of the different species acts as a good reference point during the daily weighing (Table 26.1).

RELEASE

The principle behind all wildlife care is to get the animal back to fitness and ready for release. Bats are no different but there is still little evidence of the success or failure of releasing bats.

Bats should be returned to where they were found. They will be familiar with the vicinity and should be able to return to their native roost. Young bats that have been hand-reared will probably not have a native roost site to be returned to. These can be released in a suitable area using the 'hack' system practised with birds of prey. Basically the young bats are kept confined in a large release box set about 2 m above the ground. They are fed and watered for 3–4 days and then a small entrance door at one end of the box is left open Feeding should continue until the bats are obviously not going to return.

However, they may return some considerable time later, maybe months. For this reason the hack box should be left where it is. In the meantime it can be used for other bat releases.

In order to give bats protection from diurnal predators all releases should be carried out after dusk and when the weather is fine. It is not advisable to release bats during the winter months, December to March inclusive.

LEGAL IMPLICATIONS

Bats and their roosts have complete protection under the Wildlife and Countryside Act 1981. However, a person is not committing an offence if they take into care any bat that is disabled other than by their action. Any bat taken into care must be released as soon as it is fully fit.

There has been considerable discussion on the suitability of hand-reared bats for release. The Abandonment of Animals Act 1960 legislates against the release of unsuitable animals, thus causing them unnecessary suffering. Opinions are now changing with the present attitude being that hand-reared bats can be successfully released provided the release programme offers some monitoring of their survivability.

27
Other Mammal Species

Species mentioned:
- Mole (*Talpa europaea*)
- Scottish wild cat (*Felis silvestris*)
- Common seal (*Phoca vitulina*)
- Grey seal (*Halichoerus grypus*)
- Cetacea (various species)

Part I: Terrestrial mammals

Mole

NATURAL HISTORY

The mole spends most of its life in a series of tunnels it digs underground just below the surface or over a metre down. It patrols this system taking invertebrate prey, mainly earthworms *Lumbricus terrestris*. It also stores earthworms by biting their anterior segments and storing them paralysed.

The mole is active throughout the whole day and during the whole year. In frozen or dry spells it will dig deeper following its prey down to lower levels. They are very solitary animals that only get together during mating. During the rest of the year they will aggressively drive other moles from their territory.

Numerous colour varieties occur including piebald, grey, albino and an almost golden colour (Plate 42).

To enable it to dig, the mole has a broad, flattened humerus quite unlike the humerus in any other mammal. Its forepaws are also adapted for digging being also broad and flat with five strong claws making it a very efficient excavator.

EQUIPMENT AND TRANSPORT

The only specific items needed for mole care are thick gloves and for containment a large dry glass aquarium. No lid is necessary. Moles cannot climb so can be carried in any cardboard box.

RESCUE AND HANDLING

Rescuing moles usually involves taking a victim off a cat or picking up a road casualty. Their movement above ground is frantic but not very fast so they are easily caught. However, on suitable soil they will dig and rapidly disappear from sight.

Moles do bite and although it is not a serious bite it is advisable to wear gloves. They can, without gloves, be held with their scruff secured between the thumb and index finger.

Their nose region is very sensitive and should be protected during handling or examination.

COMMON DISEASES

There is scant evidence of infectious diseases affecting moles but that is not to say that they may not be present.

Parasites

Moles can carry fleas, mites and ticks but generally they are clean of external parasites.

Internally, they can be susceptible to trematodes, protozoans and fungal infection but these will not generally affect their rehabilitation.

COMMON INCIDENTS

Mole casualties are usually picked up for one of three reasons:

(1) They are caught by cats
(2) They get injured on the roads
(3) They are found dehydrated above ground during exceptionally dry weather

COMMON INJURIES

Injuries are not normally seen in mole admittances. Cats may cause minor lacerations.

ADMISSION AND FIRST AID

Subcutaneous fluids are the norm for moles together with long-acting amoxycillin for cat attack.

CAGING

As mentioned earlier, moles can be kept in a large aquarium that should be about half full of loose soil and peat. They are extremely active spending most of their time tunnelling through the soil. Apart from a water dish, they require no other fittings, branches or ornament.

Food should be put straight on to the soil. The soil can get quite dirty and should be replaced every few days.

FEEDING

Moles are active for three periods over 24 hours. They should have access to food at all times. It is said that a mole will die if deprived of food for more than an hour.

They will take mealworms and waxworms scattered amongst the soil mix in their containers. However, they eat so much that it is both expensive and time-consuming to try to keep them fed on invertebrates. Moles can be fed on chopped mice, a single mole has been known to eat as many as 16 mice in a day. This gives some idea of their voracious appetite.

Water, of course, should be provided at all times. This may need changing regularly as it soon becomes soiled as the ever active mole passes through it on its incessant ramblings.

RELEASE

The preferred habitat for a mole is in deciduous woodland where there is no evidence of other moles. As they are released amongst the leaf litter it is advisable to stay with them until they disappear underground.

LEGAL IMPLICATIONS

Moles in care are protected from cruelty with the Protection of Animals Act 1911 and in the wild by the Wild Mammals (Protection) Act 1996.

Scottish wildcat

The Scottish wildcat is a highly secretive animal confined now to the remote highlands in Scotland (Fig. 27.1). In the wild it feeds mainly by hunting rabbits and small animals.

It is not dissimilar to a large, strong domestic tabby cat but has a larger, thicker tail with three to five dark rings and a black blunt tip. It will, unfortunately, breed with feral cats resulting in hybrids weakening the genetic strain.

Dr Andrew Kitchener of the National Museum of Scotland is deeply involved with the Scottish wildcat populations and would be happy to advise on the identification of any wildcats brought into rehabilitation (pers.comm.). What is needed are good-quality colour photographs of the animals' dorsal, ventral and lateral aspects of both sides.

In general:

(1) Wildcats should not be released until formally identified
(2) There is currently no genetic identification possible but photographs should help
(3) Hybrids, infectious or feral domestic cats should not be released in the known range of the wildcat

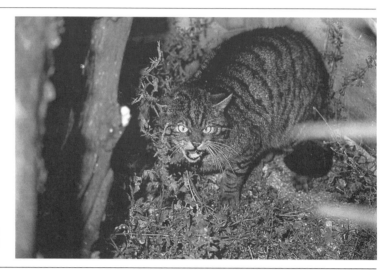

Fig. 27.1 A Scottish wildcat is more fierce and much stronger than even a feral cat.

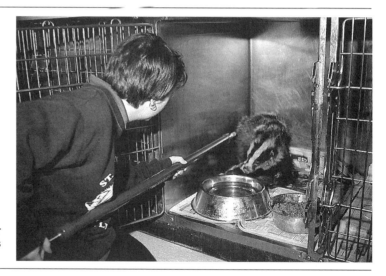

Fig. 27.2 A pole syringe can be useful for injecting unapproachable animals such as wildcats and badgers.

(4) All dead wildcats should be sent for post-mortem to the National Museum of Scotland

EQUIPMENT AND TRANSPORT

Wildcats are extremely powerful and fierce animals demanding the strongest equipment. A dog grasper is essential together with a strong carrying basket that has a crush facility. In care, the use of a pole syringe together with a broom will allow the use of injectable treatments (Fig. 27.2). Alternatively a blow pipe and darts can provide a method of remotely injecting.

RESCUE AND HANDLING

Apart from orphans, any wildcat that needs rescuing will be severely injured and disabled. To safely handle a wildcat that is not unconscious a dog grasper should be used around the neck and front leg. Do not try to scruff a wildcat as you would scruff a domestic cat. It is much stronger and can inflict serious injury with its claws as well as its teeth.

In care, it is possible to inject a wildcat with a syringe mounted on a 'pole syringe'. The technique is to let the wildcat arch itself and threaten your approach. It will usually stand erect in the back corner of its cage and spit and snarl. While attracting its attention by offering a broom to its front end the pole syringe can be gently slid into the cage and the injection given in the rump.

This technique takes a lot of time and patience but saves both the handler operative and the wildcat the trauma of handling it, if that were even possible.

COMMON DISEASES

Ectoparasites

Various parasites have been recorded from wildcats, probably as opportunists from prey species (Corbett, 1979). Species recorded have included:

- Cat flea (*Ctenocephalides felis*)
- Rabbit flea (*Spilopsyllus cuniculi*)
- Rodent flea (*Hystrichopsylla talpae*)

Ticks (*Ixodus ricinus*) and lice (*Filicola subrostuatus*) have also been recorded.

There have been few records of wildcats in care but generally ectoparasites should not be a major problem.

Endoparasites

Roundworms (*Toxicara cati*) and tapeworms (*Taenia* spp.) can be treated with standard cat remedies.

Cat diseases

One of the great worries with the spread of feral cats is the introduction to wildcat populations of feline diseases.

There is evidence that pure-bred Scottish wildcats commonly register positive for feline leukaemia virus (FeLV) and no doubt other diseases of the domestic cat can be transmitted to the wild populations (J. Lewis, pers. comm.).

All Scottish wildcats should be screened for feline diseases and not be released if they could pose a threat to the wild population.

Dental damage

Wildcats often have damaged teeth which should be remedied before they are released (Plate 43). (See also p. 96)

COMMON INCIDENCES

Scottish wildcats are very rarely near enough to human habitation to be involved in traumatic incidences. Usual occurrences are road traffic accidents and there are records of casualties caused by heather burning, traps and snares.

COMMON INJURIES

Recorded injuries are usually fractures caused by road traffic accidents, notably fractures to the jaw. In all respects the wildcat road traffic accident victim suffers similar injuries to other casualty domestic cats.

ADMISSION AND FIRST AID

Apart from an unconscious wildcat or one that is seriously debilitated, it is usually necessary to sedate the animal in order to provide intravenous fluids and medication. Once again it will be seen to present as a large aggressive domestic or feral cat and will benefit from standard cat care practices.

CAGING

The Scottish wildcat is extremely powerful and needs a really strong metal cage. The provision of a divider is essential for cleaning. Any unnecessary handling of a wildcat should be avoided.

A rehabilitation pen outside needs to be strong, high, covered and with many large branches and platforms set well above the ground.

FEEDING

Although wildcats can be provided with good-quality cat food, their diet should reflect their wild preferences. Rabbits, mice, rats and day-old chicks are taken. The latter will need a feline mineral supplement in order to provide a balanced diet.

RELEASE

Scottish wildcats should be released where they were found. However, with the problems of hybridisation, Scottish Natural Heritage (Appendix 7) will be able to advise if that location is unsuitable and can recommend alternatives.

In a new area a system of hacking will give the cat a better chance of integrating with the local fauna.

LEGAL IMPLICATIONS

Scottish wildcats are protected from cruelty as are all British mammals. They also fall under the auspices of the Dangerous Wild Animals Act (1976) as members of the Felidae.

A Dangerous Wild Animal licence is required. These can be provided, at a cost, from the Environmental Health Officer at the local Council.

The use of a blow pipe and pneumatic darts does require a Firearms Licence available at a local police station.

Part II: Sea mammals

Both these groups of animals require specialised rescue techniques, handling, holding and treatment beyond the capabilities of most practices and rescue centres.

Seals

Seals are abundant in several areas around the British coast. In these areas there is usually a group or centre specialising in seal rescue and rehabilitation.

Most casualties are seal pups with the occasional adult debilitated by disease or injury (Fig. 27.3). Their rescue is often not appropriate and if necessary needs experienced handlers so as not to get bitten.

Any sightings of a seal possibly needing rescue should be immediately referred to the local centre for assistance. The police in the area will have a list of the most suitable people to contact. It is best not to attempt a rescue but to monitor the animal until help arrives.

Cetaceans

Even more specialised than seal care is the rescue and treatment of stranded or trapped whales, dolphins or porpoises.

Any stranding or other incident can be at any point around Britain's coastline. The advice on finding a stranded or trapped cetacean is not to try to rescue it but to contact the British Divers Marine Life Rescue (BDMLR) who have estab-

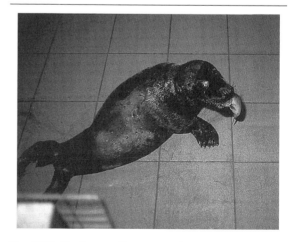

Fig. 27.3 Most casualties are seal pups.

lished a nationwide network of volunteer rescue teams (see Appendix 7). The rescue team will ask for some information and will advise which procedures to follow to steady the animal until help arrives.

For the notes on these procedures from the British Divers Marine Life Rescue *Marine Mammal Medic Handbook* (Barnett *et al.*, 1998) see Appendix 2.

28
Rearing Orphaned Wild Mammals

Every year many young mammals become separated from their mothers. It is practically unknown for a wild mother to abandon her young, although it can happen if they are seriously disturbed. Normally orphans are found because some disaster has befallen the mother or their nest is destroyed, usually during human construction or repair work.

With any wild mammal orphan taken into care the circumstances of its rescue should be considered and the opportunity taken to return it to its nursery, if that is at all possible. Otherwise the young animal will need hand-rearing and the commitment of time and patience that that requires.

All of the British terrestrial species have been reared by hand at some time or another. Various protocols are now in place based on the experience of rehabilitators. It is recommended that their practices are followed as each species has its own idiosyncrasies that need to be addressed. However, others may have their own methods that have been successful so 'if it works for you' do not change it.

Many of the accepted practices apply to more than one species so familiarity with the normal protocols can be adapted to suit any individual species.

NATURAL HISTORY

Mammals in Britain are born at various times of the year and in varying litter sizes from one in most deer to multiple births in smaller mammals. The young are either born fully furred and mobile or more commonly born without much or no fur and with their eyes and ears closed. Their mothers suckle them for various amounts of time until they are weaned on to an adult solid diet.

Being available to take on mammal orphans, it is possible to predict some arrivals but it is preferable to have a complete range of consumables and equipment ready in order to cope with whichever animal is brought in.

CONSUMABLES

In hand-rearing we seek to enable suckling, by providing milk replacers and sometimes passive immunity, until weaning leads to the release of a fully wild animal.

Milk replacers

Each species of mammal produces its own individual milk. It is not practical to obtain exactly these particular milks but substitutes can be made up of similar component parts (Table 28.1).

There are pet milks and, of course, milk products from cows, but these have generally proven to be inappropriate for use with wild mammals. All milks should be warmed otherwise the animal may not feed.

Additives to milk replacers

Some species require additional minerals or enzymes to the milk replacers, especially goats' milk (Table 28.2).

Table 28.1 Analysis of the milk of some UK mammals (after Pet-Ag).

	% solids	Protein % solids	Fat % solids	Carbohydrates % solids
Badger	18.6	38.7/38.8	33.9	18.8
Bottle-nosed dolphin	41.7	16.3	79.1	2.6
Brown rat	22.1	37.0	40.0	17.0
Fallow deer	25.3	26.0	50.0	24.0
Ferret	23.5	25.5	34.0	16.2
Fox	18.2	34.6	34.6	25.3
Grey seal	67.7	16.5	78.6	3.8
Grey squirrel	39.6	18.7	62.5	9.4
Harbour porpoise	45.8	—	89.7	2.8
Hare	32.2	31.0	46.0	5.0
Hedgehog	21.6	33.3	46.3	9.3
House mouse	29.3	31.0	45.0	10.0
Mink	21.7	26.0	33.0	21.0
Otter	38.0	28.9	63.0	0.3
Rabbit	31.2	32.0	49.0	6.0
Red deer	21.1	34.0	40.0	21.9
Red-necked wallaby	13.9	28.8	33.1	32.4
Roe deer	19.4	45.4	34.5	20.1
Sika deer	36.1	34.3	52.6	9.4
Stoat	23.5	25.5	34.0	16.2
Water shrew	35.0	28.6	57.1	0.3

Table 28.2 Milk replacers and additives.

Milk replacers

	Solids %	Protein % of	Fat % of	Carbohydrates % of
Goat	12	22	32	39
Esbilac (Pet Ag)	97	33.2	43.0	15.8
Multi Milk (Pet Ag)	97	30.0	55.0	trace
Lamlac (Volac Feeds)	60	24	24	—

Additives to milk replacers

Avipro (Vetark Animal Health) – pro-biotic
Abidec (Warner Lambert) – multivitamins
Stress (Phillips Yeast Products) – calcium/phosphorus supplement
Prolam (Schering-Plough Animal Health) – colostrum antibody supplement
Pancrex (Pharmacia & Upjohn) – digestive enzyme

Weaning foods

- Farley's Rusks (HJ Heinz)
- Plain digestive biscuits
- Pedigree Chum Puppy Food (Pedigree Masterfoods)
- A ready access to wild plants such as dandelion, chickweed and clover
- Prosecto dried insects (Haiths)
- Waxworm larvae
- Mealworms
- 'St Tiggywinkles Mammal Glop'

St Tiggywinkles Mammal Glop is mixed in bulk and is made up of:

One dog food tin of Pedigree Chum Puppy Food (Pedigree Masterfoods)
One dog food tin of water
One dog food tin of dried insects (Prosecto – Haith)
One pinch of Pancrex (Pharmacia & Upjohn) enzyme
One pinch of Vetamin & Zinc (Millpledge Pharmacenticals) multivitamins

$\frac{1}{2}$ teaspoon of Nutri-Plus (Virbac)
One pinch of Stress (Phillips Yeast Products)

This is mixed to the consistency of soft ice cream and frozen in shallow dishes with lids (Jonipax – Ashwood Timber & Plastics). The mixture is defrosted in a refrigerator before use.

HYGIENE PRODUCTS

- Trigene (Medichem International) – a combined surface cleaner and disinfectant that when used at the recommended concentration is a safe cleaning medium
- Milton (Proctor & Gamble) – for sterilising bottles, teats and feeding utensils
- Mediscrub Handscrub (Medichem International) – for personal hygiene

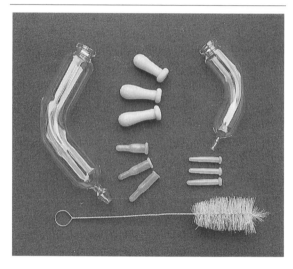

Fig. 28.1 The range of Catac kitten and puppy rearing bottles and teats suitable for wild animals.

Also cotton buds, paper towels, pet or baby wipes.
Do not use household disinfectants or detergents.

Creams and ointments

- White petroleum jelly is useful to provide relief if the animal becomes sore after urinating
- Metanium (Roche) provides: titanium dioxide, peroxide, salicylate, tannate to further relieve urine scalding.

EQUIPMENT

Feeding bottles, etc.

Obviously, different babies will require various sizes of bottles and teats to suit. Some are available at pet stores or veterinary practices, others need to be improvised but these are mainly for the smallest orphans.

Available commercially are:

- Esbilac Nursing Kits (Pet Ag) – contains a bottle, teats and a cleaning brush and is suitable for small and larger animals.
- Catac Kitten and Puppy Rearing Bottles and teats (Fig. 28.1), useful for smaller animals.

- Belcroy Premature Baby Bottle.
- Large deer may require a full-sized baby bottle and teat. Lamb-feeding bottles from agricultural merchants are also suitable.
- Pastettes (Alpha Laboratories) – these are available in a range of sizes up to the size for a squirrel. They are not practical for sterilisation and should be discarded after each feed. In use the tip of the pastette is cut off and a small Catac teat is attached.

Points to consider are:

- Hedgehog feeders can be made from:
  - A 1 ml syringe body
  - An eye dropper bulb
  - A 16 g hypodermic needle with the point cut off
  - The rubber insert from a Vacutainer blood sampling needle (Fig. 28.2)
- Some animals have a particularly strong sucking action, so it is essential that all teats are secure
- Mice, voles, shrews and bats can be fed with a small artist's paintbrush
- Shallow plastic dishes with lids for freezing prepared food (Jonipax – Ashwood Timber & Plastics) (Fig. 28.3).

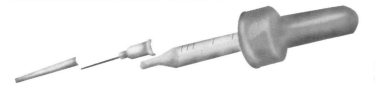

Fig. 28.2 A hedgehog baby feeder and components.

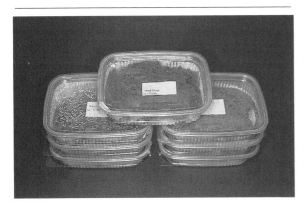

Fig. 28.3 Jonipax (Ashwood Timber & Plastics) flat dishes prevent anaerobic bacteria from flourishing in 'glop' formula.

Housing and other equipment

- Various plastic cages, boxes and aquaria
- Heat lamps which can be flexible table lamps with a 20 W, 25 W or 40 W red bulb (Fig. 28.4)
- Metal heat mats
- Scales capable of weighing in 1 g increments
- Small veterinary bedding
- Food liquidiser

PROCEDURES

On Admittance

The infant casualty as it arrives will probably be in some distress. It will be cold and possibly dehydrated, and sometimes injured and attacked by flies.

Initially it should be weighed, warmed and given warm subcutaneous fluids. Some youngsters, e.g. deer, foxes, badgers and otters, will be large enough to be infused intravenously with warmed fluids.

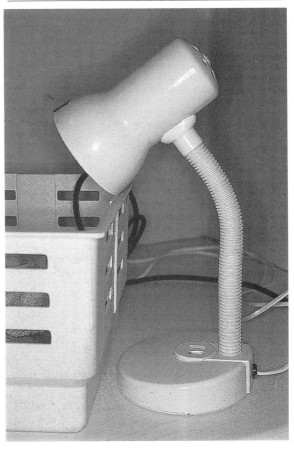

Fig. 28.4 A simple heater can be a flexible table lamp fitted with red bulbs of various wattages.

Also at this stage all babies benefit from a small amount of Pet Breeder Nutri Drops (Net-Tex) given orally. The dose rate is 0.1 ml per 90 g.

Toileting

The next priority, and one that is often forgotten, is to stimulate the animal to urinate and sometimes defecate. Most mammal young are unable to urinate without assistance. Normally their mothers will stimulate them to do this but if the youngster is orphaned it may not have been relieved for some-time. Failure to urinate can lead to fatal uraemias and most mammals will show no interest in feeding if their bladders are full.

The animal can be stimulated to urinate by rapidly, but gently, brushing a damp cotton bud or piece of paper towel over the genital area and anus. At first the animal may not respond but persevere until it does urinate. This procedure should be carried out before and after each feed. In fact deer will respond to being stimulated while they are suckling.

With smaller infants there may be an element of overflow from the bladder which may appear to be spontaneous urination. Left unchecked the bladder may not empty and the overflow will lead to urine scalding. Assume that it is overflow unless the urination is seen to be pulsing under some pressure.

Urination scalding can be relieved with either white petroleum jelly or Metanium (Roche).

First bottle feed

The next stage of rearing is to get the orphan used to bottle feeding. At first it may reject the bottle or else overindulge leading to flooding of the mouth and inhalation of the liquid. This can lead to inhalation pneumonia but there is less chance of this developing if Lectade (Pfizer) or other oral rehydration fluid is given for the first two feeds.

Generally, hold the animal tipped slightly forward as this helps prevent inhalation. Then offer up the feeding bottle to its mouth. Do not force it to drink but be patient and let a drop or two go into its mouth. Once it starts to take the liquid then it will be more receptive to milk feeding. Do make sure that the hole in the teat is not too large. In fact the most suitable orifice in a teat is a cross-shaped cut that can be easily extended if it is too small (Fig. 28.5).

Milk feeding

Once the orphan has taken those first two feeds and has been toileted, a regime of feeding can be established. Overnight feeding is not necessary

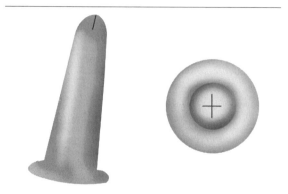

Fig. 28.5 A cross-shaped cut in the top of a teat.

except for moles, shrews, tiny mice and voles. Generally four feeds a day can be planned:

> Early morning; lunchtime; teatime and one late at night

A fifth feed should be fitted in for shrews and moles.

Some species will require one or two feeds a day. In the wild, rabbits and hares will be fed only once daily but in captivity opt for two feeds. This is because the milk used is artificial without the whole range of suitable ingredients in milk provided naturally.

It is important that the orphan is seen to swallow milk. If milk overflows from the mouth or down the nose there is a possibility that the hole in the teat is too large or just that too much milk is being given. It may also point to a split or cleft palate.

After each feed the orphan must be toileted again and its face and fur wiped clean with a baby or pet wipe.

Colostrum

Mammals have passive immunity passed to them in colostrum in their mother's milk. In most cases an orphan will have received colostrum and, except in animals like hedgehogs, will not need any more.

However, in some situations a substitute colostrum should be provided:

(1) When an animal has not received any maternal milk, e.g after it is delivered by caesarean

section. One day on neat colostrum is usually sufficient.

(2) When an animal would naturally be provided with colostrum for a longer period. For example, hedgehogs absorb colostrum for up to 41 days after birth. Mice also have the ability to receive colostrum up to 16 days after birth.

With these orphans, the first day's milk should be 50:50 colostrum mixed with the milk substitute. On the second day mixed 50:50 with the milk substitute and from then on mixed 25:75 with the milk. Mice should receive this until they are weaned while hedgehogs should receive colostrum until they are about 21 days old and starting to wean.

Hygiene

At each feed all bowls and feeding utensils should be thoroughly washed and kept in a sterilising solution such as Milton (Procter & Gamble). Any unused milk should be discarded and mixed freshly for each feed.

It is impractical to try to sterilise pastettes, which should also be discarded. It is not possible to clean them thoroughly before sterilisation. Organic matter cannot be sterilised.

It is a distinct advantage if each orphan can be fed with its own particular bottle.

Rest

In between feeds the animals must be allowed to sleep and digest their meals. A tired animal will be reluctant to feed. Also it is much easier to feed an animal that is hungry so, as long as mealtimes are adhered to, the orphan should be letting you know it is hungry and needs feeding.

All wild mammal orphans should be kept in family groups remote from any other animals, especially domestic pets, and should not be allowed to walk around on the floor either in rescue centres or houses.

Housing

Pet-carrying baskets or plastic aquaria are ideal nurseries for young animals. In these an overhead heat source can be provided with a flexible lamp fitted with a red bulb. The animals must be able to move away from the heat if they wish. A non-slip mat on the floor will stop the animals from slipping.

The use of veterinary bedding is ideal as it keeps the animals dry. Do not cover the bedding with anything and only use newspaper underneath it.

Most small mammals will appreciate a cuddly toy or piece of warm blanket to snuggle up to or under.

Weighing

A development chart will provide a record of an animal's progress and a basis for future excursions into rearing.

Each orphan should be weighed at the same time each day. Its weight should remain constant or increase. Any weight loss must be monitored and if it occurs over 48 hours then something may be going wrong. This could be caused by:

* Diarrhoea – the baby should be starved for 24 hours and only receive oral fluids (Lectade – Pfizer) in place of milk
* Infection – there may be the start of an infection warranting the use of antibiotics
* Parasites – there may be a heavy burden of worms or coccidia

THINGS THAT GO WRONG

Inhalation pneumonia

This is the main killer of orphaned mammals. Using oral rehydration fluids for the first feed prevents a lot of the problem.

If it does happen the affected animal may start to breathe heavily and even with an open mouth. An audible 'click' can sometimes be heard as it breathes. Amoxycillin by injection can help to remedy the condition and the veterinary surgeon may prescribe other respiratory drugs.

Hypothermia

An infant mammal will not feed if it is cold. Usually it should feel just warm to the touch. However too much heat can lead to hyperthermia which can very quickly be fatal.

Winding

Some of the larger infants will gulp air as well as milk replacer. This causes the very human baby complaint of 'wind'. It can usually be relieved by gently massaging or patting the back. Major wind problems may be relieved with gripe water, available at chemists for human babies.

Imprinting

This is the worst thing that can happen to an orphaned mammal. It can become totally reliant on human company or that of domestic animals and, in the end, cannot be released.

Various rules should be implemented to prevent imprinting:

(1) Never attempt to rear a mammal on its own. Seek out another fosterer who may have orphans of the same species.
(2) Do not talk to the orphans especially after weaning.
(3) Do not handle the animals other than when they are being bottle fed and toiletted.
(4) Keep particularly vulnerable animals such as fox cubs and deer from seeing humans and hearing human voices.
(5) Do not let children handle or play with young animals.

Quarantine

The only occasion when an orphan should be kept on its own is when it is first admitted. It is advisable to keep it away from established groups as it may be harbouring an infection. Usually this will show itself in 3–4 days.

Penis sucking

This happens a lot with squirrels and otters. Where it is other siblings causing the problem the affected animal should be removed and kept on its own.

Often it is the animal itself that is self-mutilating. The only way to prevent this is to fashion an Elizabethan collar out of a piece of plastic or cardboard.

SPECIES IDIOSYNCRASIES

Mice and voles

Milk: Colostrum mixed 25:75 with milk for mice until weaning. Esbilac (Pet Ag) with the brush dipped in Stress (Phillips Yeast Products) once a day.
Feeder: Paintbrush dipped in milk or a small pastette.
Frequency: Hourly from early morning until late at night. Then two hourly overnight.
Weaning: Will wean before their eyes are open, usually about 9 days after birth. Food for mice try crumbled digestive biscuits or rusks scattered on the floor. For voles try greenstuff such as chickweed, dandelion or clover.

Shrews

Milk: Esbilac (Pet Ag).
Feeder: Paintbrush dipped in milk or a small pastette.
Frequency: Avid feeders should be fed hourly both day and night.
Weaning: Wean as soon as possible on to live invertebrate food, e.g. maggots, mini-mealworms or waxworm larvae.
Notes: Shrews should have food available all the time. Their rapid metabolism requires constant nourishment.

Squirrels and dormice

Milk: Goats' milk with teat dipped in Stress (Phillips Yeast Products) once a day.
Bottle: Catac Kitten Bottle with small teat.
Frequency: Four to five feeds a day.
Weaning: At 2–3 weeks wean on to Farley's Rusks (HJ Heinz). Adult food should be a good-quality dry puppy food. Do not feed peanuts or sunflower seeds.
Notes: Squirrels can be susceptible to hypocalcaemia.

Hedgehogs

Milk: Colostrum to be added to milk up to 21 days. First day 50:50 colostrum/milk, second day 50:50 colostrum/milk, third day and for 21 days 25:75 colostrum/milk. Then 100% milk. Goats' milk is suitable.

Feeder: Use a 1 ml syringe with a Vacutainer rubber tip or pastettes which should be discarded after each feed (Fig. 28.6).

Frequency: Four to five feeds a day.

Weaning: When teeth appear at about 21 days wean on to St Tiggywinkles Mammal Glop. This should be liquidised to the consistency of soft ice-cream and frozen in shallow dishes (Jonipax – Ashwood Timber & Plastics). Glop should be allowed to defrost in a refrigerator. Do not warm it in an oven or microwave.

Always freeze 'glop' before using it – this stops bacteria multiplying before use.

Notes: Baby hedgehogs tend not to suck on the teat. The milk must be slowly fed into the mouth. It is also crucial that baby hedgehogs have overhead heat.

Weasels and stoats

Milk: Goats' milk or Esbilac (Pet Ag) are suitable for these small mustelids.

Feeder: The Catac Kitten Bottle with a small teat is ideal.

Frequency: Weasels and stoats can be fed four or five times a day.

Weaning: These animals wean very early on to chopped mice. They wean before their eyes are open.

Notes: Weasels are very easily tamed so it is crucial that handling and contact is kept to a minimum.

Badgers

Milk: Once more goats' milk or Esbilac (Pet Ag) are suitable for this species.

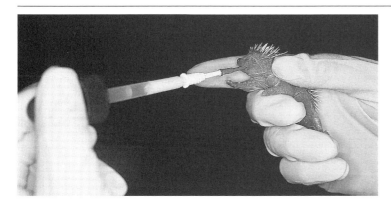

Fig. 28.6 Baby hedgehogs are fed using a feeder made from a 1 ml syringe.

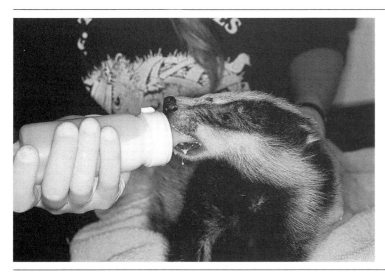

Fig. 28.7 Badger cubs are more suited to Esbilac (Pet Ag) feeding bottles.

Feeder: Being larger the Esbilac (Pet Ag) Puppy Bottles are suitable (Fig. 28.7).

Frequency: Four or five feeds daily suit this species.

Weaning: Badgers should be weaned on to dog food. Once fully weaned the badgers will feed on mice or chicks. Badgers take a long time to wean, as long as 10–12 weeks.

Notes: Badgers are easily tamed so once more handling and contact should be kept to a minimum. In fact these animals should be reared with others. They should not be reared on their own.

Winding: Badgers may gulp air and need 'burping' by gently rubbing the back as you would a human baby.

Rabbits and hares

Milk: Both can be reared on Esbilac (Pet Ag).

Bottles: Catac Puppy Bottles and small teats are ideal.

Frequency: These animals should be fed only twice a day.

Weaning: Hares are born far in advance of rabbits and wean much earlier. Dandelions and clover are suitable. Rabbits are born naked, with their eyes closed and take a little longer to wean on to the same greenstuffs.

Foxes

Milk: Goats' milk is suitable.

Feeder: The Esbilac (Pet Ag) Puppy Bottles or Belcroy Premature Baby Feeders.

Frequency: Four to five feeds a day.

Weaning: Wean on to dog food or mice and chicks.

Notes: Important to keep fox cubs from imprinting and to try to provide natural food before their eventual release in the autumn. Road kill rabbits, pheasants and other victims will provide training in the type of food they will need in the wild.

Winding: Fox cubs may need to be 'burped'.

Deer

Milk: Lamlac (Volac Feeds) ewe replacer milk seems to be to the liking of deer fawns.

Feeder: The smaller deer will take from the Esbilac (Pet Ag) bottles while larger species may need human baby bottles or lamb feeders.

Frequency: Four to five times a day

Weaning: As early as possible on to hay, dandelions leaves, chickweed and coarse goat mix.

Notes: New admissions may be difficult. The secret with deer is that only one person should feed each one. The deer should be kept in a shed away from other distractions. They will only feed while standing up and will be more receptive if they are toiletted while they are suckling, one hand holding the bottle the other hand toiletting.

Winding: Deer fawns may need to be 'burped'.

Bats

Milk: Esbilac (Pet Ag) does seem suitable for bats. Mixed 1 part powder to one part water provides a thicker, more suitable, milk substitute.

Feeder: Allow the bats to lap off a small paintbrush.

Frequency: Every two hours during the day, i.e. 7.00 AM to 11.00 PM. It is not necessary to feed overnight.

Weaning: Bats will be weaned on to the insides of mealworms squeezed so they can lap the soft contents.

Moles

Milk: Esbilac (Pet Ag) is suitable.

Feeder: Pastette.

Frequency: Every hour day and night.

Weaning: As soon as possible on to chopped mice or 'glop'.

Wildcat

Should be reared like a domestic kitten but weaned on to mice, rabbit or chicks.

It will usually stay wild.

Sea mammals

Should be referred to specialist centres (see Chapter 27).

29
Reptiles and Amphibians

Part I: Reptiles

British species seen:
- **Snakes:**   grass snake (*Natrix natrix*), adder or viper (*Vipera berus*) and smooth snake (*Coronella austriaca*)
- **Lizards:**   slow worm (*Anguis fragilis*), common lizard (*Lacerta vivipara*) and sand lizard (*Lacerta agilis*)

Other escaped exotic species of snakes, lizards, iguanas and chelonians are found and rescued. However, these are normally tropical species and require the specialised paraphernalia and veterinary attention now proliferating to cope with the various pet species. They are not truly rehabilitation candidates; they cannot be released and are therefore not covered by the rehabilitation procedures covered in this chapter.

NATURAL HISTORY

The three species of British snake are easily recognised. Only one, the adder, is poisonous; the smooth snake is a constrictor, but is now very rare. The grass snake, Britain's largest and commonest snake, is neither, it catches its prey in its mouth where the typical serpentine back-facing teeth make escape difficult. The adder will feed on small mammals and birds as will the other two species. However, the smooth snake is noted for taking lizards, especially the endangered sand lizard which shares its habitat.

The grass snake is very aquatic and is often injured visiting garden ponds hunting fish and frogs. This is the snake most often injured by its excursions into gardens and its habit of favouring compost heaps for egg-laying.

The lizards with legs, the common and sand lizard, are very fleet of foot and not often caught and injured. Some cats, however, seem to specialise in lizards probably because they happen to live near to good lizard habitat.

The slow worm is a lizard but does not possess legs. It is more often caught than the other two species presumably because it does not possess their wariness and speed of escape.

All three lizards practise autotomy wherein they can lose their tail to a predator. There is an unossified fracture plane in the mid-region of the centrum of a caudal vertebra (Davies, 1981). When caught by a predator this snaps and a portion of the tail breaks off and wriggles madly to attract the attention of the assailant. The lizard then escapes and grows a new tail.

EQUIPMENT, TRANSPORT, RESCUE AND HANDLING

Snakes and lizards, except the venomous adder, can be simply picked up if they are injured. They are, however, easily bruised where autolysis may be caused. They should be handled gently. Never pick up a lizard by its tail, it will break off.

Grass snakes when caught will emit a particularly foul-smelling liquid from their anal gland. The wearing of vinyl gloves will prevent your hands from becoming contaminated. They may make an effort to bite, but are not dangerous. They may also 'play dead'. Do not be fooled until a thorough examination has been made.

These species of snakes and lizards can be safely transported in small plastic aquaria with hinged lids in the top. They are particularly good at escaping through even the tightest gap.

Adders are quite different, they are dangerous. Although the bite of an adder is rarely fatal, it can be and can cause severe illness or discomfort. Do not get bitten. In approaching an adder do wear thick gauntlets. However, although these will offer protection from an adder's bite, the snake may damage its teeth on the heavy material even though a snake's teeth are being constantly replaced.

With the gloves on, the snake can often be simply lifted on a snake hook and deposited in something deep such as a dustbin. If the dustbin is lined with a cloth bag this can be closed with a draw string to contain the snake. A second tie can be wrapped around just below the draw string to make doubly sure of no escape. After this is secure the snake can still bite through the bag itself so do not touch it. Another method featured in the guidelines of the Joint Nature Conservation Committee is by using a foam-padded restraining stick for directing the snake into a swing-lid kitchen bin laid on its side (Griffiths & Langton, 1998). The bin is then emptied into a draw-string bag. Take particular care with any snake you do not recognise. There are many exotic pets that escape and some may be venomous. Until they are identified treat every exotic as a venomous species.

COMMON DISEASES

There are many diseases recorded in the thousands of species of reptile with many of them being described in the various excellent works on reptile disease. However, as disease diagnosis is strictly the province of the veterinary surgeon (Veterinary Surgeons Act 1966) the diseases mentioned here are those commonly encountered and accepted as conditions not strictly requiring a diagnosis per se.

CONDITIONS AFFECTING SNAKES

Hypothermia and hyperthermia

Snake and lizards are ectothermic in which their body temperature matches that of their surroundings. If they are too cold their digestion of food slows down causing regurgitation or rotting of food in the stomach leading to bacterial infection. If they are too hot then they will quickly dehydrate and dessicate. At their preferred body temperature (PBT), which is a range of temperatures between which they are comfortable, all their bodily functions operate normally.

The PBTs for British snakes (after Cooper & Jackson, 1981) are:

Grass snake	26.0°C
Adder	30.0°C
Smooth snake	27.0°C
Sand lizard	27.0°C
Slow worm	22.6°C

Any of these with a deep cloacal temperature of over 38°C (slow worm 30°C) can be classed as hyperthermic and should be cooled by immersing in cold water.

Hypothemia will automatically resolve under the gentle heat of an overhead heater suitable for reptiles.

The suggested relative humidity of any containers for common species is between 45 and 70%.

Dysecdysis

As reptiles grow their skin does not expand and so they have to shed it (ecdysis). For the shedding to go without a hitch the conditions have to be suitable. Too low or too high a humidity might prevent ecdysis – dysecdysis. The wrong environment with the lack of suitable rocks on which to rub off the old skin can cause problems as can the reptile not having bathed regularly. If the old skin is not shed it could cause constriction and resulting necrosis, particularly in lizards and tail tips.

It is possible to see a snake with dysecdysis because the old skin covering the eyes may be cloudy. Sometimes all that is needed is for the snake to bathe and be given a rock or a rough piece of wood on which to slough the old skin (Fig. 29.1). If this does not work putting the animal in between two layers of wet towel which may help the sloughing.

Another method is to rub the reptile with a series of cotton wool balls ranging from wet to dry. Working from the nose to the tail should see all the old skin removed. Particular care should be taken over the eyes. The old 'spectacles' should be moistened and slid off with damp cotton buds or the spectacles softened with hypromellose and then slid off. If that is unsuccessful refer the snake to a veterinary surgeon experienced with reptiles.

The use of adhesive tape or forceps will probably cause permanent damage to the underlying eye (Lawton, 1991).

Maladaption syndrome

This applies particularly to the grass snake. It means that the animal will not settle to captivity, will not eat and eventually does not thrive. It may be that the lighting or temperature is unsuitable. Specialised ultraviolet lighting with the spectrum of natural light (using Trulite (Durotest International) or Life-Glo (Rolf C Hagen) fluorescent lights) for

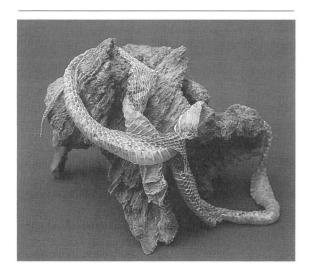

Fig. 29.1 Snakes with dysecdysis can be helped, like this grass snake, by being provided with a rough piece of wood.

a photoperiod of 12 hours on, 12 hours off may stimulate the appetite.

Generally though, grass snakes will need to be force fed if they are contained for any length of time.

The real success with all of these reptile casualties is to release them as soon as possible into a suitable habitat.

COMMON INCIDENTS

Cat attack

The domestic cat will capture lizards including slow worms and small snakes, usually grass snakes.

Medication should be with amoxycillin at 22 mg/kg by mouth 1–2 times daily or 10 mg/kg intramuscularly daily as long as the animal is at its PBT. It is suggested that amoxycillin alone is often ineffective in reptiles unless given with aminoglycosides (Bishop, 1998). The addition of amikacin (Amikin – Bristol-Myers) at 5 mg/kg can be effective.

Injections should be given into the front third of the body so that the drug is not transported directly to the kidneys via the renal portal vein (Frye, 1991).

Netting

Grass snakes are fond of visiting garden ponds. Often the pond is covered with netting to protect fish from herons. Grass snakes can get tangled in the netting causing damage to the scales and skin. After they are cut free any wounds should be bathed with saline.

Pressure necrosis may develop but usually the snake can be released after 5 days observation and broad-spectrum antibiotic cover with enrofloxacin (Baytril 2.5% – Bayer) at 5 mg/kg by mouth daily.

COMMON INJURIES

Bite wounds

Apart from those wounds inflicted by cats, grass snakes often get attacked by dogs. The bite wounds are usually severe with underlying damage to internal organs and the skeletal frame. The wounds can be cleaned with saline and sutured taking particular care of the internal organs.

Damage to the skeleton, particularly the spine, may not be fatal. A veterinary surgeon familiar with reptile injury will be able to advise on treatment or euthanasia.

Antibiotic cover should be based on amoxycillin to counter the bacteria carried on the dog's teeth.

Implement wounds

People will attack snakes with sticks, spades or even just the feet. The injuries are usually of the skin, internal organs or skeletal frame. Referral for an experienced prognosis, as made for bite wounds, is recommended for all seriously injured snakes.

Autotomy in lizards

This is the ability a lizard has to shed its tail. The resulting wound will not require suturing as a new tail will regenerate. This new tail may not be as slender and pointed as the original tail. Any closure of the wound could result in abnormal growth.

ADMISSION AND FIRST AID

Dehydration

The main first-aid procedure with snakes is to provide fluids. Dehydration in snakes is noticeable by a wrinkling of the skin and the classic tenting.

The snake should be weighed and the degree of dehydration estimated. Snakes can show a 20% dehydration but mostly it is better to assume a 5–10% of bodyweight deficit.

Three routes of administration are available:

(1) *Oral route.* Either Hartmann's solution or Lectade (Pfizer) can be given by a small stomach tube. The lubricated tube is slid into the stomach which is approximately one-third of the distance from the nose to the cloaca. The dose is 2% of bodyweight given twice daily (Marshall, 1993). It may take some days to fully rehydrate a snake.

(2) *Subcutaneous route.* With a 25 g hypodermic needle fitted on to a syringe, fluids can be given along the medial line on the side of the body. The siting should be about one-third of the body length between the nose and the cloaca. Fluids are administered in a forward direction (Fig. 29.2).

A seriously debilitated snake could be boosted with a subcutaneous bolus of amino acids and vitamins (Duphalyte – Fort Dodge Animal Health) at 2% of bodyweight. In injecting reptiles the needle should be slid under the scales not through them.

(3) *Intracoelomic route.* Warm fluid may be given into the body cavity either by injection or an intravenous catheter for prolonged fluid therapy. As this is entry into the body cavity the author thinks this method, though very effective, should be the province of the veterinary surgeon.

PROGNOSIS

A good knowledge of reptile anatomy is essential as some damage to the internal organs is irretrievable.

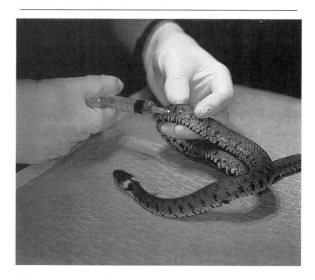

Fig. 29.2 A grass snake can receive fluids subcutaneously along its side.

CAGING

Snakes and lizards are best kept in either plastic or glass aquaria with a lid ventilated with small holes. The base should be covered with newspaper or paper towel making it much easier to keep the set up clean.

A sick or injured reptile will benefit from an overhead ceramic heat lamp at one end of the aquarium. This should be controlled by a thermostat to maintain a temperature between 25 and 30°C. Slow worms should be maintained at 20–25°C. The complete heating and thermostat kit is available at most large pet stores.

Water must be provided, especially for grass snakes who like to completely immerse themselves. Pieces of bark will allow the animals to hide away.

Lighting should be with an ultraviolet light suitable for reptiles and providing a full spectrum of natural light. A 'Trulite' (Durotest International), 'Reptisun' (Zoo-Med Laboratories) or 'Iguana Light' (Zoo-Med Laboratories) bulb within 30 cm of the reptile will certainly assist its recovery. The bulbs will have to be replaced every 9 months.

FEEDING

Snakes are going to be reluctant to feed but may take dead brown mice, slightly warmed and moved around in front of them on a piece of string.

Lizards will take flies, maggots or crickets dusted with a calcium/phosphorus supplement (Cricket Diet Calci-Paste – International Zoo Veterinary Group; Nutrobal – Vetark Animal Health).

Slow worms naturally feed on the small grey slug *Limax agrestis* easily found in gardens under rocks or pieces of wood. This food is readily taken and is the food of choice for captive slow worms.

RELEASE

All these reptiles should be released where they were found provided that the habitat is suitable.

In particular grass snakes do tend to live near water and can be released, not near a garden pond, but near to a stream or small river.

Smooth snakes and sand lizards are very rare and any casualties should definitely be released where there are others of their species. Advice can be obtained from English Nature (Appendix 7).

LEGAL IMPLICATIONS

Reptiles in captivity are protected by the Protection of Animals Act 1911.

Adders are classed as dangerous wild animals by virtue of being members of the Viperidae. To keep one in captivity requires a licence under the Dangerous Wild Animals Act 1976. This can be obtained from the local District Council.

Part II: Amphibians

Native species:

- **Frogs:**   common frog (*Rana temporaria*).

- **Toads:**   common toad (*Bufo bufo*) and natterjack toad (*B. calamita*).

- **Newts:**   great crested newt (*Triturus cristatus*), Smooth (or common) newt (*T. vulgaris*) and palmate newt (*T. helveticus*).

Introduced species:
Pool frog (*R. lessonae*), marsh frog (*R. ridibunda*), edible frog (hybrid of pool and marsh frogs) (*R. esculenta*), tree frog (*Hyla arborea*) and North American bull frog (*R. catesbeiana*).

NATURAL HISTORY

Amphibians need water in which to breed. They return to familiar waters in the spring having spent the rest of the year on dry land.

The mating of frogs and toads is by the males clinging to the females in a grip called amplexus. The males grow black pads on their fore feet to obtain a more secure grip (nuptial pads). Male toads croak when they are touched, presumably to let other male toads know their sex.

The eggs of frogs are laid in clumps, those of toads in strings and those of newts singly under the leaves of water plants. They all go through a stage as tadpoles and then metamorphose into the adult animal.

All species frequent gardens even if they have no water feature. Often a toad will become a familiar resident living under its own particular rock and emerging to catch various invertebrates.

Amphibians in this country practise a simple form of hibernation. Usually it is on dry land under a rock or buried in the ground. Frogs may sometimes 'hibernate' in the mud at the bottom of ponds.

EQUIPMENT, HANDLING, RESCUE AND TRANSPORT

When amphibians are in captivity they should be kept in a glass or plastic vivarium or aquarium. In there they should have access to dry land as well as to water.

Amphibians have moist and permeable skin and can be damaged by being picked up with a dry, dirty hand. Before handling wash the hands thoroughly in water with no soap or detergent and keep the hands wet for handling. Even more suitable are unpowdered vinyl gloves.

For transporting amphibians they should be provided with a cool, ventilated, waterproof box in which they can rest on damp vegetation or a clean damp sponge. Tadpoles should only be transported immersed in water.

Most rescues are after garden accidents or, in the case of newts, when they are found hibernating in the most unlikely places.

Each spring toads migrate to their mating ponds along the same routes that have been used for centuries. Unfortunately many of these routes cross busy roads. Many hundreds of toads get killed or maimed. They can be rescued or helped across the road by organised teams. The phenomenon only lasts for a few wet nights in spring.

COMMON DISEASES

There is still little known about the ongoing diseases affecting amphibian populations. In fact over the last few years research has been carried out into which epizootics are killing masses of frogs every year. Any mass die-offs should be recorded for Froglife (see Appendix 7) who are maintaining British records of herpetofauna incidents.

Some diseases, given below, are well known and have been seen for many years.

Red leg in frogs

Red leg is a common bacterial infection caused by *Aeromonas hydrophila*. It is known as 'red leg' because of the red lesions seen on the hind legs and underneath.

Sometimes many animals will be found dead for no apparent reason while others may present terminal neurological signs, spasms or vomiting.

Aeromonas hydrophila may be part of a frog's normal bacteria load so isolation of it is not a guarantee for diagnosis (Williams, 1991). It is highly contagious and will kill all of the frogs in a pond. Some protection can be provided by moving surviving frogs into clean water and replacing the pond water and contents.

In captivity a weak solution of saline (0.6%) will provide some disinfection.

'Red leg' will also describe symptoms of other diseases which the veterinary surgeon may wish to investigate as an alternative diagnosis.

Iridovirus-like agent from frogs

During 1993 many frog deaths were referred to the Central Veterinary Laboratory. Of 17 carcasses examined, 16 had evidence of iridovirus-like particles, the first time these had been reported from the common frog (Drury *et al.*, 1995).

Once again deaths of this nature should be referred to Froglife (Appendix 7) for guidance.

Salt poisoning

Toads on their migratory treks often cross roads that have been recently salted. A team of volunteer rescuers in Madingley, Cambs, reported toads suffering from a reddish skin discoloration and disorientation sometimes resulting in the toads stumbling and hitting their chins on the road. Washing the toads in clean water remedied most of those affected but 19, the most heavily salted, died (Foster, 1997).

Hydrops

This is where lymph accumulates in the dorsal lymph sacs and sometimes in the coelom. According to Williams (1991), the aetiology is unknown and the fluid accumulates again after aspiration. The condition is reported in anulans (tail-less frogs and toads) but the author has seen a similar condition in a smooth newt, one of the Caudata (with tails).

Subcutaneous emphysema

Frogs have also been presented bloated with air and unable to swim (Plate 44). No cause has been established.

The air can be aspirated with a syringe and small gauge needle. It may well reoccur but will eventually return to normal.

COMMON INCIDENTS

Garden accidents

Accidents in the garden are the most common source of amphibian casualties, especially frogs. They have a habit of sitting out in long grass and consequently get caught in mowers or strimmers.

Newts are found in dry situations such as under paving slabs or sheds. People think they should be in water but after breeding they, like the other amphibians, will venture on to dry land for most of the year and for hibernation.

Road accidents

Hundreds of toads do get killed every year on their migration treks across roads. Some, however, do manage to survive and are often picked up and brought into care.

Cat attacks

Cats do not seem to prey on amphibians as much as other animals and perhaps they have learnt the hard way that toads secrete an evil-tasting substance through their skin making them particularly unpalatable. Frogs and newts do, however, get caught and are sometimes rescued alive and brought into care.

COMMON INJURIES

Skin lacerations

These are usually suffered by frogs involved in garden accidents. They are often on the legs accompanied by fractures and other soft tissue damage (Plate 45). They can be sutured with 4.0–6.0 absorbable sutures with a swaged-on cutting needle (Vicryl – Ethicon).

A frog's skin is surprisingly tough to suture and frogs are particularly slippery and difficult to control. For suturing it is best to anaesthetise them. The simplest anaesthetic for use with amphibians is tricaine mesilate (MS222 – Thomson and Joseph). MS222 is dissolved in water at a concentration of 25–1000 g/l. The frog is placed in the solution up to its nostrils. It is observed and once flaccid should be removed from the water and placed on a cool, damp sponge for any procedure. Depth of anaesthesia can be maintained by occasionally syringing the anaesthetic solution over the frog or conversely to lighten the anaesthesia syringing it with oxygenated water.

Provided the lacerations are not debilitating, the frog could be released after 2 days, preferably into a pond area in a garden. A quick release is necessary because common frogs do not fare that well in captivity.

Fractures

Both frogs and toads are presented with limb fractures and jaw fractures. They do take a long time to heal but limb fractures can be immobilised with a range of methods including Vet-Lite (Runlite) splinting, extracutaneous fixation or intramedullary pinning.

Jaw fractures will need suturing, preferably with surgical wire.

Amputees

Toads cope well with the loss of one leg, although they should only be released in a known garden pond area.

Frogs are less likely to cope with amputations and should be humanely destroyed if subject to the loss of a leg.

Newts will possibly generate a new leg to replace the one that is missing.

Tongue injuries in anurans

Both frogs and toads have their tongues hinged at the front of their mouths. These they flick forward to catch their prey. The tongue is often traumatised when a jaw is injured. It can be sutured using Vicryl (Ethicon) but may be inoperative post trauma.

Without the use of the tongue the frog or toad would not be able to feed. Frogs who have lost the use of their tongues should be humanely destroyed but toads can often be taught to feed from the hand and can be kept in captivity in a suitable environment.

Eye injuries

Frogs and toads not only use their eyes to seek out prey, they also use them to push food from their mouths into their oesophagus. Obviously a blind amphibian should be humanely destroyed but the animal can probably exist as long as one eye is functioning. There is the question of focusing on prey with only one eye but amphibians do seem to cope.

The author has seen a frog with one eye firmly grown inside its mouth that had obviously coped in the wild for some time before it was caught by a cat. However, strangely enough the frog could see with the eye in its mouth and had adjusted its prey-catching ability to counter the disadvantage (Plate 46).

ADMISSION AND FIRST AID

Euthanasia

The essence of triage is that some casualties have no prognosis and should be humanely destroyed.

Euthanasia is particularly difficult to achieve with amphibians using just an overdose of barbiturates. Because of the erratic nature of barbiturates in amphibians it is most humane to deeply anaes-thetise the animal with gaseous anaesthesia and then provide the overdose by the intracardiac or intracoelomic routes.

Decapitation, freezing or pithing with a needle inserted into the foramen magnum are not now acceptable (UFAW/WSPA, 1989).

Fluid therapy

Hartmann's solution laced with 10% amino acids and vitamins (Duphalyte – Fort Dodge Animal Health) can be provided subcutaneously at 10% of bodyweight.

Antibiotics

A range of antibiotics has been used with amphibians and is well documented (Bishop, 1998).

Enrofloxacin (Baytril 2.5% – Bayer) at 5–10 mg/kg by month or subcutaneously is a broad-spectrum antibiotic we have used without any obvious side effects.

CAGING

Amphibians are best kept in glass or plastic aquaria. A ventilated lid is essential as newts have the ability to climb glass. Ultraviolet lighting and a dark heat source will hasten the healing processes. The PBT for native amphibians should be lower than that required for reptiles. Heating should provide a temperature of not higher than 20–23°C.

Although these are amphibians, they do not necessarily need to be kept in water. In particular toads and newts often favour a dry environment but still need access to water to immerse themselves. Frogs tend to be more aquatic and will spend most of their time in water.

FEEDING

These animals will only take moving live prey invertebrates. These are available at most pet stores as mealworms, waxworms, crickets, red worms and clean maggots. To feed them they should be put into a fridge for 15 minutes to cool them and slow them down. They are then dusted with a calcium/

phosphorus supplement (Mealworm or Cricket Diet Calci-Paste – International Zoo Veterinary Group; Nutrobal – Vetark Animal Health) and put near to the animal so that it can register their movement when they warm up.

Toads will readily take waxworm larvae. Newts will take small worms and waxworm larvae. Frogs may take crickets or any of the other foods but will probably not feed.

RELEASE

Once again these animals, especially toads, are best released where they were found. If that is not suit-able then they can be released near any garden pond.

Great crested newts are now very rare and should be returned to their original location as should natterjack toads.

LEGAL IMPLICATIONS

The only proviso affecting amphibian rehabilitation is not to release non-native species and not to take or possess healthy great crested newts or natterjack toads.

Appendix 1
Bat Conservation Trust Guidelines on Handling Bats

Important information about bats and rabies

Following the recent incident of a Daubenton's bat in the UK carrying a rabies-related virus (European Bat Lyssavirus 2), we are obliged to revise certain aspects of the advice to people handling bats to give renewed encouragement to people to submit fresh dead bats to the Central Veterinary Laboratory (CVL). The BCT remains in contact with all relevant national authorities and these guidelines have been produced in discussion with them.

1. Vaccination

It is now the Department of Health's recommendation that people regularly handling bats should be vaccinated against rabies. We are including in this category all licence holders and those regularly taking in sick and injured bats. Arrangements for receiving vaccination (free of charge) will be sent to all licence holders individually; for bat carers the *Bat Care News* mailing list will be used. If you know of anybody this would miss please let BCT know.

As a general precaution people should avoid being bitten (using leather gloves or gloves of equivalent protection). Any bat bite should be thoroughly cleansed with soap and water. Liquid Savlon is appropriate for cleansing in the field. Advice should be sought from your doctor about the need for post-exposure prophylactic treatment if the bat was sick or behaving oddly.

2. Submission of fresh dead bats to Central Veterinary Laboratory

The fact that nearly 1900 bats have already been submitted before this incident and the experiences of our colleagues elsewhere in Europe have been invaluable in allaying much public and professional anxiety. Nevertheless, only 22 Daubenton's bats have been tested. We would encourage an increase in the rabies surveillance carried out by CVL by the submission of more fresh dead bats. To that end, in consultation with CVL and MAFF, we recommend:

(i) All dead bats should be sent by first-class mail to the CVL as soon as possible (but not on Friday). If there is a delay in posting, keep in a refrigerator (4–6°C) until the bat can be collected or posted. Rabies related virus can be isolated from frozen or decomposing material, but the chances are enhanced in fresh unfrozen specimens.

(ii) If euthanasia is agreed this can be carried out by a vet using gaseous anaesthetic and barbiturates. Other methods are available but should avoid breaking the skin or skull.

(iii) Samples should be accompanied by details of date, source and circumstances of finding (Appendix 4). If there is reason to be suspicious of the animal call your local MAFF Animal Health Office before despatching the bat.

(iv) Packaging must comply with the Post Office regulations for pathological material. Carcasses should be packed in a tightly sealed container with absorbent material, sealed inside a leak-proof container or bag and placed in a rigid container and surrounded by absorbent material. This should be securely fastened and placed in a stout envelope or padded bag. The package must be marked 'Pathological specimen; Fragile with Care' and sent by first-class post to CVL. Packages should be clearly marked with a large red 'R' next to the address.

(v) The package should be directed to Rabies Diagnostics, Central Veterinary Laboratory, Woodham Lane, New Haw, Addlestone, Surrey KT15 3NB. Some bat groups have had an arrangement with their local Veterinary Officers of their local MAFF Animal Health Office regarding collection for delivery to CVL.

(vi) As in other countries, the identification of all bats submitted to CVL is confirmed by one appropriate bat specialist (currently myself) and the material is subsequently passed to one of our national museums (mostly to Liverpool or Edinburgh).

3. Advice to the public who find grounded bats

For the present we have to advise that the public do not handle grounded bats. It may be possible for a bat group member to visit to examine the bat and retrieve it if appropriate. The local MAFF Animal Health Office (or its equivalent in Northern Ireland, Eire,

Isle of Man and Channel Islands) should be contacted if the bat is behaving abnormally or aggressively and for which no explanation of its behaviour is readily available. It should be remembered that there are hazards to both animals and humans in inexperienced people handling any wild animal. We should, however, establish whether the bat has bitten anybody – if so, then we should consider encouraging the finder to collect the bat (using stout gloves or a heavy cloth) into a box where it can be examined later. General advice about the container and the provision of a shallow dish of water, etc., should be continued.

If a bat has bitten a member of the public seek medical attention. The bat should be retained in captivity for at least 2 weeks, or euthanasia applied, depending on the assessed risk. Post-exposure treatment should be considered after discussion with a doctor or GP.

The BCT office holds a list of all Great Britain MAFF Animal Health Offices and their equivalents elsewhere and has details of appropriate health offices.

4. Taking bats in captivity
We see no reason to revise our approach to the taking of bats into captivity.

MAFF confirms that any bat that is still alive after any necessary treatment and care, can be considered safe to release as soon as it is in a fit state in other respects.

5. Daubenton's bats in captivity
We appeal for data on Daubenton's bats taken into captivity since 1990.

We would be grateful for knowledge of the number taken into captivity and details of their release or death, highlighting any that have been retained for more than 1 year (and that might therefore be regarded as tested and negative).

All bats that die in captivity should be submitted to CVL as soon as possible.

If you require further information or advice please let me know.

A.M. Hutson
Conservation Officer, BCT

Bat Conservation Trust
15 Cloisters House
8 Battersea Park Road
London
SW8 4SG
Bat Helpline: 020 7627 8822

Appendix 2

British Divers Marine Life Rescue (BDMLR)
Guidelines for Response to Cetacean Strandings

Cetacean anatomy

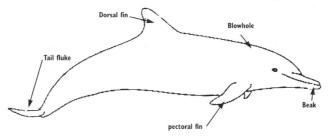

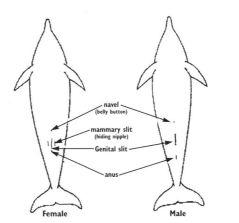

Dawson S.M. The NZ Whale and Dolphin Digest

Initial response to cetacean stranding reports on the telephone

ASK FOR DETAILS

- Species size and number (if species not known, size and appearance).
- Contact details (who reported by / contact tel. no.).
- Exact location (nearest town / name of beach / location on beach / access to beach).
- Conditions at the scene (weather / sea state / tide state / level of disturbance).
- Condition of cetacean (alive or dead / no. of breaths per minute / any wounds / skin condition / obvious dipping of lumbar muscles or neck? / period of time observed).
- Position of cetacean (in sun or shade / in or above the surf / on rocks, shingle or sand).
- Any attempts made to refloat? (if so, how was it done and how long was taken over it).

ADVICE TO GIVE OUT:

- Support the animal in an upright position and dig trenches under the pectoral fins.
- Cover the animal with wet sheets or towels (even seaweed) and keep it moist by spraying or dousing with water.

NB the blowhole should not be covered, and care should be taken to avoid any water or sand entering it.

- All contact, noise and disturbance should be kept to a minimum.

Taken with permission from: *Marine Mammal Medic Handbook* (Barnett *et al.*, 1998)

Appendix 3
Birds on Schedule 4 of the Wildlife and Countryside Act 1981 (as of May 1998)

Common name	Scientific name
Bunting, Cirl	*Emberiza cirlus*
Bunting, Lapland	*Calcarius lapponicus*
Bunting, Snow	*Plectrophenax nivalis*
Buzzard, Honey	*Pernis apivorus*
Eagle, Adalbert's	*Aquila adalberti*
Eagle, Golden	*Aquila chrysaetos*
Eagle, Great Phillipine	*Pithecophaga jefferyi*
Eagle, Imperial	*Aquila heliaca*
Eagle, New Guinea	*Harpyopsis novaeguineae*
Eagle, White-tailed	*Haliaeetus albicilla*
Chough	*Pyrrhocorax pyrrhocorax*
Crossbills (all species)	*Loxia* spp.
Falcon, Barbary	*Falco pelegrinoides*
Falcon, Gyr	*Falco rusticolus*
Falcon, Peregrine	*Falco peregrinus*
Fieldfare	*Turdus pilaris*
Firecrest	*Regulus ignicapillus*
Fish-Eagle, Madagascar	*Haliaeetus vociferoides*
Forest-falcon, Plumbeous	*Micrastur plumbeus*
Goshawk	*Accipiter gentilis*
Harrier, Hen	*Circus cyaneus*
Harrier, Marsh	*Circus aeruginosus*
Harrier, Montagu's	*Circus pygargus*
Hawk, Galapagos	*Buteo galapagoensis*
Hawk, Grey-backed	*Leucopternis occidentalis*
Hawk, Hawaiian	*Buteo solitarius*
Hawk, Ridgway's	*Buteo ridgwayi*
Hawk, White-necked	*Leucopternis lacernulata*
Hawk-Eagle, Wallace's	*Spizaetus nanus*
Hobby	*Falco subbuteo*
Honey-Buzzard, Black	*Henicopernis infuscata*
Kestrel, Lesser	*Falco naumanni*
Kestrel, Mauritius	*Falco punctatus*
Kite, Red	*Milvus milvus*
Merlin	*Falco columbarius*
Oriole, Golden	*Oriolus oriolus*
Osprey	*Pandion haliaetus*
Redstart, Black	*Phoenicurus ochruros*
Redwing	*Turdus iliacus*
Sea-Eagle, Pallas'	*Haliaeetus leucoryphus*
Sea-Eagle, Steller's	*Haliaeetus pelagicus*
Serin	*Serinus serinus*

Serpent-Eagle, Andaman	*Spilornis elgini*
Serpent-Eagle, Madagascar	*Eutriorchis astur*
Serpent-Eagle, Mountain	*Spilornis kinabaluensis*
Shorelark	*Eremophila alpestris*
Shrike, Red-backed	*Lanius collurio*
Sparrowhawk, New Britain	*Accipiter brachyurus*
Sparrowhawk, Gundlach's	*Accipiter gundlachii*
Sparrowhawk, Imitator	*Accipiter imitator*
Sparrowhawk, small	*Accipiter nanus*
Tit, Bearded	*Panurus biarmicus*
Tit, Crested	*Parus cristatus*
Warbler, Cetti's	*Cettia cetti*
Warbler, Dartford	*Sylvia undata*
Warbler, Marsh	*Acrocephalus palustris*
Warbler, Savi's	*Locustella luscinioides*
Woodlark	*Lullula arborea*
Wryneck	*Jynx torquilla*

Any bird one of whose parents or other lineal ancestor was a bird of a kind specified in the above list.

Appendix 4

The Veterinary Certificate Required for Birds Registered with the Department of the Environment, Transport and the Regions (DETR)

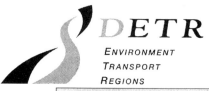

VETERINARY SURGEON'S CERTIFICATE CONFIRMING DISABILITY OF A BIRD

(to be completed in block capitals by a <u>currently practising veterinary surgeon</u> - please continue on a separate sheet if required)

---

1. KEEPER'S DETAILS

a) Name of keeper: ....

b) Address: ....

....

.... Postcode: ....

2. SPECIES OF BIRD

a) Scientific name: ....

....

b) Common name: ....

....

---

3. IDENTIFYING MARKINGS

a) Close ring / cable tie / Swiss ring / other ring numbers / markings:

....

b) Leg which ring/cable tie is fitted to: Left ☐   Right ☐

c) Microchip number: ....

d) Microchip make: (please ✓ the appropriate box)

Identichip	☐	Trovan	☐
Avid	☐	Other *	☐

* If other please state below:

....

....

e) Please scan the bird with an appropriate microchip reader, and note below the area where the chip is implanted: (i.e. left pectoral etc.)

....

f) Sex: (please ✓ the appropriate box)

Male	☐	Female	☐
Unknown	☐		

g) Age: (please ✓ the appropriate box)

Juvenile	☐	Adult	☐
Unknown	☐		

Specific age (if known): ....(years)................(months)

---

4. BIRD'S HISTORY

a) Date the bird was taken into care: ....(day) .... (mth) .... (yr)

b) Was the bird examined by a vet when initially taken into care? Yes ☐   No ☐

If Yes, please provide the vet's details:

Vet's name: ....

Practice address:...

c) Initial injuries/disabilities:..

....

....

....

....

....

....

d) Was the bird x-rayed? Yes ☐   No ☐

If Yes, what was the diagnosis?

....

....

e) Initial treatment given:..

....

....

....

....

....

....

....

5. BIRD'S CURRENT HEALTH

a) What are the bird's current injuries/disabilities: (in particular any musculo/skeletal/ophthalmic injuries, and behavioural abnormalities)

....

....

....

....

....

b) Do you believe that further treatment or investigation (i.e. x-ray, surgery etc.) would aid the bird's   Yes ☐   No ☐
chances of full recovery or release?

If Yes, please provide details of the treatment you recommend:

....

....

....

....

c) In your opinion, are these injuries/disabilities permanent?   Yes ☐   No ☐

If No, when should this bird be reassessed by a veterinary surgeon with a view to release?   .... (day) .... (mth) .... (yr)

d) In your opinion, would displaying the bird to the public cause it unnecessary   Yes ☐   No ☐
stress and risk further injury/disablement?

If yes, please provide your reasons below:

....

....

....

....

....

....

6. CONCLUSION	**7. VETERINARY SURGEON'S DETAILS**
a) I believe this bird should continue to be treated for its injuries and/or disabilities and reassessed at a later date, with a view to possible release to the wild. Yes ☐ No ☐	Vet's name: .... Vet's qualifications: .... Practice address: ....
b) I believe this bird has permanent injuries/disabilities which prevent its release to the wild. Yes ☐ No ☐	....Postcode:................... Telephone: (...............) .... Fax: (..............) ....

8. DECLARATION BY THE CONSULTING VETERINARY SURGEON

Vets/keepers are reminded that wild birds may only be kept in captivity for the purpose of tending injuries, and once the bird becomes fit it must be released. Failure to release a fit bird is an offence under the Wildlife and Countryside Act 1981.

I declare that the information given in sections 1 to 7 above are true and correct to the best of my knowledge and belief:

Name: ....   Date:..

Signed: ....

Please return completed certificate to:
Wildlife Crime and Inspectorate Branch, Department of the Environment, Transport and the Regions,
Room 8/10, Tollgate House, Houlton Street, Bristol BS2 9DJ
Tel: 0117 987 8148   Fax: 0117 987 8393

Appendix 5

Suggested Record Sheet to Accompany Bat Samples to the Central Veterinary Laboratory

Appendix 3 to AHC 96/
Ministry of Agriculture Fisheries and Food
Scottish Office Agriculture, Environment and
Fisheries Department
Welsh Office Agriculture Department

```
Laboratory Use Only


R/
BAT
Data rec'd
```

BAT SAMPLES FOR RABIES SCREENING

SUBMITTING OFFICE

1. SPECIES, AGE and SEX:
2. DATE and TIME FOUND:
3. DATE and TIME OF DEATH: NATURAL/KILLED
    (Estimate if not known)

4. LOCATION (Give map reference if possible)
5. CIRCUMSTANCES OF FINDING
6. SYMPTOMS
7. GENERAL CONDITION
8. GIVE DETAILS OF ANY BITING
    OR SCRATCHING INCIDENTS
    INVOLVING HUMANS OR ANIMALS

SIGNED   DATE

Please send to:

Rabies Diagnostics
Central Veterinary Laboratory
New Haw
Addlestone
Surrey KT15 3NB Tel: 019323 41111
Copy to: VA (Rabies) Tolworth TJ and VA Pentland House or
Cathays Park if appropriate

BAT 1 (Rev. 1996)

Appendix 6
Selected Rehabilitation Supplies and Suppliers

Avian bone splints; intraosseous needles
Cook Veterinary Products, Cook (UK) Ltd, Monroe House, Letchworth, Herts, SG6 1LN

Bat detectors; bat boxes – woodcrete
Alana Ecology Ltd, The Old Primary School, Church Street, Bishop's Castle, Shropshire, SY9 5AE

Catching equipment
MDC Products Ltd, Unit 11, Titan Court, Luton, Beds, LU4 8EF

Esbilac (Pet Ag)
Kruuse UK Ltd, Unit 17, Moor Lane Industrial Estate, Sherburn in Elmet, North Yorkshire, LS25 6ES

General rehabilitation supplies
Wildlife Hospital Trading Ltd, Aston Road, Haddenham, Bucks, HP17 8AF
Tel: 01844 292292

Hagen Products
Available from pet stores

Humane squirrel traps
Okasan Ltd, 6 Stake Lane, Farnborough, Hants, GU14 8NP

Materials handling products for swan pens and flooring
Powell Mail Order Ltd, Unit 1 Heol Aur, Dafen Industrial Park, Llanelli, SA14 8QN

Mealworms; waxworms; crickets; additives
The Mealworm Co. Ltd, Houghton Road, North Anston Trading Estate, Sheffield, S25 4JJ

Metal heat mats
Pet Nap, 4 Hartham Lane, Biddestone, Chippenham, Wilts, SN14 7EA

Nutrobal; Avipro
Vetark Animal Health, PO Box 60, Winchester, SO23 9XN

Pet Breeder Nutri Drops; puppy colostrum
Net-Tex Ltd, Priestwood, Harvel, Nr. Meopham, Kent, DA13 0DA

Plastic bird rings
AC Hughes Ltd, 1 High Street, Hampton Hill, Middx, TW12 1NA

Poly-Aid
The Birdcare Company, Unit 9, Spring Mill Industrial Estate, Avening Road, Nailsworth, Glos, GL6 0BU

Prosecto dried insects; most bird seeds
John E Haith, Park Street, Cleethorpes, Lincs, DN35 7NF

Skeletons
John Dunlop Osteological Supplies, 12 Tideway, Littlehampton, West Sussex, BN17 6QT

Stainless steel kennels
Shorline Ltd, Unit 39a/39b, Vale Business Park, Llandow, Cowbridge, South Glamorgan, CF71 7PF

Trigene
Medichem International, PO Box 237, Sevenoaks, Kent, TN15 6ZS

Appendix 7
Useful Addresses in Wildlife Rehabilitation

Bat Conservation Trust
15 Cloisters House, 8 Battersea Park Road, London, SW8 4BG

British Divers Marine Life Rescue
39 Ingram Road, Gillingham, Kent, ME7 1SB
Rescue Hotline Tel: 01634 281680

Countryside Council for Wales
Plas Penrhos, Ffordd Penrhos, Bangor, Gwynnedd, LL57 2LQ

Department of Environment, Transport and the Regions (DETR)
Tollgate House, Houlton Street, Bristol, BS2 9DJ

English Nature
Northminster House, Peterborough, PE1 1HA

Environment Agency
Rio House, Waterside Drive, Aztec West, Almondsbury, Bristol, BS32 4HD
Emergency Hotline Tel: 0800 807060

European Wildlife Rehabilitation Association
c/o Wildlife Hospital Trust, Aston Road, Haddenham, Bucks, HP17 8AF

Froglife
Mansion House, 27/28 Market Place, Halesworth, Suffolk IP19 9AY

Institute of Zoology
Regents Park, London, NW1 4RY

International Zoo Veterinary Group
Keighley Business Centre, South Street, Keighley, West Yorks, BD21 1AG

Dr A. Kitchener, National Museum of Scotland's
Chambers Street, Edinburgh, EH1 1JF

Mammal Society
15, Cloisters House, 8 Battersea Park Road, London, SW8 4BG

Ministry of Agriculture, Fisheries and Food, Wildlife Incident Unit
Central Science Laboratory, Sand Hutton, York, YO4 1LZ
Poisons Hotline Tel: 0800 321 600

National Federation of Badger Groups
15 Cloisters House, 8 Battersea Park Road, London, SW8 4BG

Operation Chough
Paradise Park, Hayle, Cornwall, TR27 4HY

St Tiggywinkles, Wildlife Hospital Trust
Aston Road, Haddenham, Bucks, HP17 8AF
E-mail: tiggys@globalnet.co.uk
Website: http://www.sttiggywinkles.org.uk
Tel: 01844 292292

Scottish Natural Heritage
2–5 Anderson Place, Edinburgh, EH6 5NP

Swan Sanctuary
Field View, Pooley Green, Egham, Surrey, TW20 8AT
Tel: 01784 431667

Veterinary Poisons Information Service
Medical Toxicology Unit, Avonley Road, London, SE14 5ER
Tel: 020 7635 9195
Fax: 020 7771 5309
or
The General Infirmary, Great George Street, Leeds, LS1 3EX
Tel: 0113 245 0530
Fax: 0113 244 5849

Wildlife Information Network
The Royal Veterinary College, Royal College Street, London, NW1 0TU

References and Further Reading

Anon (1994) Viral haemorrhagic disease confirmed in wild rabbits (News and Reports). *Veterinary Record*, **135**, 342.

Barlow, R.M. (1986) Capture myopathy. In: *Management and Diseases of Deer*, (ed. T.L. Alexander), pp. 130–31. Veterinary Deer Society, London.

Barnard, S.M. (1995) *Bats in Captivity*. Wild Ones Animal Books, Springville, CA.

Barnett, J., Knight, A. & Stevens, M. (1998) *Marine Mammal Medic Handbook*. British Divers Marine Life Rescue, Gillingham, Kent.

Bennet, R.A. & Kuzma, A.B. (1992) Fracture management in birds. *Journal of Zoo and Wildlife Medicine*, **23**(1), 5–38.

Bishop, Y. (1998) *The Veterinary Formulary*, 4th edn. Pharmaceutical Press, London.

Boydell, P. (1997) *Survey of Ocular Disease in Birds of Prey in the UK*. Proceedings of the 4th Conference of the European Committee of the Association of Avian Veterinarians, Loughborough, Leics.

Bray, J.P. (undated) *The Biology of Wound Healing and the Practical Care of Wounds*. Queen's Veterinary School Hospital, Cambridge.

Brown, B. (1994) Bats and ectoparasites. *Bat Care News*, June, 2–8.

Brown, M. (1994) Baby bat release structure. *Bat Care News*, December, 13–14.

Brown, M. (1994) Baby bats. *Bat Care News*, June, 8–9.

Brown, M. (1995) Sticky wing. *Bat Care News*, September, 10–11.

BVNA (1994–95) *Fracture Management and Bandaging for Veterinary Nurses*. British Veterinary Nursing Association, London.

Capucci, L., Nardin, A. & Lavuzza, A. (1997) Seroconversion in an industrial unit of rabbits infected with a non-pathogenic rabbit haemorrhagic disease-like virus. *Veterinary Record*, **140**, 647–50.

Coles, B.H. (1997) *Avian Medicine and Surgery*, 2nd edn. Blackwell Science, Oxford.

Cooper, J.E. (1979) Parasites. In: *First Aid and Care of Wild Birds*, (eds J.E. Cooper & J.T. Eley), pp. 140–49. David & Charles, Newton Abbot, Devon.

Cooper, J.E. (1993) Pathological Studies on the Barn Owl. *Raptor Medicine*. Chiron Publications, Keighley, Yorks.

Cooper, J.E. & Jackson, O.F. (1981) *Diseases of the Reptilia*. Academic Press, London.

Cooper, P.E. & Penaliggon, J. (1997) Use of Frontline Spray on rabbits. *Veterinary Record*, **140**, 535.

Corbet, G.B. & Harris, S. (1991) *The Handbook of British Mammals*, 3rd edn. Blackwell Scientific Publications, Oxford.

Corbett, L.K. (1979) Feeding ecology and social behaviour of wildcats (*Felis silvestris*) and domestic cats (*Felis catus*) in Scotland. PhD thesis, University of Aberdeen.

Crissey, S.D. (1998) *Handling Fish Fed to Fish Eating Mammals*. United States Department of Agriculture, Washington, DC.

Davies, P.M.C. (1981) Anatomy and physiology. In: *Diseases of the Reptilia*, (eds J.E. Cooper & O.F. Jackson), pp. 9–73. Academic Press, London.

Divers, S.J. (1996) Ultraviolet lights for reptiles. *Veterinary Record*, **138**, 627–8.

Drury, S.E.N., Gough, R.E. & Cunningham, A.A. (1995) Isolation of an iridovirus-like agent from common frogs (*Rana temporaria*). *Veterinary Record*, **137**, 72–3.

Duff, J.P., Scott, A. & Kegmer, I.F. (1996) Parapox virus infection of the grey squirrel. *Veterinary Record*, **138**, 527.

Evans, L. (1993) First Aid Wound and Fracture Treatment for Birds. *Wildlife Rehabilitation Today*, **5**(2), 34–8.

Flecknell, P.A. (1991) Rabbits In: *Manual of Exotic Pets*, (ed P.H. Beynon & J.E. Cooper), pp. 69–81. British Small Animal Veterinary Association, Cheltenham.

Foster, J. (1997) Salty Toads Turn Red, Bump Chins. *BBC Wildlife Magazine*, **15**(3), 62.

Frazer, D. (1983) *Reptiles and Amphibians in Britain*. Bloomsbury Books, London.

Frink, L. (1989) The basics of oiled bird rehabilitation *Wildlife Rehabilitation Today*, **1**(2), 4.

Frink, L. (1993) Anatomy of an oil spill response *Wildlife Rehabilitation Today*, **5**(2), 27–31.

Froglife. Unusual Frog Mortality. *Froglife Advice Sheet 7*. Froglife, Halesworth, Suffolk.

Frost, L.M. (1999) Hand-rearing orphaned or deserted neonate or young hedgehogs. In: *Proceedings of the 3rd*

International Hedgehog Workshop of the European Hedgehog Research Group, (ed. N. Reeve), p. 18. Roehampton Institute, London.

Frye, F.L. (1991) Biomedical and Surgical Aspects of Captive Reptile Husbandry, 2nd edn. Kreiger, Malabar, India.

Gallagher, J. & Nelson, J. (1979) Causes of ill health and natural death in badgers in Gloucestershire. Veterinary Record, 105, 546–51.

Gorrel, C. (1996) Teeth trimming in rabbits and rodents. Veterinary Record, 139, 528.

Goulden, S. (1995) Botulism in water birds. Veterinary Record, 137, 328.

Greenwood, A.G. (1979) Poisons. In: First Aid and Care of Wild Birds, (eds J.E. Cooper & J.T. Eley), pp. 150–73. David & Charles, Newton Abbot, Devon.

Greenwood, A.G. & Barnett, K.C. (1980) The investigation of the visual defects in raptors. In: Recent Advances in the Study of Raptor Diseases, (eds J.E. Cooper & A.G. Greenwood), pp. 131–5. Chiron Publications, Keighley, Yorks.

Gregory, M.W. & Stocker, L.R. (1991) Hedgehogs. In: Manual of Exotic Pets, (eds P.H. Beynon & J.E. Cooper), pp. 63–8. British Small Animal Veterinary Association, Cheltenham, Glos.

Greig, A., Stevenson, K., Percy V., Pirie, A.A., Grant, J.M. & Sharp, J.M. (1997) Paratuberculosis in wild rabbits. Veterinary Record, 140, 141–3.

Griffiths, R.A. & Langton, T. (1998) Catching and handling of reptiles. In: Herpetofauna Workers' Manual, (eds J. Gent & S. Gibson), pp. 33–43. Joint Nature Conservation Committee, Peterborough, Cambs.

Harcourt-Brown, F. (1998) Pet rabbits. Part 4. Looking after their teeth. Veterinary Practice Nurse, 10(4), 4–8.

Harden, J. (1996) Trichomoniasis in raptors, pigeons and doves Journal of Wildlife Rehabilitation, 19(1), 8–17.

Harris, S., Jeffries, D. & Cheeseman, C. (1994) Problems with badgers?, 3rd edn. RSPCA, Horsham, W. Sussex.

Helliwell, L. (1993) Nutrition of captive bats. Bat Care News, September, 2–4.

Joseph, V. (1996) Aspergillosis: the silent killer. Journal of Wildlife Rehabilitation, 19(3), 15–18.

King, A.S. & McLelland, J. (1984) Birds, Their Structure and Function. Baillière Tindall, Eastbourne, E. Sussex.

Kirkwood, J.K. (1991) Wild mammals. In: Manual of Exotic Pets, (eds P.H. Beynon & J.E. Cooper), pp. 122–49. British Small Animal Veterinary Association, Cheltenham, Glos.

Kirkwood, J.K., Holmes, J.P. & Macgregor, S. (1995) Garden bird mortalities. Veterinary Record, 136, 372.

Klem, D. Jnr (1989) Bird – window collisions. The Wilson Bulletin, 101(4), 606–20.

Lambrechts, N. (1995) Wound management and care. In: Proceedings of the SASOL Symposium on Wildlife Rehabilitation, (ed. B.L. Penzhorn), pp. 130–34. South African Veterinary Association, Onderstepoort, South Africa.

Lane, D.R. & Cooper, B. (1994) Veterinary Nursing (formerly Jones's Animal Nursing, 5th edn). Elsevier Science, Oxford.

Lawton, M.P.C. (1991) Lizards and snakes. In: Manual of Exotic Pets, (eds P.H. Beynon & J.E. Cooper), pp. 244–60. British Small Animal Veterinary Association. Cheltenham, Glos.

Lewis, J.C.M. (1992) Resuscitation. Presented at the Congress of the European Wildlife Rehabilitation Association, 31 October–1 November, Thame, Oxon. European Wildlife Rehabilitation Association, Haddenham, Bucks.

Lewis, J.C.M. (1998) Badgers for vets. UK Vet, 2, Nos. 2, 3, 4.

Lollar, A. & Schmidt-French, B. (1998) Captive Care and Medical Reference for the Rehabilitation of Insectivorous Bats. Bat World, Mineral Wells, TX.

McLelland, J. (1990) A Colour Atlas of Avian Anatomy. Wolfe Publishing, London.

Malley, D. (1996) Teeth trimming in rabbits and rodents. Veterinary Record, 139, 603.

Marshall, C. (1993) Reptiles for Veterinary Nurses. British Veterinary Nursing Association, London.

Matthews, K.A. (1996) Veterinary Emergency and Critical Care. Lifelearn, Guelph, Ontario.

Mead, C.J. (1991) Seabird mortality as seen through ringing. Ibis, 113, 418.

Mean, R.J. (1998) The prevalence and pathology of the helminth parasites of the British Hedgehog (Erinaceus europaeus). MPhil thesis, School of Biological Sciences, Univerisity of Portsmouth and Wildlife Hospital Trust, Haddenham, Bucks.

Michell, A.R. (1985) What is shock? Journal of Small Animal Practice, 26, 719–38.

Morgan, R.V. (1985) Manual of Small Animal Emergencies. Churchill Livingstone, New York, NY.

Morris, P. (1999) Studies of released hedgehogs, what next? In: Proceedings of the 3rd International Hedgehog Workshop of the European Hedgehog Research Group, (ed. N. Reeve), p. 13. Roehampton Institute, London.

Munro, R., Wood, A. & Martin, S. (1995) Treponemal infection in wild hares. Veterinary Record, 136, 78–9.

Murray, M.J. (undated) Fluid Therapy and Administration in Wildlife Care. Skills Seminar VIII – International Wildlife Rehabilitation Council, Suisun, CA.

Neal, E.G. (1977) Badgers. Blandford Press, Poole, Dorset.

Neff, T. (1997) Emaciation in raptors. In: Proceedings of the 1997 Conference – From Science to Reality. A Bridge to the 21st Century, (ed. M.D. Reynolds), pp. 197–200. International Wildlife Rehabilitation Council, Concord, CA.

Ness, M. (1997) The art and science of fracture repair. Veterinary Practice Nurse, 9(4), 26–7.

Otto, C.M., Kaufman, G. & McCrowe, D.T. (1989) Intraosseous infusion of fluids and therapeutics. The Compendium on Continuing Education for the Practicing Veterinarian, 11(4), 421–31.

Oxenham, M. (1991) Ferrets. In: Manual of Exotic Pets, (eds P.H. Beynon & J.E. Cooper), pp. 97–110. British

Small Animals Veterinary Association, Cheltenham, Glos.

Penman, S. & Ciapparelli, L. (1990) Endodontic disease. In: *Manual of Small Animal Dentistry*, (eds C.E. Harvey & H. Simon Orr), pp. 73–83. British Small Animal Veterinary Association, Cheltenham, Glos.

Penman, S. & Harvey, C.E. (1990) Periodontal disease. In: *Manual of Small Animal Dentistry*, (eds C.E. Harvey & H. Simon Orr), pp. 37–48. British Small Animal Veterinary Association, Cheltenham, Glos.

Perrins, C. (1987) *Birds of Britain & Europe*. Collins, London.

Plunkett, S.J. (1993) *Emergency Procedures for the Small Animal Veterinarian*. WB Saunders, Philadelphia, PA.

Pukas, A. (1999) Death lurks as the crow flies. *The Express*, 6 February, p. 33.

Racey, P.A. (undated) Keeping, handling and releasing. In: *The Bat Worker's Manual*, (ed. A.J. Mitchell-Jones), pp. 36–41. Nature Conservancy Council, Peterborough, Cambs.

Redig, P.T. (1979) Infectious diseases. In: *First Aid and Care of Wild Birds*, (eds J.E. Cooper & J.T. Eley), pp. 118–39. David & Charles, Newton Abbot, Devon.

Reeve, N. (1994) *Hedgehogs*. T. & A.D. Poyser, London.

Reichenbach-Klinke, H. & Elkan, E. (1965) *The Principal Diseases of Lower Vertebrates. Diseases of Amphibians*. TFH Publications, Hong Kong.

Reynolds, M. (undated) *Operation Chough*. Paradise Park, Hayle, Cornwall.

Ritchie, B.W., Otto, C.M., Latimer, K.S. & Crowe, D.T. (1990) A technique of intraosseous cannulation for intravenous therapy in birds. *The Compendium on Continuing Education for the Practicing Veterinarian*, **12**(1), 55–8.

Rosen, M. (1971) Botulism. In: *Infections and Parasitic Diseases of Wild Birds*, pp. 100–17. University Press, Ames, IA.

Routh, A. (1992) The bat – European Microchiroptera. Considerations for their successful rehabilitation. *Presented at the Congress of the European Wildlife Rehabilitation Association*, 31 October–1 November, Thame, Oxon. European Wildlife Rehabilitation Association, Haddenham, Bucks.

Routh, A. & Sleeman, J.M. (1995) Greenfinch mortalities (letter). *Veterinary Record*, **136**, 500.

Rudge, A.J.B. (1984) *The Capture and Handling of Deer*. Nature Conservancy Council, Peterborough.

Sainsbury, A.W. (1997) Veterinary care of squirrels. *UK Vet*, **2**(6), 40; **3**(1), 56.

Sainsbury, A.W. & Gurnell, J. (1995) An investigation into the health and welfare of red squirrels (*Sciurus vulgaris*), involved in re-introduction studies. *Veterinary Record*, **137**, 367–70.

Samour, J.H., Bailey, T.A. & Cooper, J.E. (1995) Trichomoniasis in birds of prey (Order Falconiformes) in Bahrain. *Veterinary Record*, **136**, 358–62.

Sandys-Winsch, G. (1984) *Animal Law*, 2nd edn. Shaw & Sons, London.

Sharp, B.E. (1996) Post-release survival of oiled, cleaned seabirds in North America. *Ibis*, **138**, 222–8.

Shaw, E. (1990) Diagnosis and treatment of 'sick gull syndrome'. *Journal of Wildlife Rehabilitation*, **13**(2), 3–5.

Simpson, V.R. (1997) Health status of otters (*Lutra Lutra*) in south-west England based on post mortem findings. *Veterinary Record*, **141**, 191–7.

Sims, M. (1997) Strictly for the birds. *Veterinary Practice Nurse*, **9**(1), 320–33.

Sims, S. (1983) Use of IV fluids in small wild birds. *Journal of Wildlife Rehabilitation*, **6**(3), 5–6.

Stebbings, R. (1993) *Which Bat Is It?* The Mammal Society, London.

Stocker, L.R. (1987) *The Complete Hedgehog*. Chatto & Windus, London.

Stocker, L.R. (1991a) *Code of Practice for the Rescue, Treatment, Rehabilitation and Release of Sick and Injured Wildlife*. Wildlife Hospital Trust, Aylesbury, Bucks.

Stocker, L.R. (1991b) *The Complete Garden Bird*. Chatto & Windus, London.

Stocker, L.R. (1992) *St Tiggywinkles Wildcare Handbook*. Chatto & Windus, London.

Stocker, L.R. (1994a) Rescue and Rehabilitation of Badgers in Britain. *Journal of Wildlife Rehabilitation*, **17**(3), 12–16.

Stocker, L.R. (1994b) *The Complete Fox*. Chatto & Windus, London.

Stocker, L.R. (1995) Wild mammals seen in general practice. *Presented at the 1993 meeting of the British Veterinary Zoological Society, London*, 4 December 1993.

Stocker, L.R. (1996) Respite for rehabilitators who handle deer. *Wildlife Rehabilitation Today*, **7**, 4.

Stocker, L.R. (1997) Feedback on euthanasia. *Bat Care News*, June, 11–12.

Stocker, L.R. (1998) *Medication For Use In The Treatment of Hedgehogs* (Erinaceus europaeus). Wildlife Hospital Trust, Aylesbury, Bucks.

Stocker, L.R. (1999) Incidents adversely affecting the hedgehog (*Erinaceus europaeus*): its rescue and rehabilitation in the United Kingdom. In: *Proceedings of the 3rd International Hedgehog Workshop of the European Hedgehog Research Group*, (ed. N. Reeve), p. 17. Roehampton Institute, London.

Taylor, P.M. (undated) *Fluid Therapy in Animals: A Practical Guide*. Hoecst UK Ltd, Milton Keynes.

UFAW/WSPA [World Society for the Protection of Animals] (1989) Euthanasia of amphibians and reptiles. *Report of a Joint UFAW/WSPA Working Party*. Universities Federation for Animal Welfare, Potters Bar, Herts.

Vindevogel, H. & Duchatel, J.P. (1985) *Understanding Pigeon Paramyxovirosis*. Natural Granen NV, Schoten, Belgium.

Welsh, V. (1981) *Immobilisation of Simple and Compound Fractures in Mammals*. Wildlife Rehabilitation Council, Walnut Creek, CA.

Welsh, V. (1983) *Immobilisation of Simple and Compound Fractures in Songbirds and Raptors*. Wildlife Rehabilitation Council, Walnut Creek, CA.

Whitby, J.E., Johnstone, P., Parsons, G., King, A.A. & Hutson, A.M. (1996) Ten-year survey of British bats for the existence of rabies. *Veterinary Record*, **139**, 491–3.

White, J. (1990) Current treatments for anemia in oil-contaminated birds. In: *The Effects of Oil on Wildlife* from: The Oil Symposium October 1990, (eds J. White & L. Frink), pp. 67–72. International Wildlife Rehabilitation Council, Suisun, CA.

Williams, D.L. (1991) Amphibians. In: *Manual of Exotic Pets*, (eds P.H. Beynon & J.E. Cooper), British Small Animal Veterinary Association, Cheltenham, Glos.

Wobeser, G.A. (1981) *Diseases of Wild Waterfowl*. Plenum Press, New York, NY.

Wynne, J. (1998) Management of dehydration in nestling birds. *Journal of Wildlife Rehabilitation*, **11**(2), 13–14.

Index

Figures are referenced by italic page numbers; plate numbers are given in bold.